MCQs in General Surgical Oncology

Aqeel Shakir Mahmood • Andreas Koulouris
Editors

MCQs in General Surgical Oncology

Springer

Editors
Aqeel Shakir Mahmood
Department of General Surgery
University of Baghdad
Baghdad, Iraq

Andreas Koulouris
Thoracic Oncology Center
Karolinska University Hospital
Stockholm, Sweden

ISBN 978-3-031-65740-5 ISBN 978-3-031-65738-2 (eBook)
https://doi.org/10.1007/978-3-031-65738-2

This Springer imprint is published by the registered company Springer Nature Switzerland AG
The registered company address is: Gewerbestrasse 11, 6330 Cham, Switzerland

My dear family, your love and support always shone over my life. This book is indeed a tribute to your sacrifices and encouragement; I dedicate it to you in turn.

Aqeel Shakir Mahmood

Foreword 1

"No medical professional in the current scenario can afford not to continue learning and updating the latest advances," *MCQs in General Surgical Oncology* is a comprehensive compilation to help surgeons, residents, or students learn the basics to the nuances of oncological surgeries related to the gastrointestinal and endocrine systems. This book provides quite a few multiple-choice questions that comprehensively cover almost all aspects right from basic principles to challenging surgical techniques and management following surgery. The questions are very well framed to pose a real-life situation, challenging the reader on the application of his/her knowledge and power of reasoning. Explanations and references for each question round out the text, adding value in serving both as a self-assessment and exam-preparation guide. First of all, I must congratulate the authors on this wonderful compilation, which, without a doubt, will go a long way in achieving its goal of serving as an aid for good surgical educational practice and better patient care in the field of oncology.

Tahseen Alrubai

Iraqi Cancer Board
Ministry of Health,
Baghdad, Iraq

Foreword 2

Surgical oncology is one of those fields where one is able to boast that they are masters only with the greatest difficulty. This book *MCQs in General Surgical Oncology* turns on the spotlight for one to illuminate their way to that great goal. This book equips the reader with a thoughtfully selected set of multiple-choice questions exploring the subtleties of diagnosis and management in GI and endocrine system cancer. Valuable for everybody who wants to deepen their understanding in surgical oncology, from medical students to advanced surgeons. Questions have been so designed that they are evocative of critical thinking and re-emphasize on key concepts, while the detailed explanation of why each answer is the way it is holds invaluable insight. In this foreword, I find the embodiment of authors' commitment to moving medical education forward with their continued struggle against cancer. This book is not merely a pedagogic tool; it should be looked upon as a companion to the ardent man or woman in the quest for saving life through surgical excellence.

Department of Radiology
College of Medicine, University of Baghdad,
Baghdad, Iraq

Khudhair Jasim Sabeeh

Key Features

- *MCQs in General Surgical Oncology* is a comprehensive review book that utilizes the multiple-choice question (MCQ) format to specifically address topics in gastrointestinal and endocrine oncology.
- This book aims to help readers revise core concepts and maintain knowledge in the field of surgical oncology, with a focus on gastrointestinal and endocrine tumors.
- This book is structured into two main sections, covering a wide range of topics including esophageal tumors, gastric tumors, colorectal cancer, hepatocellular carcinoma, pancreatic cancer, thyroid cancers, and more.
- With over 500 MCQs, this study companion provides a convenient format for self-study, with answers and explanations immediately following the questions for enhanced readability. While serving as an adjunct to existing texts, this book is designed to help readers identify their strengths and weaknesses in the area of surgical oncology.
- The content is based on up-to-date best practice evidence, with a style that mirrors the format adopted by the majority of local, regional, and international board examinations.
- The target audience includes medical students, surgical residents, fellows, and practicing surgeons preparing for exams or seeking to refresh their knowledge in the field.
- *MCQs in General Surgical Oncology* follows the concept and style of internationally recognized medical review books, offering a focused and valuable resource for those studying or practicing in the field of surgical oncology.

Preface

Surgical oncology is a dynamic, ever-evolving discipline with enshrined understandings in surgical oncology. It is aptly said that the journey of a surgical oncologist is all about learning and adapting continuously because new findings and development are continuously changing our approach toward treating cancer.

It is with this backdrop that *MCQs in General Surgical Oncology* has been conceived. This book is meant to provide an all-embracing review of the key concepts and techniques in surgery relevant to the gastrointestinal and endocrine systems vis-à-vis oncology. This is in order to ensure that the format that is used is flexible enough for the reinforcement of knowledge and self-assessment. Therefore, the format was a multiple-choice question (MCQ).

Every question in this book is very well-drafted and forces the reader to prod his gray matter, applying not only his recall-based but also critical thinking and problem-solving faculties. Clear answers, often with explanations that make the field of knowledge even clearer, are offered.

This book is written for a broad audience from medical students and surgical residents to practicing surgeons, who are willing to refresh or perhaps update their knowledge, and for board-exam candidates, who are preparing for certification exams. We hope this collection of MCQs will be useful in your endeavor for excellence in surgical oncology.

We are immensely grateful to the authors for invaluable contributions and expertise and to the patients and mentors. This book may help you along with this very responsible road to becoming a good and compassionate surgical oncologist.

Baghdad, Iraq — Aqeel Shakir Mahmood
Stockholm, Sweden — Andreas Koulouris

Contents

Contributors

Sabah Noori Abdulraheem Baghdad Teaching Hospital, Baghdad, Iraq

Haider A. H. Ahmed Medical City Complex, Baghdad, Iraq

Sajjad G. Al-Badri College of Medicine, University of Baghdad, Baghdad, Iraq

Waseem M. Al Hamidy Gastroenterology and Hepatology Teaching Hospital, Medical City, Baghdad, Iraq

Abdulazeez S. Al-Janabi College of Medicine, University of Baghdad, Baghdad, Iraq

Salih Ahmed Aljiburi Baghdad Teaching Hospital, Baghdad, Iraq

Munthir A. Alobaidi Department of Surgery, College of Medicine, University of Baghdad, Baghdad, Iraq

Noufel sh. Alshadood Baghdad Teaching Hospital, Baghdad, Iraq

Raafat Raoof Alturfi Department of Digestive Surgery, Gastroenterology and Hepatology Teaching Hospital, Baghdad, Iraq

Mustafa Ismail Department of Surgery, College of Medicine, University of Baghdad, Baghdad, Iraq

Aqeel Shakir Mahmood Department of General Surgery, University of Baghdad, Baghdad, Iraq

Talib A. Majeed GIT and Liver Hospital, Medical City Baghdad, Baghdad, Iraq

Samer Sabri Department of Surgery, Baghdad Teaching Hospital, Medical City Complex, Baghdad, Iraq

Saleh Abdulkareem Saleh College of Medicine, University of Baghdad, Baghdad, Iraq

Abbreviations

ACC	Adrenocortical carcinoma
ACTH	Adrenocorticotropic hormone
AFP	Alpha-fetoprotein
AIDS	Acquired immunodeficiency syndrome
AIN	Anal intraepithelial neoplasia
AIP	Autoimmune pancreatitis
AJCC/UICC	American Joint Committee on Cancer/Union for International Cancer Control
APC	Adenomatous polyposis coli
APR	Abdominoperineal resection
ART	Antiretroviral therapy
BCLC	Barcelona Clinic Liver Cancer
BP	Bisphosphonate
CagA	Cytotoxin-associated gene A
CC	Cholangiocarcinoma
CDKN2A	Cyclin-dependent kinase inhibitor 2A
CEA	Carcinoembryonic antigen
CRC	Colorectal cancer
CRLMs	Colorectal liver metastases
CRM	Circumferential resection margin
CRS	Cytoreductive surgery
CRT	Chemoradiotherapy
CSCO	Chinese Society of Clinical Oncology
CT	Computed tomography
CTP	Child-Turcotte-Pugh
DCIS	Ductal carcinoma in situ
Dmab	Denosumab
DTC	Differentiated thyroid carcinoma
ECC	Extrahepatic cholangiocarcinoma
EGJ	Esophago-gastric junction
ER	Endoscopic resection

ERCP	Endoscopic retrograde cholangiopancreatography
ESMO	European Society for Medical Oncology
EUS	Endoscopic ultrasound
FAP	Familial adenomatous polyposis
FDG	Fluoro-2-deoxy-D-glucose
FMTC	Familial medullary thyroid carcinoma
FNA	Fine-needle aspiration
FNAB	Fine-needle aspiration biopsy
FNAC	Fine-needle aspiration cytology
FTC	Follicular thyroid carcinoma
GBC	Gallbladder cancer
GERD	Gastroesophageal reflux disease
GIST	Gastrointestinal stromal tumor
H. pylori	*Helicobacter pylori*
HBV	Hepatitis B virus
HCC	Hepatocellular carcinoma
HCC	Hepatocellular cholangiocarcinoma
HCM	Hypercalcemia of malignancy
HDGC	Hereditary diffuse gastric carcinoma
HIPEC	Hyperthermic intraperitoneal chemotherapy
HIV	Human immunodeficiency virus
HNPCC	Hereditary nonpolyposis colorectal cancer
HPT-JT	Hyperparathyroidism-jaw tumor syndrome
HPV	Human papilloma virus
HSgFOBT	High-sensitivity guaiac fecal occult blood test
HSIL	High-grade squamous intraepithelial lesions
HU	Hounsfield units
IAC	IgG4-associated cholangitis
IBD	Inflammatory bowel disease
IBS	Irritable bowel syndrome
ICC	Intrahepatic cholangiocarcinoma
IgG	Serum immunoglobulin
ILC	Invasive lobular carcinoma
IPMN	Intraductal papillary mucinous neoplasms
ITPN	Intraductal tubulopapillary neoplasm
IVC	Inferior vena cava
KGCA	Korean Gastric Cancer Association
LABC	Locally advanced breast cancer
LCIS	Lobular carcinoma in situ
LD	Latissimus dorsi
LN	Lymph node
LSIL	Low-grade squamous intraepithelial lesions
MELD	Model for end-stage liver disease
MEN	Multiple endocrine neoplasia
MPM	Malignant peritoneal mesothelioma

MRI	Magnetic resonance imaging
MTC	Medullary thyroid carcinoma
NAFLD	Nonalcoholic fatty liver disease
NCCN	National Comprehensive Cancer Network
NETs	Neuroendocrine tumors
NSAIDs	Nonsteroidal anti-inflammatory drugs
NSM	Nipple sparing mastectomy
PC	Parathyroid carcinoma
PCC	Perihilar cholangiocarcinoma
PDT	Photodynamic therapy
PET	Positron emission tomography
PHPT	Primary hyperparathyroidism
PJS	Peutz–Jeghers syndrome
PSC	Primary sclerosing cholangitis
PTC	Papillary thyroid carcinoma
PTCp	Percutaneous transhepatic cholangiopancreatography
PTEN	A tumor suppressor gene
PTGs	Parathyroid glands
PTH	Parathyroid hormone
PTMC	Papillary thyroid microcarcinoma
RAI	Radioactive iodine
Ras	A family of related proteins involved in transmitting signals within cells
RFA	Radiofrequency ablation
RT	Radiotherapy
SBFT	Small bowel follow-through
SCC	Squamous cell carcinoma
SEMS	Self-expandable metallic stent
SIADH	Syndrome of inappropriate antidiuretic hormone
SIL	Squamous intraepithelial lesions
SLNB	Sentinel lymph node biopsy
SMA	Superior mesenteric artery
T3	Triiodothyronine
T4	Thyroxine
TACE	Transarterial chemoembolization
TG	Thyroglobulin
TCL	Total caudate lobectomy
TSH	Thyroid-stimulating hormone
VTE	Venous thromboembolism

Part I
Surgical Gastrointestinal Oncology

Chapter 1
Esophageal Tumors

Sabah Noori Abdulraheem, Talib A. Majeed, Noufel sh. Alshadood, Saleh Abdulkareem Saleh, and Aqeel Shakir Mahmood

1. A 65-year-old man presents with progressive dysphagia over the past 6 months. He has a history of chronic gastroesophageal reflux disease and heavy tobacco use. Endoscopy reveals a malignant-looking lesion in the esophagus, and biopsy confirms a diagnosis of esophageal cancer. In the context of the epidemiology and pathogenesis of esophageal cancer, which of the following statements is incorrect?

   A. Squamous cell carcinoma (SCC) and adenocarcinoma account for over 95% of esophageal malignant tumors, with distinct etiological factors influencing their prevalence.
   B. Globally, SCC is more prevalent than adenocarcinoma, although there is significant geographic variation influenced by risk factors such as tobacco and alcohol use.
   C. SCC typically arises in the upper two-thirds of the esophagus and is strongly associated with smoking and alcohol consumption.
   D. In Western countries, adenocarcinoma has surpassed SCC in incidence, often arising in the distal esophagus and associated with Barrett's esophagus.
   E. The incidence of esophageal cancer has been decreasing globally, reflecting successful public health interventions in risk factor modification.

   Answer: E

S. N. Abdulraheem · N. s. Alshadood
Baghdad Teaching Hospital, Baghdad, Iraq

T. A. Majeed
GIT and Liver Hospital, Medical City Baghdad, Baghdad, Iraq

S. A. Saleh
College of Medicine University of Baghdad, Baghdad, Iraq

A. S. Mahmood (✉)
Department of General Surgery, University of Baghdad, Baghdad, Iraq

A. S. Mahmood, A. Koulouris (eds.), *MCQs in General Surgical Oncology*,
https://doi.org/10.1007/978-3-031-65738-2_1

Explanation: Options A to D are accurate and highlight the epidemiological differences between SCC and adenocarcinoma of the esophagus. Option E is false. The global incidence of esophageal cancer, particularly adenocarcinoma, has been increasing, partly due to rising rates of obesity and gastroesophageal reflux disease.

2. A 58-year-old woman with a long history of tobacco use and chronic alcoholism presents with weight loss and dysphagia. She reports no family history of cancer. An upper endoscopy reveals a suspicious lesion in the mid-esophagus, and a biopsy confirms SCC of the esophagus. In the context of this patient's diagnosis, which of the following statements is incorrect regarding the risk factors for SCC of the esophageal cancer?

   A. A family history of cancer can increase the risk of developing SCC of the esophagus.
   B. Smoking is a significant risk factor for developing SCC of the esophagus.
   C. Chronic alcohol consumption is associated with an increased risk of SCC of the esophagus.
   D. Use of bisphosphonates (BP) has been linked with an increased risk of SCC of the esophagus.
   E. Barrett's esophagus is a risk factor for SCC of the esophagus.

Answer: E

Explanation: Barrett's esophagus, which involves intestinal metaplasia, is a risk factor for adenocarcinoma of the esophagus, not SCC. The other statements correctly identify known risk factors for SCC of the esophagus, although the association with BP is less definitive compared to smoking and alcohol.

3. A 62-year-old man, a heavy smoker with a long history of dietary habits that include high red meat and hot beverage consumption, presents with symptoms suggestive of esophageal cancer. His dietary history is being reviewed as part of the risk assessment and counseling. In the context of this patient's risk profile, which of the following statements is incorrect regarding dietary risk factors of esophageal cancer?

   A. Increased intake of red meat, particularly when processed or cooked at high temperatures, has been associated with an increased risk of esophageal cancer due to the formation of carcinogenic compounds.
   B. High selenium intake, contrary to its antioxidant properties, is linked with an increased risk of esophageal cancer.
   C. Regular consumption of extremely hot tea has been implicated in esophageal mucosal injury, potentially increasing the risk of esophageal cancer.
   D. Low zinc intake, contributing to impaired DNA repair and mucosal defense, has been associated with an elevated risk of esophageal cancer.
   E. Low folate intake, leading to disruptions in DNA methylation and repair, is a recognized risk factor for esophageal cancer development.

Answer: B

Explanation: Contrary to the assertion in the question, low selenium levels are a risk factor for esophageal cancer, and selenium supplementation has been associated with a reduced risk. The other options accurately describe dietary factors that have been linked to an increased risk of esophageal cancer.

4. A 63-year-old patient with a history of heavy smoking and alcohol consumption presents with dysphagia and significant weight loss. An endoscopy reveals a lesion in the mid-thoracic esophagus, and biopsy confirms SCC. The oncology team is discussing the patient's diagnosis in light of common characteristics and presentations of SCC of the esophagus. In the context of this patient's diagnosis, which of the following statements is incorrect regarding SCC of the esophagus?

   A. LN metastases are present in at least 75% of patients at the time of initial diagnosis, indicating the aggressive nature of this cancer.
   B. Carcinoma in situ in the esophagus typically progresses to invasive SCC over a period of 2 to 4 years.
   C. The most common locations for SCC of the esophagus are the upper and mid-thoracic segments, correlating with this patient's lesion.
   D. Esophageal carcinoma, including SCC, tends to present with multifocal lesions, necessitating thorough evaluation of the entire esophagus.
   E. Ulcerative lesions with extensive infiltration of the adjacent esophageal wall represent the most common macroscopic finding in SCC of the esophagus.

Answer: E

Explanation: Macroscopically, the most common form of SCC of the esophagus is fungating intraluminal growths (60%), not ulcerative lesions with extensive infiltration (25%). The other statements correctly describe aspects of SCC of the esophagus: high prevalence of LN metastases at diagnosis, progression timeline from carcinoma in situ to invasive cancer, common locations of tumors, and the tendency for multifocality.

5. A 67-year-old man with a long-standing history of smoking and alcohol use presents with progressive dysphagia, particularly to solid foods, and recent unexplained weight loss. Given his risk factors and symptoms, the medical team suspects esophageal cancer and plans a comprehensive diagnostic workup. In the context of this patient's clinical presentation, which of the following statements is incorrect regarding the presentation of esophageal cancer?

   A. Dysphagia, a hallmark symptom of esophageal cancer, typically manifests when approximately 90% of the esophageal lumen is obstructed by the tumor.
   B. Dysphagia is generally the most common presenting symptom in patients with esophageal cancer, often indicating advanced disease.
   C. In cases of proximal and middle esophageal tumors, bronchoscopy may be indicated to assess for potential airway involvement.

D. Implementing a widespread screening program for esophageal cancer is not considered cost-effective due to the relatively low prevalence and the specificity of risk factors.
E. Positron emission tomography (PET) scan, offering metabolic information, is often superior to computed tomography (CT) in assessing the extent of esophageal cancer and detecting distant metastases.

Answer: A

Explanation: Dysphagia in esophageal cancer typically occurs when approximately two-thirds of the esophageal lumen is obstructed, not 90%. The other options are accurate: dysphagia is a common presenting symptom, bronchoscopy may be necessary for tumors in certain locations, screening programs are not widely implemented for esophageal cancer, and PET scans can provide more detailed information compared to CT scans in certain aspects of staging.

6. A 62-year-old woman with a long history of GERD presents with recent worsening of her symptoms. She mentions a new onset of dyspepsia and has lost weight over the past few months. Her family history is notable for gastrointestinal cancer. The clinical team is considering further investigations to rule out serious underlying conditions. In the context of this patient's presentation, which of the following statements is incorrect regarding alarm features of GERD?

A. New onset of dyspepsia in a patient aged 60 years or older warrants further investigation due to the increased risk of malignancy in this age group.
B. Iron-deficiency anemia, which may indicate chronic gastrointestinal bleeding, is a significant alarm feature in patients with GERD.
C. Odynophagia, or painful swallowing, is an alarming symptom that can indicate severe esophageal inflammation or malignancy.
D. Gastrointestinal cancer in a first-degree relative not related to the patient's current symptoms is considered an alarm feature in GERD.
E. Anorexia, particularly when associated with unintentional weight loss, is an alarming symptom that may indicate a more serious underlying pathology in GERD patients.

Answer: D

Explanation: While having a first-degree relative with gastrointestinal cancer is an important consideration in the overall assessment, it is not directly considered an alarm feature of GERD unless it specifically relates to the patient's symptoms. The other options accurately describe alarm features that necessitate further evaluation to rule out serious conditions such as esophageal cancer.

7. A 60-year-old man with a history of chronic gastroesophageal reflux disease (GERD) for over 15 years presents for a routine checkup. He has been on long-term proton pump inhibitor therapy and occasionally takes nonsteroidal anti-inflammatory drugs (NSAIDs) for joint pain. An endoscopy reveals changes

suggestive of Barrett's esophagus. In the context of this patient's condition, which of the following statements is incorrect about Barrett's esophagus?

A. Barrett's esophagus is two to threefold more common in men than in women.
B. NSAIDs are a risk factor for Barrett's esophagus.
C. The mean age at diagnosis of Barrett's esophagus is approximately 55 years.
D. *Helicobacter pylori* (*H. pylori*) infection is a protective factor against Barrett's esophagus.
E. Goblet cells are one of the hallmarks of Barrett's esophagus.

Answer: B

Explanation: NSAIDs, particularly COX-2 inhibitors, have been shown to have antiproliferative and pro-apoptotic effects in Barrett's esophagus-associated esophageal adenocarcinoma cell lines and may even have a role in chemoprevention. They are not a risk factor for Barrett's esophagus. The other options accurately describe characteristics and associations of Barrett's esophagus.

8. A 63-year-old man presents with progressive dysphagia and weight loss. He has a history of iron-deficiency anemia and reports a family history of esophageal cancer. His physical examination reveals hyperkeratosis on his palms and soles. An esophagogastroduodenoscopy (EGD) is scheduled to investigate the possibility of esophageal cancer. In the context of this patient's presentation, which of the following statements is incorrect regarding conditions associated with esophageal cancer?

A. Tylosis, a rare genetic disorder characterized by hyperkeratosis, is strongly associated with a high risk of esophageal cancer.
B. Plummer-Vinson syndrome, characterized by iron-deficiency anemia and esophageal webs, increases the risk of SCC of the esophagus.
C. Zenker's diverticula, pouches forming at the upper part of the esophagus, are linked with an increased risk of esophageal cancer.
D. Vitamin B12 deficiency has been shown to be associated with an increased risk of esophageal cancer.
E. Howel-Evans syndrome, a rare genetic condition, is associated with an increased risk of esophageal cancer.

Answer: D

Explanation: While deficiencies of certain B vitamins (B1, B3, B6, B9) have been associated with a decreased risk of esophageal cancer, vitamin B12 supplementation, not deficiency, has been linked with an increased risk of esophageal cancer. Zenker's diverticula are not directly associated with an increased risk of esophageal cancer but may cause symptoms similar to esophageal malignancies.

9. A 55-year-old man with a long-standing history of heartburn and GERD undergoes a routine endoscopy. The endoscopy reveals erosive esophagitis and areas suspicious for Barrett's esophagus. A treatment plan including acid suppression therapy and further diagnostic procedures is being formulated. In the context of

this patient's case, which of the following statements is incorrect regarding the screening of Barrett's esophagus?

A. In patients with erosive esophagitis on initial endoscopy, a repeat endoscopy is recommended after a 3-month course of acid suppression therapy.
B. Two to four biopsies should be performed during endoscopy to provide sufficient material for histologic and molecular interpretation.
C. Endoscopic resection (ER) can be utilized for the management of high-grade dysplasia found in Barrett's esophagus.
D. Approximately 40% of patients diagnosed with esophageal adenocarcinoma do not have a prior history of heartburn.
E. The maximum and circumferential extent of the affected area are reliable markers in the diagnosis of Barrett's esophagus.

Answer: B

Explanation: The correct protocol for biopsies in Barrett's esophagus involves taking multiple biopsies, specifically six to eight, using standard-size endoscopy forceps to provide sufficient specimens for accurate histologic and molecular interpretation. The other statements correctly describe practices and observations associated with the screening and management of Barrett's esophagus.

10. A 50-year-old man, recently diagnosed with esophageal cancer located at the junction of the middle and lower thirds of the esophagus, is being evaluated for potential surgical resection. The surgical team discusses the pattern of lymphatic spread to plan the extent of lymph node (LN) dissection. In the context of this patient's diagnosis, which of the following statements is incorrect regarding the lymphatic drainage of the esophagus?

A. The cervical esophagus predominantly drains to the neck and supraclavicular lymph nodes.
B. The upper thoracic esophagus drains to the nodes on the innominate artery, ligamentum arteriosum, paraesophageal, and paratracheal nodes.
C. The middle thoracic esophagus primarily drains to the tracheobronchial, paraesophageal, and pulmonary hilar lymph nodes.
D. The lower thoracic esophagus drains to the paraesophageal and diaphragmatic lymph nodes.
E. The esophagogastric junction (EGJ) drains to the superior mesenteric lymph nodes.

Answer: E

Explanation: The EGJ drains to the lymph nodes on the left gastric, celiac, common hepatic, and splenic arteries, as well as to the paracardiac and lesser curvature nodes, not to the superior mesenteric lymph nodes. Understanding the lymphatic drainage is crucial for planning surgical resection and predicting the potential routes of metastatic spread in esophageal cancer.

11. A 58-year-old man diagnosed with esophageal cancer is undergoing staging to determine the extent of the disease. The multidisciplinary team, including

surgical oncologists, discusses the relevance of LN involvement and the use of various diagnostic tools for accurate staging. In the context of this patient's cancer staging, which of the following statements is incorrect regarding the staging of esophageal cancer?

A. N2 designation in esophageal cancer staging refers to metastasis in three to six regional lymph nodes, which significantly impacts treatment planning and prognosis.
B. The specific region of nodal spread is a key determinant in the prognosis of esophageal cancer, influencing both therapeutic approach and expected outcomes.
C. Endoscopic ultrasound (EUS) is considered the most accurate technique for locoregional staging of invasive esophageal cancer, particularly for assessing tumor depth and nearby LN involvement.
D. To confirm the diagnosis and assess the extent of esophageal cancer, a minimum of seven biopsies is recommended during endoscopic examination.
E. The presence of distant metastasis in esophageal cancer is a critical factor, often resulting in an overall survival rate of less than 5%.

Answer: B

Explanation: Current understanding and evidence suggest that the number of involved lymph nodes, rather than their specific location, has greater prognostic importance in esophageal cancer, particularly after chemoradiotherapy (CRT). The other options accurately reflect aspects of esophageal cancer staging, including the role of EUS and the impact of metastasis on survival.

12. A 48-year-old woman with a long history of GERD is being evaluated for her persistent symptoms despite lifestyle modifications and medical therapy. She provides a detailed dietary history and mentions various medications she is taking for other health issues. In the context of this patient's ongoing management for GERD, which of the following statements is incorrect regarding the causes of GERD?

A. Transient lower esophageal sphincter relaxations, which are the primary mechanism in many patients with GERD, can be exacerbated by factors like fatty foods and certain medications.
B. Consumption of fermented foods, erroneously thought by some to balance gastrointestinal pH, does not contribute to the pathophysiology of GERD.
C. Impaired esophageal acid clearance, due to ineffective esophageal peristalsis or anatomical abnormalities, is a significant contributor to prolonged acid exposure in GERD.
D. Hiatus hernia, especially when large, can disrupt the normal pressure gradient between the stomach and esophagus, exacerbating reflux symptoms.
E. Estrogen, particularly in high doses or in hormone replacement therapy, has been implicated in reducing lower esophageal sphincter pressure, thus potentially aggravating GERD symptoms.

Answer: B

Explanation: While specific dietary items such as fatty foods, chocolate, and peppermint, along with caffeine, alcohol, smoking, and various drugs, can exacerbate reflux by inducing lower esophageal sphincter (LES) hypotension, there is no evidence that fermented foods play a direct role in the causation of GERD. The other options accurately describe mechanisms and factors that contribute to GERD.

13. A 55-year-old patient with esophageal cancer has completed neoadjuvant CRT. The tumor was initially staged as T3N1M0. The multidisciplinary oncology team is discussing the patient's eligibility for esophagectomy based on the current staging and response to CRT. In the context of this patient's treatment plan, which of the following statements is incorrect regarding the indications for esophagectomy following neoadjuvant chemotherapy or CRT in esophageal cancer?

    A. Esophagectomy is typically not indicated for patients with clinical T1N0M0 lesions, as these are usually treated solely with surgery without the need for CRT.
    B. Patients with thoracic esophageal cancer demonstrating full-thickness (T3) involvement are considered candidates for esophagectomy following neoadjuvant CRT.
    C. EGJ tumors with full-thickness (T3) involvement are typically managed with esophagectomy after neoadjuvant CRT, depending on the response to treatment.
    D. Patients with T4a disease showing isolated invasion into the pericardium may be considered for esophagectomy post-CRT, depending on the extent of local invasion and response to therapy.
    E. Patients with T4a disease and isolated invasion into the diaphragm can be considered for esophagectomy following CRT, based on a multidisciplinary evaluation of the tumor's responsiveness and resectability.

Answer: A

Explanation: Clinical T1N0M0 lesions in esophageal cancer are typically treated with esophagectomy alone, as neoadjuvant CRT is not usually indicated for such early-stage tumors. The other options correctly describe scenarios where esophagectomy following neoadjuvant CRT may be considered, based on the extent of tumor invasion and response to initial treatment.

14. A surgical oncology team is evaluating a 60-year-old patient with Barrett's esophagus and high-grade dysplasia for surgical intervention. The discussion revolves around the suitability of transhiatal esophagectomy, considering the patient's condition and the anatomical location of the disease. In the context of this surgical planning, which of the following statements is incorrect regarding transhiatal esophagectomy?

    A. Transhiatal esophagectomy is performed without a thoracotomy, making it a less invasive option compared to transthoracic approaches.

B. This approach is associated with improved safety regarding the cervical anastomosis, as it avoids thoracic incisions and related complications.
C. Transhiatal esophagectomy is particularly advantageous for the removal of the entire esophagus, especially in cases involving long-segment Barrett's esophagus or when clear margins are a concern.
D. The procedure carries an increased risk of inadvertent injury to the tracheobronchial tree due to limited direct visualization during dissection.
E. Transhiatal esophagectomy allows for comprehensive dissection of middle esophageal tumors with adequate visualization and access.

Answer: E

Explanation: Transhiatal esophagectomy has a limited ability to adequately dissect middle esophageal tumors due to the approach's restricted visualization and access in this area. The other options accurately describe the characteristics of transhiatal esophagectomy, including its non-thoracotomy approach, cervical anastomosis safety, suitability for extensive esophageal resection, and the risks associated with limited visualization.

15. The surgical oncology team is considering a transthoracic esophagectomy for a 57-year-old patient with mid-thoracic esophageal cancer. The team discusses the benefits and risks of this approach, especially in terms of lymphadenectomy, locoregional recurrence, and postoperative complications. In the context of this surgical decision-making, which of the following statements is incorrect regarding transthoracic esophagectomy?

A. Transthoracic esophagectomy allows for more deliberate and thorough lymphadenectomy, which is beneficial for achieving clear margins and assessing nodal status.
B. This approach is associated with lower rates of locoregional recurrences due to extensive surgical resection and LN clearance.
C. Transthoracic esophagectomy is characterized by a lower incidence of pulmonary complications compared to other surgical approaches for esophageal cancer.
D. The procedure enables preservation of the membranous portions of the tracheobronchial tree, minimizing the risk of injury to these structures.
E. Transthoracic esophagectomy is associated with higher morbidity and mortality, primarily due to the risks of anastomotic leaks and the extensive nature of the surgery.

Answer: C

Explanation: Transthoracic esophagectomy actually has a higher incidence of pulmonary complications due to the invasiveness of the thoracic approach and the associated pulmonary manipulation. The other options correctly describe aspects of transthoracic esophagectomy, including the advantages of extensive lymphadenectomy, lower locoregional recurrence rates, and the increased risks of morbidity and mortality.

16. A 59-year-old patient with locally advanced esophageal cancer is being evaluated for CRT. The tumor is located in the mid-esophagus, and the patient has significant dysphagia. The oncology team discusses the optimal CRT strategy, taking into account the tumor's location, molecular characteristics, and the patient's overall condition.

    In the context of this patient's treatment planning, which of the following statements is incorrect regarding CRT of esophageal cancer?

    A. When treating tumors located above the carina, the supraclavicular fossae are typically included in the radiation field to address potential lymphatic spread.
    B. For distal esophageal and EGJ tumors, the radiation field generally covers the celiac axis to encompass regional lymph nodes.
    C. The cornerstone of chemotherapy in CRT for esophageal cancer often involves fluoropyrimidine or taxane-based regimens, selected based on tumor characteristics and patient tolerance.
    D. Trastuzumab combined with chemotherapy is now the preferred treatment for localized HER2-positive gastroesophageal junction tumors in CRT settings.
    E. In cases of metastatic esophageal cancer, palliative care including interventions for malignant dysphagia remains a crucial aspect of treatment to maintain quality of life.

Answer: D

Explanation: Trastuzumab in combination with chemotherapy is currently preferred for metastatic HER2-positive EGJ tumors, not necessarily for localized disease. The other options accurately describe various aspects of CRT for esophageal cancer, including radiation field considerations, chemotherapy regimens, and palliative care approaches.

17. During a surgical planning meeting, a 54-year-old patient with esophageal cancer is being discussed. The tumor is located in the middle third of the esophagus, and the team is considering various esophagectomy techniques, evaluating the suitability of different reconstructive options and the implications for lymphadenectomy. In the context of this patient's surgical planning, which of the following statements is incorrect regarding esophagectomy?

    A. If the stomach is not a viable option for reconstruction, the colon may be utilized as an alternative conduit.
    B. In cases where the jejunum is used for reconstruction, an anastomosis with the carotid artery is sometimes indicated for adequate blood supply.
    C. A tri-incisional esophagectomy approach may be indicated if there is a sufficient margin on the upper esophageal sphincter, allowing for complete tumor resection.
    D. The Ivor-Lewis transthoracic esophagectomy is typically used for resecting cancers in the middle third of the esophagus, providing optimal proximal margins.

E. The three-incisional technique enables the surgeon to perform a thorough two-field lymphadenectomy under direct vision, with a cervical esophagogastric anastomosis being a key feature of this approach.

Answer: D

Explanation: The Ivor-Lewis transthoracic esophagectomy is actually more suited for cancers in the lower third of the esophagus, not the middle third, due to limitations in achieving adequate proximal margins. The other options correctly describe aspects of esophagectomy: alternative conduits for reconstruction, the use of the jejunum and its vascular considerations, the indications for tri-incisional esophagectomy, and the advantages of the three-incisional technique.

18. The surgical oncology team is discussing the optimal surgical approach for a 56-year-old patient diagnosed with adenocarcinoma at the EGJ. The tumor's location and characteristics are being evaluated in the context of the Siewert classification to determine the most appropriate surgical strategy. In the context of this patient's surgical planning, which of the following statements is incorrect regarding esophagectomy in relation to the Siewert classification?

A. For patients with Siewert type II tumors, an Ivor-Lewis esophagectomy is often the recommended approach, considering the tumor's proximity to the EGJ.
B. Siewert type I adenocarcinoma typically originates in the distal esophagus, often associated with Barrett's esophagus.
C. Type III adenocarcinoma originates from a subcardial gastric location, infiltrating the EGJ and distal esophagus from below.
D. Siewert type II adenocarcinoma generally arises from the cardia or directly at the EGJ, necessitating a specific surgical approach.
E. Patients with Siewert type I tumors are typically treated with a total gastrectomy combined with a transhiatal resection of the distal esophagus and extensive lymphadenectomy.

Answer: E

Explanation: Siewert type III tumors, not type I, are the ones typically managed with a total gastrectomy combined with a transhiatal resection of the distal esophagus and extensive lymphadenectomy. Siewert type I tumors are generally treated with esophagectomy due to their location in the distal esophagus. The other options correctly describe the surgical approaches based on the Siewert classification of EGJ adenocarcinomas.

19. In a postoperative review meeting, a surgical oncology team is discussing the case of a 60-year-old patient who recently underwent an esophagectomy. The patient experienced several complications, prompting a review of common and uncommon complications associated with this procedure. In the context of postoperative care for esophagectomy patients, which of the following statements is incorrect regarding complications of esophagectomy?

A. Pulmonary complications, including pneumonia and respiratory failure, are the most frequently observed complications following an esophagectomy.
B. The occurrence of pneumonia post-esophagectomy is an independent risk factor for increased postoperative mortality.
C. Atrial fibrillation, while concerning, is a rare complication in the postoperative period of an esophagectomy.
D. The risk of venous thromboembolism (VTE) following an esophagectomy is estimated to be between 1.5 and 2.4%, necessitating vigilant prophylactic measures.
E. In cases of unilateral vocal cord paralysis post-esophagectomy, management may involve vocal cord injection to improve voice quality and prevent aspiration.

Answer: C

Explanation: Atrial fibrillation is not a rare complication; it is reported to occur in up to 20% of patients undergoing an esophagectomy. The other statements are accurate: pulmonary complications are common, pneumonia increases mortality risk, VTE is a significant concern post-esophagectomy, and vocal cord injection may be required for unilateral vocal cord paralysis.

20. A 68-year-old patient with advanced esophageal cancer is being evaluated for endoscopic palliative measures due to inoperability and significant dysphagia. The multidisciplinary team discusses various endoscopic palliation options, considering their efficacy, potential complications, and the need for repeat interventions. In the context of this patient's palliative care, which of the following statements is incorrect regarding endoscopic palliation of esophageal cancer?

A. Esophageal stenting, particularly with self-expandable metal stents, is the most commonly used method for palliation of malignant dysphagia in esophageal cancer.
B. The development of an esophago-respiratory fistula is a potential delayed adverse event following the placement of an esophageal stent.
C. Most malignant esophageal strictures can be safely dilated to 16 or 17 mm across several sessions to alleviate dysphagia.
D. Repeat dilatation of malignant esophageal strictures is typically required every 2 to 4 months to maintain luminal patency.
E. Photodynamic therapy (PDT), an alternative palliative treatment, is less commonly utilized than self-expandable metal stents due to its specific indications and availability.

Answer: D

Explanation: Repeat dilatation for malignant esophageal strictures is usually required more frequently, typically every 2 to 4 weeks, rather than months, due to the rapid progression of the disease and the tendency for strictures to recur. The other statements accurately reflect the current practices and considerations in the endoscopic palliation of esophageal cancer.

21. A 62-year-old patient who recently underwent an esophagectomy presents with chylothorax in the postoperative period. The surgical oncology team is discussing the management options and potential interventions, considering the patient's current clinical status and the severity of the chylothorax. In the context of managing this patient's postoperative complication, which of the following statements is incorrect regarding postoperative chylothorax in esophagectomy?

    A. Prophylactic ligation of the thoracic duct during esophagectomy is generally not beneficial in preventing chylothorax.
    B. Chylothorax occurs in approximately 1–2% of esophagectomy cases, representing a significant postoperative complication.
    C. Surgical intervention for chylothorax is typically considered if conservative measures fail to resolve the condition within 7 to 14 days.
    D. Conservative management of chylothorax often includes a low-fat diet supplemented with medium-chain triglycerides and diuretic therapy.
    E. If left untreated, chylothorax can result in a mortality rate of up to 50% due to its severe impact on respiratory and nutritional status.

Answer: A

Explanation: Intraoperative prophylactic ligation of the thoracic duct has been shown to reduce the incidence of chylothorax following esophagectomy. The other options correctly describe various aspects of chylothorax post-esophagectomy: its incidence rate, indications for surgical intervention, conservative management strategies, and the potential for high mortality if not adequately treated.

22. The surgical oncology team is discussing various esophagectomy techniques for a 55-year-old patient with mid-esophageal cancer. The team is weighing the benefits and risks of different reconstruction methods and their associated complications. In the context of selecting an appropriate esophagectomy technique for this patient, which of the following statements is incorrect?

    A. Not all esophageal perforations necessitate surgical repair; some may be managed conservatively depending on the size and clinical context.
    B. The colon transposition graft procedure for esophageal reconstruction is associated with the highest morbidity and mortality rates among the various options.
    C. The gastric pull-up procedure generally allows for the quickest return to oral feeding postoperatively compared to other reconstruction methods.
    D. Bronchorrhea is considered the most disabling complication specifically of two-field esophagectomy.
    E. The radial forearm free flap, used in esophageal reconstruction, is particularly susceptible to ischemic injury due to its vascular supply characteristics.

Answer: D

Explanation: Bronchorrhea is actually the most disabling complication of three-field esophagectomy, not two-field esophagectomy. This complication arises from extensive LN dissection in the neck, thorax, and abdomen. The other statements correctly address various aspects of esophagectomy techniques: the management of esophageal perforations, morbidity and mortality associated with colon transposition, advantages of gastric pull-up, and the risk of ischemic injury in radial forearm free flap procedures.

23. During a multidisciplinary meeting, a surgical oncology team discusses a challenging case of a 55-year-old patient with an esophageal tumor. The tumor's location in relation to key anatomical landmarks of the esophagus is crucial for planning the surgical approach. In the context of this case discussion, which of the following statements is incorrect about the anatomy of the esophagus?

    A. The esophagus is located in the posterior mediastinum.
    B. The recurrent laryngeal nerves typically ascend in a groove at the junction of the trachea and esophagus.
    C. The esophagus extends from the level of the sixth cervical vertebra to the tenth thoracic vertebra.
    D. The esophagus constricts at the cricopharyngeus muscle, the bronchoaortic constriction, and the EGJ.
    E. The EGJ is the most common site of esophageal perforation.

Answer: C

Explanation: The esophagus actually extends from the level of the seventh cervical vertebra to the 11th thoracic vertebra. The other statements correctly describe aspects of esophageal anatomy important for surgical planning and understanding esophageal pathologies.

24. A 45-year-old patient is undergoing an esophagectomy for esophageal cancer. The surgical oncology team is meticulously navigating the complex anatomy surrounding the esophagus to ensure a successful and complication-free procedure. In the context of this intricate surgical procedure, which of the following statements is incorrect about the anatomy of the esophagus?

    A. Laimer's triangle, located adjacent to the esophagogastric junction, is superior to Killian's triangle, found at the pharyngoesophageal junction.
    B. The esophageal hiatus, a diaphragmatic opening for the esophagus, is positioned superiorly compared to the aortic hiatus, which transmits the aorta and thoracic duct.
    C. The thoracic duct, a critical structure for lymphatic drainage, ascends to the left of the esophagus, joining the venous system at the junction of the left subclavian and internal jugular veins.
    D. The left vagus nerve, following its course around the aortic arch, provides anterior vagal trunk fibers that contribute to the esophageal plexus.
    E. The right vagus nerve, known for its path behind the esophagus and primary right bronchus, forms the posterior vagal trunk which contributes to the posterior esophageal plexus.

Answer: A

Explanation: Laimer's triangle is not superior to Killian's triangle; in fact, both are located at the same level, each at different parts of the esophagus. Killian's triangle is at the pharyngoesophageal junction, while Laimer's triangle is adjacent to the esophagogastric junction. The other options, while complex, accurately describe the intricate anatomical relationships around the esophagus that are crucial during esophageal surgeries.

25. A 58-year-old patient who underwent esophagectomy for esophageal cancer 6 months ago is being followed up in clinic. The patient had a history of SCC and received a combination of surgery and radiation therapy. The oncology team is reviewing the patient's posttreatment outcomes and discussing common issues encountered in similar cases. In the context of this patient's posttreatment follow-up, which of the following statements is incorrect regarding outcomes after esophageal cancer treatment?

    A. Surgical bypass is seldom utilized for unresectable esophageal carcinoma due to limited efficacy and the presence of less invasive palliative options.
    B. The development of reflux esophagitis following low intrathoracic esophagogastric anastomosis is rare, as most patients with esophageal carcinoma have limited life expectancy post-surgery.
    C. Radical transthoracic esophagectomy with en bloc dissection of lymph node-bearing tissues has not demonstrated a survival advantage over transhiatal esophagectomy.
    D. Although SCC of the esophagus is generally considered radiosensitive, radiation therapy alone rarely achieves a cure in most patients.
    E. Endoscopic laser fulguration, used for palliative treatment of esophageal tumors, achieves symptomatic improvement in up to 75% of patients.

Answer: B

Explanation: Contrary to the traditional teaching, the development of reflux esophagitis after low intrathoracic esophagogastric anastomosis is a significant concern, even in patients with esophageal carcinoma. These patients can experience severe reflux symptoms and dysphagia from benign stenosis. The other options accurately describe various aspects of esophageal cancer treatment outcomes: limited role of surgical bypass, comparison of radical transthoracic and transhiatal esophagectomies, the efficacy of radiation therapy in SCC, and the success rate of endoscopic laser fulguration.

26. A 42-year-old patient presents with dysphagia and mild chest pain. An endoscopy reveals a submucosal mass in the esophagus, and subsequent investigations suggest a benign neoplasm, likely a leiomyoma. The surgical oncology team discusses the management options and the general characteristics of benign esophageal neoplasms. In the context of this patient's diagnosis, which of the following statements is incorrect regarding benign esophageal neoplasms?

    A. Benign tumors of the esophagus are relatively rare, constituting less than 1% of all esophageal neoplasms.

B. Asymptomatic leiomyomas can often be managed with observation and followed up with periodic barium esophograms and endoscopic ultrasonography.
C. Leiomyomas in the esophagus characteristically occur in patients between 50 and 70 years of age.
D. Benign esophageal tumors smaller than 5 cm in size infrequently cause symptoms and are often found incidentally.
E. Leiomyomas are the most common type of benign intramural tumor found in the esophagus.

Answer: C

Explanation: Leiomyomas typically occur in a younger age group, characteristically between 20 and 50 years of age, not 50 to 70 years as stated. The other options correctly describe aspects of benign esophageal neoplasms: their rarity, management approach for asymptomatic leiomyomas, symptomatology related to tumor size, and the prevalence of leiomyomas as benign esophageal tumors.

27. In a multidisciplinary team meeting, a 68-year-old patient with end-stage esophageal cancer is being discussed. The patient has undergone chemoradiation and is experiencing significant dysphagia. The team reviews various aspects of management and prognosis for patients in similar stages of esophageal cancer. In the context of this patient's condition and treatment, which of the following statements is incorrect regarding end-stage esophageal cancer?

A. Patients with dysphagia secondary to esophageal cancer who are treated with radiation can generally expect symptomatic relief to last for approximately 2–3 months.
B. Surgery following chemoradiation induction is typically recommended to occur after 6 months.
C. The general 5-year relative survival rate for esophageal cancer in the United States is around 21%.
D. Esophageal cancer is responsible for over 15,000 deaths annually in the United States.
E. More than one-third of esophageal cancer cases are metastasized at the time of diagnosis.

Answer: B

Explanation: Surgery after chemoradiation induction for esophageal cancer is typically planned for 6 to 8 weeks following the completion of therapy, not after 6 months. The other statements correctly reflect aspects of end-stage esophageal cancer: the duration of symptomatic relief from radiation therapy for dysphagia, the general 5-year survival rate, the annual mortality rate, and the proportion of cases presenting with metastasis at diagnosis.

Bibliography

1. Baquet CR, Commiskey P, Mack K, Meltzer S, Mishra SI. Esophageal cancer epidemiology in blacks and whites: racial and gender disparities in incidence, mortality, survival rates and histology. J Natl Med Assoc. 2005;97(11):1471–8. PMID: 16334494; PMCID: PMC2594901.
2. Hvid-Jensen F, Pedersen L, Drewes AM, Sørensen HT, Funch-Jensen P. Incidence of adenocarcinoma among patients with Barrett's esophagus. N Engl J Med. 2011;365(15):1375–83. https://doi.org/10.1056/NEJMoa1103042.
3. Steevens J, van den Brandt PA, Goldbohm RA, Schouten LJ. Selenium status and the risk of esophageal and gastric cancer subtypes: The Netherlands Cohort Study. Gastroenterology. 2010;138(5):1704–13. Epub 2009 Dec 16. https://doi.org/10.1053/j.gastro.2009.12.004.
4. Yang H, Lin Z, Lin Y, He F, Liu S, Zhang Z, Wang J, Xie Q, Chen Y, Chen W, Hu Z. Risk factors of esophageal squamous cell cancer specific for different macroscopic types. Nutr Cancer. 2020;72(8):1336–44. Epub 2020 Mar 11. https://doi.org/10.1080/01635581.2020.1733623.
5. Zwischenberger JB, et al. Esophagus. In: Townsend Jr CM, Beauchamp RD, Evers BM, Mattox KL, editors. Sabiston textbook of surgery, vol. 1120. 17th ed. Philadelphia: Elsevier; 2004. p. 1123.
6. Shetty A, Balaraju G, Shetty S, Pai CG. Diagnostic utility of alarm features in predicting malignancy in patients with dyspeptic symptoms. Indian J Gastroenterol. 2021;40(2):183–8. Epub 2021 Apr 8. PMID: 33830441; PMCID: PMC8187202. https://doi.org/10.1007/s12664-021-01155-x.
7. Buttar NS, Wang KK, Anderson MA, Dierkhising RA, Pacifico RJ, Krishnadath KK, Lutzke LS. The effect of selective cyclooxygenase-2 inhibition in Barrett's esophagus epithelium: an in vitro study. J Natl Cancer Inst. 2002;94(6):422–9. https://doi.org/10.1093/jnci/94.6.422.
8. Ma JL, Zhao Y, Guo CY, Hu HT, Zheng L, Zhao EJ, Li HL. Dietary vitamin B intake and the risk of esophageal cancer: a meta-analysis. Cancer Manag Res. 2018;10:5395–410. PMID: 30464635; PMCID: PMC6225909. https://doi.org/10.2147/CMAR.S168413.
9. Graham DY, Schwartz JT, Cain GD, Gyorkey F. Prospective evaluation of biopsy number in the diagnosis of esophageal and gastric carcinoma. Gastroenterology. 1982;82(2):228–31.
10. National Comprehensive Cancer Network. NCCN guidelines version 1.2012: esophageal and esophagogastric junction cancers. Vancouver: NCCN; 2012. www.nccn.org. Accessed 21 May 2012.
11. Zhang HL, Chen LQ, Liu RL, Shi YT, He M, Meng XL, Bai SX, Ping YM. The number of lymph node metastases influences survival and International Union against cancer tumor-node-metastasis classification for esophageal squamous cell carcinoma. Dis Esophagus. 2010;23(1):53–8. Epub 2009 Apr 15. https://doi.org/10.1111/j.1442-2050.2009.00971.x.
12. Fox M, Gyawali CP. Dietary factors involved in GERD management. Best Pract Res Clin Gastroenterol. 2023;62–63:101826. Epub 2023 Feb 17. https://doi.org/10.1016/j.bpg.2023.101826.
13. Wu AJ, Goodman KA. Clinical tools to predict outcomes in patients with esophageal cancer treated with definitive chemoradiation: are we there yet? J Gastrointest Oncol. 2015;6(1):53–9. PMID: 25642338; PMCID: PMC4294820. https://doi.org/10.3978/j.issn.2078-6891.2014.099.
14. Chang AC, Ji H, Birkmeyer NJ, Orringer MB, Birkmeyer JD. Outcomes after transhiatal and transthoracic esophagectomy for cancer. Ann Thorac Surg. 2008;85(2):424–9.
15. Stiles BM, Altorki NK. Traditional techniques of esophagectomy. Surg Clin North Am. 2012;92(5):1249–63.
16. Bang YJ, Van Cutsem E, Feyereislova A, et al. Trastuzumab in combination with chemotherapy versus chemotherapy alone for treatment of HER2-positive advanced gastric or gastro-oesophageal junction cancer (ToGA): a phase 3, open-label, randomized controlled trial. Lancet. 2010;376(9742):687–97.
17. Chang AC, Ji H, Birkmeyer NJ, Orringer MB, Birkmeyer JD. Outcomes after transhiatal and transthoracic esophagectomy for cancer. Ann Thorac Surg. 2008;85(2):424–9. https://doi.org/10.1016/j.athoracsur.2007.10.007.

18. Zhang S, Orita H, Fukunaga T. Current surgical treatment of esophagogastric junction adenocarcinoma. World J Gastrointest Oncol. 2019;11:567–78.
19. Murthy SC, Law S, Whooley BP, Alexandrou A, Chu KM, Wong J. Atrial fibrillation after esophagectomy is a marker for postoperative morbidity and mortality. J Thorac Cardiovasc Surg. 2003;126(4):1162–7. https://doi.org/10.1016/s0022-5223(03)00974-7.
20. Yoda Y, Yano T, Kaneko K, Tsuruta S, Oono Y, Kojima T, Minashi K, Ikematsu H, Ohtsu A. Endoscopic balloon dilatation for benign fibrotic strictures after curative nonsurgical treatment for esophageal cancer. Surg Endosc. 2012;26(10):2877–83. Epub 2012 Apr 28. https://doi.org/10.1007/s00464-012-2273-9.
21. Kamaleddine I, Hendricks A, Popova M, Schafmayer C. Adequate management of postoperative complications after esophagectomy: a cornerstone for a positive outcome. Cancers (Basel). 2022;14(22):5556. PMID: 36428649; PMCID: PMC9688292. https://doi.org/10.3390/cancers14225556.
22. Shirinzadeh A, Talebi Y. Pulmonary complications due to esophagectomy. J Cardiovasc Thorac Res. 2011;3(3):93–6. Epub 2011 Aug 20. PMID: 24250962; PMCID: PMC3825331. https://doi.org/10.5681/jcvtr.2011.020.
23. Rice TW, Kelsen D, Blackstone EH, et al. Esophagus and esophagogastric junction. In: Amin MB, editor. AJCC Cancer Staging Manual. 8th ed. Chicago: AJCC; 2017. p. 185. Corrected at 4th printing, 2018.
24. Oezcelik A, DeMeester SR. General anatomy of the esophagus. Thorac Surg Clin. 2011;21(2):239–97, x. https://doi.org/10.1016/j.thorsurg.2011.01.003.
25. Nishimura K, Tanaka T, Tanaka Y, Matono S, Murata K, Shirouzu K, Fujita H. Reflux esophagitis and columnar-lined esophagus after cervical esophagogastrostomy (following esophagectomy). Dis Esophagus. 2010;23(2):94–9. Epub 2009 Jul 31. https://doi.org/10.1111/j.1442-2050.2009.00998.x.
26. O'Hanlon DM, Clarke E, Lennon J, Gorey TF. Leiomyoma of the esophagus. Am J Surg. 2002;184(2):168–9. https://doi.org/10.1016/s0002-9610(02)00905-4.
27. Rampado S, Bocus P, Battaglia G, Ruol A, Portale G, Ancona E. Endoscopic ultrasound: accuracy in staging superficial carcinomas of the esophagus. Ann Thorac Surg. 2008;85(1):251–6. https://doi.org/10.1016/j.athoracsur.2007.08.021.
28. Watanabe M, Otake R, Kozuki R, Toihata T, Takahashi K, Okamura A, Imamura Y. Recent progress in multidisciplinary treatment for patients with esophageal cancer. Surg Today. 2020;50(1):12–20. Epub 2019 Sep 18. Erratum in: Surg Today. 2020 Apr;50(4):425. PMID: 31535225; PMCID: PMC6952324. https://doi.org/10.1007/s00595-019-01878-7.

Chapter 2
Gastric Tumors

Salih Ahmed Aljiburi, Munthir A. Alobaidi, Raafat Raoof Alturfi, Saleh Abdulkareem Saleh, and Aqeel Shakir Mahmood

1. A 55-year-old male presents with weight loss and epigastric pain. Endoscopy reveals a gastric ulcer, and biopsy confirms adenocarcinoma. His family history is significant for gastric cancer in his father. Based on this case and your knowledge of gastric cancer epidemiology, identify the incorrect statement:

   A. Gastric cancer is the fifth most common malignancy globally, with higher prevalence in East Asia, Eastern Europe, and South America.
   B. The majority of cases (>70%) are diagnosed in developing countries, often presenting at advanced stages.
   C. The incidence of gastric cancer is higher in men than in women, with a male-to-female ratio of approximately 2:1.
   D. In high-incidence countries, distal gastric carcinomas are more common, while in low-incidence countries, proximal tumors predominate.
   E. *H. pylori* infection is a significant risk factor, especially in early-onset cases and those with a family history of gastric cancer.

   Answer: A

S. A. Aljiburi
Baghdad Teaching Hospital, Baghdad, Iraq

M. A. Alobaidi
Department of Surgery, College of Medicine, University of Baghdad, Baghdad, Iraq

R. R. Alturfi
Department of Digestive Surgery, Gastroenterology and Hepatology Teaching Hospital, Baghdad, Iraq

S. A. Saleh
College of Medicine University of Baghdad, Baghdad, Iraq

A. S. Mahmood (✉)
Department of General Surgery, University of Baghdad, Baghdad, Iraq

A. S. Mahmood, A. Koulouris (eds.), *MCQs in General Surgical Oncology*,
https://doi.org/10.1007/978-3-031-65738-2_2

Explanation: While option A is partially correct in stating that gastric cancer has a higher prevalence in certain regions, it inaccurately ranks gastric cancer as the fifth most common malignancy globally. Gastric cancer is actually the third most common malignancy.

2. A 63-year-old female with a history of chronic gastritis presents with progressive dysphagia and weight loss. An endoscopic biopsy confirms gastric adenocarcinoma. Considering global epidemiological trends of gastric cancer, identify the incorrect statement:

   A. Gastric cancer incidence is higher in regions with more temperate or colder climates, reflecting geographic variations in risk factors.
   B. Over the past four decades, there has been a significant worldwide decline in the incidence of gastric cancer, attributed to improved dietary and health practices.
   C. Gastric cancer ranks as the third most deadly cancer globally, following lung and colorectal cancers.
   D. Gastric cancer accounts for approximately 1 in 12 of all cancer-related deaths, underscoring its significant impact on global health.
   E. Annually, gastric cancer is diagnosed in approximately one million individuals worldwide, highlighting its substantial prevalence.

Answer: C

Explanation: Gastric cancer is actually the fourth leading cause of cancer deaths globally, after lung, colorectal, and liver cancers.

3. A 50-year-old male with a long-standing history of gastroesophageal reflux disease and recent onset of anemia is diagnosed with gastric cancer. His dietary history reveals a preference for smoked and pickled foods. Considering his diagnosis, identify the incorrect risk factor for gastric cancer:

   A. *H. pylori* infection, which is strongly associated with both intestinal and diffuse types of gastric cancer.
   B. Consumption of salt-preserved foods, which has been linked to gastric mucosal injury and subsequent carcinogenesis.
   C. Exposure to nitroso compounds, commonly found in processed and preserved meats, contributing to gastric carcinogenesis.
   D. Obesity, particularly central obesity, which is associated with an increased risk of cardia gastric cancer.
   E. High consumption of citrus fruits, which, due to their high acid content, may exacerbate gastritis and contribute to carcinogenesis.

Answer: E

Explanation: High consumption of fruits is generally considered a protective factor against gastric carcinoma due to their antioxidant properties and fiber content. The other options correctly identify established risk factors for gastric cancer. This question includes a subtle distraction (high citrus fruit consumption) which is plausible but not supported by current evidence as a risk factor for gastric cancer.

4. A 58-year-old female with a history of smoking and chronic gastritis, currently undergoing treatment for *H. pylori* infection, is diagnosed with early-stage gastric cancer. Reflecting on her history and the known risk factors for gastric cancer, identify the incorrect risk factor:

   A. Smoking, which is a well-established risk factor for gastric cancer due to its carcinogenic effects on the gastric mucosa.
   B. GERD, which can lead to Barrett's esophagus and an increased risk of gastric cardia cancer.
   C. Chronic alcohol use, associated with increased gastric mucosal damage and a heightened risk of gastric cancer.
   D. Long-term use of nonsteroidal anti-inflammatory drugs (NSAIDs), known to reduce the risk of gastric cancer, especially in patients with a history of *H. pylori*-associated ulcers.
   E. Infection with Epstein-Barr virus (EBV), implicated in a subset of gastric cancers, particularly those with lymphoepithelioma-like features.

Answer: D

Explanation: Contrary to the claim in the option, regular use of NSAIDs is associated with a protective effect against the development of gastric carcinoma, especially in patients with gastric ulcers related to *H. pylori* infection. The other options correctly identify known risk factors for gastric cancer.

5. A 62-year-old man with a 10-year history of intermittent dyspepsia presents with recent onset of weight loss and epigastric pain. Endoscopic biopsy confirms a diagnosis of gastric adenocarcinoma, and *H. pylori* infection is detected. Considering the role of *H. pylori* in gastric cancer, identify the incorrect statement about its association with gastric carcinoma:

   A. *H. pylori* infection is considered the strongest known risk factor for the development of gastric cancer, initiating a cascade of mucosal changes.
   B. The pathogenesis involves *H. pylori*-induced chronic gastritis, leading to mucosal atrophy, intestinal metaplasia, and progression to neoplasia.
   C. The VacA toxin, produced by *H. pylori*, is the primary virulence factor implicated in the direct development of gastric carcinoma.
   D. *H. pylori* infection may cause oxidative DNA damage, which contributes to the neoplastic transformation of gastric mucosal cells.
   E. *H. pylori* is implicated in the development of both intestinal-type and diffuse-type gastric cancers, affecting different gastric regions.

Answer: C

Explanation: While the VacA toxin of *H. pylori* is a significant virulence factor, it is the strain of *H. pylori* containing the cytotoxin-associated gene A (CagA) that carries the greatest risk for gastric carcinoma development. The other options accurately reflect the role of *H. pylori* in the pathogenesis of gastric cancer.

6. A 40-year-old woman with a family history of gastric cancer undergoes genetic counseling. Her father and aunt were diagnosed with diffuse gastric cancer at

ages 45 and 48, respectively. She is concerned about her risk for hereditary diffuse gastric cancer (HDGC). Based on your knowledge of HDGC, identify the incorrect statement:

A. Individuals with HDGC have a lifetime risk exceeding 70% for developing diffuse gastric cancer.
B. HDGC is often caused by mutations in the CDH1 tumor suppressor gene, leading to an increased risk of developing this cancer.
C. Female carriers of the mutation also face an elevated risk of developing lobular breast cancer.
D. The main management strategies for HDGC include prophylactic total gastrectomy or intensive endoscopic surveillance.
E. Familial HDGC is defined as having at least two family members diagnosed with diffuse gastric cancer before the age of 50, or three close relatives diagnosed at any age.

Answer: E

Explanation: Familial HDGC is defined as having two or more family members diagnosed with diffuse gastric cancer before the age of 50, or one member diagnosed before 50 and another at any age, or three close relatives diagnosed at any age

7. A 67-year-old male with a history of chronic gastritis undergoes gastrectomy for gastric cancer. Histopathological examination reveals poorly differentiated adenocarcinoma. Reflecting on the Lauren classification of gastric cancer, identify the incorrect statement:

A. The Lauren classification categorizes gastric tumors based on microscopic appearance into two main subtypes: intestinal and diffuse.
B. The diffuse type of gastric cancer is more commonly seen in older males and is characterized by poorly cohesive cells.
C. Regardless of the local extent of the disease, poorly differentiated cancers, as seen in the diffuse type, generally have a poorer prognosis.
D. The pathogenesis of gastric cancer involves epigenetic changes such as DNA methylation, histone modifications, and chromosomal rearrangements.
E. Lauren classification plays a significant role as a prognostic indicator and influences the surgical strategy in gastric cancer treatment.

Answer: B

Explanation: Diffuse-type gastric cancer is more commonly seen in younger individuals and has a higher frequency in females, not predominantly in older males as stated. The other options accurately describe aspects of the Lauren classification and its implications in the pathogenesis, prognosis, and treatment of gastric cancer.

8. A 72-year-old male presents with weight loss, abdominal pain, and iron-deficiency anemia. Gastroscopy reveals a mass in the gastric antrum, and biopsy

confirms intestinal-type gastric carcinoma. Considering the characteristics of intestinal-type gastric cancer, identify the incorrect statement:

A. Tumor cells in intestinal-type gastric carcinoma adhere together, forming distinct tubular or glandular structures.
B. This cancer subtype is more prevalent in males and is typically diagnosed in older age groups.
C. Despite its specific histological features, intestinal-type gastric carcinoma generally has a poorer prognosis.
D. Intestinal-type gastric carcinoma is often associated with lymphatic and vascular invasion, contributing to its metastatic potential.
E. The gastric antrum is the most common site for intestinal-type gastric carcinoma, correlating with specific epidemiological patterns.

Answer: C

Explanation: Intestinal-type gastric carcinoma, characterized by well-formed glandular structures, generally has a better prognosis compared to the diffuse type, especially when diagnosed at an early stage. The other options accurately describe the histopathological and clinical characteristics of intestinal-type gastric carcinoma.

9. A 45-year-old female, with no significant past medical history, presents with early satiety and abdominal bloating. An endoscopy reveals linitis plastica, and biopsies confirm a diagnosis of diffuse-type gastric cancer. Evaluating your knowledge about this subtype, identify the incorrect statement:

A. The tumor cells in diffuse-type gastric cancer characteristically lack adhesion, infiltrating the stroma either as single cells or in small clusters.
B. A hallmark feature is the presence of signet ring cells, where intracellular mucus displaces the nucleus to the periphery.
C. This cancer subtype is characterized by a lack of gland formation, with tumor cells invading surrounding tissues.
D. Diffuse-type gastric cancer tends to occur more frequently in younger individuals and has a slight predilection for females.
E. Diffuse-type gastric cancer predominantly affects the gastric fundus, presenting with distinct clinical features from other types.

Answer: E

Explanation: Diffuse-type gastric cancer most commonly affects the body of the stomach, not the fundus. This subtype is known for its worse prognosis and shorter duration of symptoms compared to intestinal-type gastric cancer. The other options correctly describe the pathological features and demographic tendencies of diffuse-type gastric cancer.

10. A 40-year-old individual with a family history suggestive of hereditary diffuse gastric cancer (HDGC) syndrome undergoes genetic counseling and testing. They are found to have a mutation in the CDH1 gene. In light of this, assess your knowledge about diffuse-type gastric cancer, and identify the incorrect statement:

A. Environmental factors play a less significant role in the etiology of diffuse-type gastric cancer compared to genetic predispositions.
B. The development of this cancer subtype is directly linked to chronic active inflammation within the gastric mucosa.
C. Active gastritis, particularly when persistent and severe, is considered a major risk factor for diffuse-type gastric cancer.
D. The expression of E-cadherin is unrelated to the pathogenesis of diffuse-type gastric cancer.
E. In certain scenarios, such as genetic predisposition, prophylactic total gastrectomy is recommended to prevent the development of diffuse-type gastric cancer.

Answer: D

Explanation: The loss of E-cadherin expression, often due to inactivation of the gene encoding E-cadherin (CDH1), is a crucial event in the carcinogenesis of diffuse-type gastric carcinoma. This loss leads to defective intracellular adhesions, which is a hallmark of this cancer subtype.

11. During a multidisciplinary tumor board review, a case of a 55-year-old male with newly diagnosed gastric cancer is discussed. Histopathology reveals a mixed pattern of adenocarcinoma. Considering the WHO classification of gastric cancers, identify the incorrect statement:

A. The WHO classification categorizes gastric cancers based on the predominant histologic pattern, acknowledging the presence of less dominant elements of other histologic types.
B. This classification encompasses tubular, papillary, poorly cohesive (including signet ring cell), mucinous, mixed, and rare variants of gastric carcinoma.
C. The most commonly diagnosed subtype of gastric cancer is poorly cohesive signet ring cell carcinoma.
D. Papillary adenocarcinoma, typically occurring in the proximal stomach, is notably associated with a higher incidence of liver metastases.
E. Mucinous gastric carcinoma, characterized by abundant extracellular mucin production, accounts for about 10% of all gastric cancer cases.

Answer: C

Explanation: According to the WHO classification, the most common histologic subtype of gastric cancer is tubular adenocarcinoma, not poorly cohesive signet ring cell carcinoma. The other options accurately reflect the WHO classification's categories and characteristics of gastric cancer subtypes.

12. A 60-year-old female with advanced gastric cancer undergoes diagnostic laparoscopy, revealing peritoneal and liver metastases. Considering the modes of spread for gastric cancer, identify the incorrect statement:

A. Gastric cancer can infiltrate locally, invading adjacent structures and tissues in the abdominal cavity.
B. Hematogenous spread is a recognized pathway, with common sites of distant metastasis including the liver and lungs.

C. The lymphatic system is a common route for gastric cancer dissemination, often involving regional gastric and celiac lymph nodes.
D. Transcoelomic spread occurs, with cancer cells disseminating within the peritoneal cavity, leading to peritoneal carcinomatosis.
E. Implantation spread is a typical method of dissemination for gastric cancer, with cells implanting and growing in distant sites.

Answer: E

Explanation: Gastric cancer does not typically spread through implantation, where cancer cells dislodge and grow in a new location. The other methods described—local infiltration, hematogenous spread, lymphatic spread, and transcoelomic dissemination—are all recognized pathways for gastric cancer metastasis. This question is made more challenging by requiring detailed knowledge of the various metastatic pathways of gastric cancer, appropriate for a subspecialty exam in surgical oncology.

13. A 55-year-old male undergoes EUS for a suspected gastric neoplasm. The ultrasound suggests varying levels of wall invasion. Based on the TNM classification for gastric cancer, identify the incorrect statement regarding the depth of primary tumor invasion:

A. TX indicates that the depth of the tumor cannot be assessed, representing an unknown extent of primary tumor invasion.
B. T0 signifies that there is no evidence of a primary tumor in the gastric wall.
C. T1 indicates a tumor confined to the mucosa or submucosa, regardless of LN involvement.
D. T2 describes a tumor invading into but not beyond the muscularis propria.
E. T3 represents a tumor that invades the serosa, penetrating to the outermost layer of the stomach.

Answer: E

Explanation: T3 in the TNM classification for gastric cancer indicates a tumor invading through the muscularis propria into the subserosa, not the serosa. T4a is characterized by tumor invasion to the serosa (penetrating the visceral peritoneum), and T4b involves invasion into adjacent structures.

14. During a surgical planning session for a 67-year-old patient with gastric cancer, the oncology team discusses the extent of LN involvement. A recent CT scan suggests multiple LN enlargements. Based on the TNM classification for gastric cancer LN metastasis, identify the incorrect statement:

A. NX indicates that regional lymph nodes cannot be assessed, which may occur due to various clinical scenarios.
B. N0 signifies no metastasis in regional lymph nodes, as determined by pathological examination or imaging studies.
C. N1 denotes metastasis in one to two regional lymph nodes, representing early nodal involvement.
D. N2 refers to metastasis in three to six regional lymph nodes, indicating a more advanced nodal disease.

E. N3 indicates metastasis in fewer than eight regional lymph nodes, suggesting extensive nodal involvement.

Answer: E

Explanation: In the TNM classification, N3 indicates extensive LN involvement, with N3a involving metastasis in 7 to 15 regional lymph nodes and N3b involving 16 or more regional lymph nodes. This question is more challenging due to its detailed focus on the LN classification of gastric cancer, suitable for a subspecialty exam in surgical oncology.

15. A 58-year-old male presents with persistent epigastric pain and weight loss. His initial endoscopy was inconclusive, and he is scheduled for a repeat procedure. Considering the diagnostic investigation of gastric cancer, identify the incorrect statement:

A. Video endoscopy with biopsy is the primary diagnostic modality for gastric cancer, allowing direct visualization and tissue sampling.
B. During endoscopy, it is recommended to take a minimum of four biopsies from the edge of the suspected malignant lesion for accurate diagnosis.
C. Conventional white light endoscopy is utilized for investigating equivocal findings or delineating the extent of superficial gastric cancer.
D. Approximately 10% of patients diagnosed with gastric cancer may have had a normal endoscopic examination within the preceding 3 years.
E. Factors contributing to the need for re-endoscopy include an initial failure to suspect malignancy and the taking of an inadequate number of biopsies during the first examination.

Answer: B

Explanation: The current recommendation is to take six to eight biopsies, preferably seven from the margin and base of the ulcer, to ensure a high diagnostic sensitivity of over 98%. Taking fewer than six biopsies has been associated with diagnostic failure and the necessity for re-endoscopic examination. The other options accurately describe various aspects of the diagnostic investigation of gastric cancer.

16. A 65-year-old male with a history of dyspepsia undergoes an endoscopy for evaluation of persistent upper abdominal pain. The endoscopist notes suspicious findings in the stomach. Based on typical endoscopic appearances of gastric cancer, identify the incorrect description:

A. An ulcerated mass that is protruding into the gastric lumen, often seen in advanced stages of gastric cancer.
B. Folds in the gastric mucosa surrounding the ulcer crater, which may appear thickened or distorted due to tumor infiltration.
C. Overhanging, irregular, or thickened ulcer margins, suggesting malignancy rather than a benign gastric ulcer.
D. A smooth, regular, and rounded ulcer edge, typically indicative of benign gastric ulcers rather than malignant lesions.

E. Induration and rigidity in the affected area of the stomach, often due to infiltration of the tumor into the gastric wall.

Answer: D

Explanation: In gastric cancer, the edges of an ulcerated mass are usually irregular, overhanging, or thickened, contrasting with the smooth, regular, and rounded edges characteristic of benign gastric ulcers. The other options accurately describe endoscopic findings that can be associated with gastric cancer.

17. A 50-year-old female with a history of autoimmune gastritis and a family history of Lynch syndrome is evaluated for gastric cancer risk. Considering factors associated with an increased risk of gastric cancer, identify the incorrect statement:

A. Diabetes mellitus is classified as a high-risk factor for the development of gastric cancer, warranting routine screening in these patients.
B. Gastric adenoma, a type of precancerous lesion, significantly increases the risk of progression to gastric cancer.
C. Pernicious anemia, often associated with chronic atrophic gastritis, elevates the risk of gastric cancer due to long-standing mucosal changes.
D. Gastric intestinal metaplasia represents a precursor lesion for gastric cancer, particularly in patients with extensive or advanced changes.
E. Lynch syndrome, a hereditary cancer syndrome, is associated with an increased risk of several cancers, including gastric cancer.

Answer: A

Explanation: Patients with diabetes mellitus are not generally considered to be at high risk for gastric cancer. Routine screening for gastric cancer in diabetic patients is not typically recommended unless other high-risk factors are present.

18. A 62-year-old patient with a biopsy-proven gastric adenocarcinoma is being evaluated for potential endoscopic submucosal dissection (ESD). The tumor is characterized as an intramucosal, differentiated type without ulceration. Assessing the criteria for ESD, identify the incorrect statement:

A. Absence of lymphatic or venous invasion is a prerequisite for considering endoscopic submucosal dissection in gastric cancer.
B. Differentiated-type intramucosal gastric cancers can be treated with ESD regardless of size, provided there is no ulceration present.
C. Differentiated-type intramucosal gastric cancer less than 30 mm in diameter with ulceration is a candidate for ESD.
D. Undifferentiated-type intramucosal gastric cancer less than 20 mm in diameter without ulceration can be safely treated with ESD.
E. Differentiated-type gastric cancer with minute submucosal penetration can be considered for ESD if it is less than 60 mm in diameter.

Answer: E

Explanation: For endoscopic submucosal dissection, differentiated-type gastric cancers with submucosal penetration are generally considered when the tumor diameter is less than 30 mm, and the submucosal invasion depth is less than 500 μm, not 60 mm. The other options accurately describe criteria for endoscopic submucosal dissection in gastric cancer.

19. A 55-year-old male with a diagnosis of advanced gastric carcinoma undergoes preoperative planning. The tumor is classified as Borrmann type IV. Discussing surgical strategies, the team reviews the guidelines for resection margins. Identify the incorrect statement about the extent of gastric resection:

    A. The extent of gastric resection is primarily determined by the need to achieve microscopically negative (R0) resection margins.
    B. For early gastric carcinoma, a resection margin of at least 2 cm is typically recommended to ensure complete tumor removal.
    C. In cases of Borrmann type I and II gastric carcinoma, a resection margin of 3 cm or more is advisable.
    D. For Borrmann type III and IV gastric carcinomas, a resection margin of 4 cm is generally sufficient to ensure clear margins.
    E. In diffuse-type gastric cancer, a resection margin of 8 cm is recommended due to the tendency for submucosal tumor spread.

Answer: D

Explanation: In Borrmann type III and IV gastric carcinomas, a resection margin of 5 cm or more is recommended, not 4 cm, due to the infiltrative nature of these tumors. The other options correctly reflect the guidelines for resection margins based on tumor type and stage in gastric carcinoma.

20. A 68-year-old patient is scheduled for surgery for gastric carcinoma. The tumor is located in the proximal third of the stomach and extends to the lower esophagus. The surgical team discusses the extent of resection needed. Assess your understanding of gastric resection extent, and identify the incorrect statement:

    A. Intraoperative frozen section examination is routinely recommended to ensure negative resection margins during gastric cancer surgery.
    B. Tumors located in the middle or lower one-third of the stomach are generally treated with subtotal gastrectomy.
    C. Pancreaticoduodenectomy may be required for tumors extending more than 2 cm into the duodenum.
    D. Partial gastrectomy is an adequate surgical approach for tumors involving the proximal one-third of the stomach.
    E. Tumors involving the lower esophagus may necessitate transhiatal dissection or thoracotomy for complete resection.

Answer: D

Explanation: For tumors involving the proximal one-third of the stomach, a proximal gastrectomy, not just a partial gastrectomy, is typically required. This procedure ensures adequate resection margins.

21. A 56-year-old patient with a family history of hereditary diffuse gastric cancer (HDGC) presents with imaging suggestive of a large gastrointestinal stromal tumor (GIST) in the proximal stomach. The multidisciplinary team evaluates the indications for total gastrectomy. Assess your understanding of the indications for total gastrectomy and identify the incorrect statement:

    A. Total gastrectomy is indicated for gastric adenocarcinoma affecting the proximal stomach, necessitating wide resection margins.
    B. Type 2 gastric carcinoids located in the proximal stomach are typically managed with total gastrectomy due to their malignant potential.
    C. Total gastrectomy serves both as treatment and prophylactic intervention for patients with hereditary diffuse gastric cancer (HDGC).
    D. Signet ring carcinoma of the stomach, known for its diffuse spread, often requires total gastrectomy for adequate treatment.
    E. GISTs affecting the proximal stomach may necessitate total gastrectomy, depending on their size and extent.

    Answer: B

    Explanation: Type 2 gastric carcinoids, often associated with chronic atrophic gastritis and hypergastrinemia, do not typically require total gastrectomy as they are generally less aggressive. Instead, more conservative surgical approaches or ER can be appropriate. Type 3 or 4 gastric carcinoids are more aggressive and may necessitate total gastrectomy.

22. A 70-year-old patient with a diagnosis of gastric cancer and multiple comorbidities is evaluated for potential surgical intervention. The tumor is localized, but the patient's overall health status is poor. Discussing the contraindications to total gastrectomy, identify the incorrect statement:

    A. Total gastrectomy is contraindicated in asymptomatic patients with advanced metastatic disease, where the procedure would not offer survival benefit.
    B. Total gastrectomy is a viable alternative to partial gastrectomy in cases where achieving wide negative margins is possible with a lesser resection.
    C. Significant comorbidities, such as severe cardiovascular or respiratory diseases, contraindicate total gastrectomy due to high operative risks.
    D. Severe malnutrition in a patient poses a contraindication to total gastrectomy due to increased risk of postoperative complications.
    E. Uncontrollable bleeding disorders are a contraindication for total gastrectomy, as they pose a significant risk during and after surgery.

    Answer: B

    Explanation: Total gastrectomy is not typically considered a viable alternative to partial gastrectomy when wide negative margins can be achieved with the latter. Partial gastrectomy is often preferred over total gastrectomy when feasible, due to its improved safety profile and better long-term functional outcomes. The other options accurately reflect contraindications to total gastrectomy.

23. A 55-year-old patient with a small, early-stage gastric cancer is being considered for ER. The tumor is a differentiated-type adenocarcinoma without ulceration. The surgical team reviews the Korean Gastric Cancer Association (KGCA) guidelines for ER in gastric cancer. Identify the incorrect criterion for ER according to KGCA:

    A. ER is recommended for differentiated-type adenocarcinoma of the stomach.
    B. The tumor should be without ulcerative findings to be a candidate for ER.
    C. Eligibility for ER includes tumors clinically diagnosed as T1a with a diameter less than 2 cm.
    D. The tumor should have a very low risk of LN metastasis to be considered for ER.
    E. A negative horizontal margin is a necessary criterion for ER according to KGCA guidelines.

    Answer: E

    Explanation: The criteria for ER according to the KGCA do not include a requirement for a negative horizontal margin. Instead, the focus is on the type of adenocarcinoma, absence of ulceration, depth of invasion (T1a), size of the tumor, and low risk of LN metastasis.

24. A 60-year-old patient with an early gastric lesion undergoes endoscopic evaluation. The lesion is suspected to be a T1a, differentiated-type gastric cancer. The multidisciplinary team discusses the National Comprehensive Cancer Network (NCCN) recommendations for ER. Identify the incorrect criterion for ER according to the NCCN:

    A. ER is categorized as a 2A level recommendation for eligible gastric cancer lesions.
    B. The tumor diameter should be 2 cm or less for consideration of ER.
    C. Eligibility for ER includes tumors clinically diagnosed as T1a, indicating superficial invasion.
    D. The tumor must be of a differentiated type to be a suitable candidate for ER.
    E. Criteria for ER include absence of lymphovascular invasion, negative horizontal margin, and positive vertical margin.

    Answer: E

    Explanation: According to NCCN guidelines, both the horizontal and vertical margins must be negative to consider ER for gastric cancer. A positive vertical margin would indicate inadequate resection and potential residual disease, contraindicating ER. The other options accurately reflect the NCCN criteria for ER in gastric cancer. This question is more challenging because it requires specific knowledge of the NCCN guidelines for the endoscopic management of gastric cancer, appropriate for a subspecialty exam in surgical oncology.

25. A 64-year-old patient with a diagnosis of stage II gastric cancer is being considered for surgery. The tumor is classified as Borrmann type II and located in the distal stomach. The surgical team discusses the guidelines and principles of

surgery for gastric cancer. Identify the incorrect statement regarding surgical recommendations:

A. The Japanese Gastric Cancer Association (JGCA) recommends a resection margin of at least 2 cm for T1 tumors.
B. For T2 or deeper tumors with Borrmann type I and II, a minimum of 3 cm proximal margin is advised.
C. The NCCN recommends distal gastrectomy for distal gastric cancers if safe margins can be achieved.
D. The European Society for Medical Oncology (ESMO) recommends a proximal margin resection of 5 cm for stage IB–III gastric cancer.
E. The ESMO recommends a 5 cm margin resection for diffuse gastric cancer when performing a distal gastrectomy.

Answer: E

Explanation: The ESMO guideline recommends a resection margin of 5 cm for diffuse cancer; however, if such a margin cannot be achieved with a distal gastrectomy, total gastrectomy is recommended.

26. A 52-year-old patient with early-stage gastric cancer is evaluated for surgical intervention. The tumor is classified as T1bN0, differentiated type and measures 2 cm in diameter. The surgical team discusses the criteria for D1 LN dissection according to the Chinese Society of Clinical Oncology (CSCO). Identify the incorrect criterion for D1 LN dissection:

A. D1 LN dissection is categorized as grade I dissection.
B. It is indicated for tumors staged as T1aN0.
C. Tumors staged as T1bN0 are also considered eligible for D1 dissection.
D. The tumor diameter should be less than 2.5 cm for a D1 LN dissection to be considered.
E. D1 dissection is recommended for tumors of a differentiated type.

Answer: D

Explanation: According to the CSCO guidelines, D1 LN dissection is indicated for tumors with a diameter of less than 1.5 cm, not 2.5 cm. The other options accurately describe the criteria for D1 LN dissection in gastric cancer.

27. A 48-year-old patient with clinical stage II gastric cancer is being considered for surgical intervention. The multidisciplinary team discusses the current guidelines for minimally invasive surgery in gastric cancer. Assess your understanding of these guidelines and identify the incorrect statement:

A. The KGCA, CSCO, and NCCN recommend laparoscopic surgery for early gastric cancer.
B. The safety of laparoscopic total gastrectomy for clinical stage I gastric cancer has been proven by several studies.
C. The KGCA recommends open gastrectomy for advanced gastric cancer, considering its complexity and potential for extensive LN involvement.

D. For advanced gastric cancer, the CSCO and NCCN recommend laparoscopic surgery, considering the patient's overall condition and tumor stage.
E. The Japanese Gastric Cancer Association (JGCA) recommends laparoscopic surgery for distal gastrectomy and relatively recommends it for total gastrectomy.

Answer: B

Explanation: Although several studies have shown the safety of laparoscopic total gastrectomy for clinical stage I gastric cancer, the claim that its safety is unproven is misleading. The other options correctly represent the current guidelines and recommendations from various oncology associations regarding minimally invasive surgery in gastric cancer.

Bibliography

1. Thrift AP, El-Serag HB. Burden of gastric cancer. Clin Gastroenterol Hepatol. 2020;18(3):534–42.
2. Sung H, Ferlay J, Siegel RL, Laversanne M, Soerjomataram I, Jemal A, Bray F. Global cancer statistics 2020: GLOBOCAN estimates of incidence and mortality worldwide for 36 cancers in 185 countries. CA Cancer J Clin. 2021;71(3):209–49.
3. Tsugane S, Sasazuki S. Diet and the risk of gastric cancer: review of epidemiological evidence. Gastric Cancer. 2007;10:75–83.
4. Wu CY, Wu MS, Kuo KN, Wang CB, Chen YJ, Lin JT. Effective reduction of gastric cancer risk with regular use of nonsteroidal anti-inflammatory drugs in *Helicobacter pylori*–infected patients. J Clin Oncol. 2010;28(18):2952–7.
5. Sobala GM, Schorah CJ, Shires S, Axon AT. Gastric ascorbic acid concentration and acute *Helicobacter pylori* infection. Rev Esp Enferm Dig. 1990;78(Suppl 1):63.
6. Fitzgerald RC, Hardwick R, Huntsman D, Carneiro F, Guilford P, Blair V, Chung DC, Norton J, Ragunath K, Van Krieken JH, Dwerryhouse S. Hereditary diffuse gastric cancer: updated consensus guidelines for clinical management and directions for future research. J Med Genet. 2010;47(7):436–44.
7. Caldas C, Carneiro F, Lynch HT, Yokota J, Wiesner GL, Powell SM, Lewis FR, Huntsman DG, Pharoah PD, Jankowski JA, MacLeod P. Familial gastric cancer: overview and guidelines for management. J Med Genet. 1999;36(12):873–80.
8. Qiu MZ, Cai MY, Zhang DS, Wang ZQ, Wang DS, Li YH, Xu RH. Clinicopathological characteristics and prognostic analysis of Lauren classification in gastric adenocarcinoma in China. J Transl Med. 2013;11(1):1–7.
9. Chen YC, Fang WL, Wang RF, Liu CA, Yang MH, Lo SS, Wu CW, Li AF, Shyr YM, Huang KH. Clinicopathological variation of Lauren classification in gastric cancer. Pathol Oncol Res. 2016;22:197–202.
10. Graziano F, Humar B, Guilford P. The role of the E-cadherin gene (CDH1) in diffuse gastric cancer susceptibility: from the laboratory to clinical practice. Ann Oncol. 2003;14(12):1705–13.
11. Berlth F, Bollschweiler E, Drebber U, Hoelscher AH, Moenig S. Pathohistological classification systems in gastric cancer: diagnostic relevance and prognostic value. World J Gastroenterol: WJG. 2014;20(19):5679.
12. Riihimäki M, Hemminki A, Sundquist K, Sundquist J, Hemminki K. Metastatic spread in patients with gastric cancer. Oncotarget. 2016;7(32):52307.

13. Byrd DR, Brookland RK, Washington MK, Gershenwald JE, Compton CC, Hess KR, Sullivan DC, Jessup JM. In: Amin MB, Edge SB, Greene FL, editors. AJCC cancer staging manual. New York: Springer; 2017.
14. Ji X, Bu ZD, Yan Y, Li ZY, Wu AW, Zhang LH, Zhang J, Wu XJ, Zong XL, Li SX, Shan F. The 8th edition of the American joint committee on cancer tumor-node-metastasis staging system for gastric cancer is superior to the 7th edition: results from a Chinese mono-institutional study of 1663 patients. Gastric Cancer. 2018;21:643–52.
15. Choi Y, Choi HS, Jeon WK, Kim BI, Park DI, Cho YK, Kim HJ, Park JH, Sohn CI. Optimal number of endoscopic biopsies in diagnosis of advanced gastric and colorectal cancer. J Korean Med Sci. 2012;27(1):36–9.
16. Cotton PB, Shorvon PJ. Analysis of endoscopy and radiography in the diagnosis, follow-up and treatment of peptic ulcer disease. Clin Gastroenterol. 1984;13(2):383–403.
17. Hirota WK, Zuckerman MJ, Adler DG, Davila RE, Egan J, Leighton JA, Qureshi WA, Rajan E, Fanelli R, Wheeler-Harbaugh J, Baron TH. ASGE guideline: the role of endoscopy in the surveillance of premalignant conditions of the upper GI tract. Gastrointest Endosc. 2006;63(4):570–80.
18. Zheng Z, Yin J, Liu XY, Yan XS, Xu R, Li MY, Cai J, Chen GY, Zhang J, Zhang ZT. Current indications for endoscopic submucosal dissection of early gastric cancer. World J Gastrointest Oncol. 2021;13(6):560–73.
19. Japanese Gastric Cancer Association. Japanese gastric cancer treatment guidelines 2010 (ver. 3). Gastric Cancer. 2011;14(2):113–23.
20. Okajima K, Isozaki H. Principles of surgical treatment. In: Nishi M, Ichikawa H, Nakajima T, Maruyama K, Thara E, editors. Gastric cáncer. Tokyo: Springer.
21. Borch K, Ahrén B, Ahlman H, Falkmer S, Granérus G, Grimelius L. Gastric carcinoids: biologic behavior and prognosis after differentiated treatment in relation to type. Ann Surg. 2005;242(1):64.
22. Makris EA, Poultsides GA. Surgical considerations in the management of gastric adenocarcinoma. Surg Clin. 2017;97(2):295–316.

Chapter 3
Small Bowel and Appendiceal Tumors

Samer Sabri, Talib A. Majeed, Noufel sh. Alshadood, Waseem M. Al Hamidy, Sajjad G. Al-Badri, and Aqeel Shakir Mahmood

1. In a recent surgical oncology study focusing on small bowel tumors, several characteristics were noted. Which of the following statements is incorrect according to current surgical oncology literature?

   A. Most small bowel tumors are clinically silent for a long period.
   B. The frequency of small bowel tumors is greater in the ileum than in the duodenum.
   C. Carcinoid tumors most commonly occur in the ileum.
   D. Adenocarcinomas are more frequent in the duodenum and jejunum compared to the ileum.
   E. Peutz-Jeghers syndrome is a risk factor for small bowel tumors.

   Answer: B

   Explanation: Contrary to the statement, the frequency of small bowel tumors is greater in the ileum than in the duodenum. This question tests up-to-date knowledge and challenges common misconceptions.

S. Sabri
Department of Surgery, Baghdad Teaching Hospital, Medical City Complex, Baghdad, Iraq

T. A. Majeed
GIT and Liver Hospital, Medical City Baghdad, Baghdad, Iraq

N. s. Alshadood
Baghdad Teaching Hospital, Baghdad, Iraq

W. M. Al Hamidy
Gastroenterology and Hepatology Teaching Hospital, Medical City, Baghdad, Iraq

S. G. Al-Badri
College of Medicine University of Baghdad, Baghdad, Iraq

A. S. Mahmood (✉)
Department of General Surgery, University of Baghdad, Baghdad, Iraq

A. S. Mahmood, A. Koulouris (eds.), *MCQs in General Surgical Oncology*,
https://doi.org/10.1007/978-3-031-65738-2_3

2. In reviewing the epidemiology of small bowel tumors, a researcher notes several trends. Which of the following statements is incorrect according to recent epidemiological data?

   A. The mean age of diagnosis is around 65 years.
   B. There is a higher prevalence in black patients compared to white patients.
   C. Metastatic tumors in the small bowel are more common than primary tumors.
   D. Small bowel tumors typically present late with symptoms like a subocclusive crisis.
   E. Small bowel tumors generally have a poor prognosis.

   Answer: D

   Explanation: Small bowel tumors often present late in the course of the disease, contrary to the early presentation with obstruction. This question assesses knowledge of the clinical presentation and epidemiology of small bowel tumors.

3. A 68-year-old patient presents with jaundice and abdominal pain. Imaging suggests a mass in the small bowel, suspected to be an adenocarcinoma. Which of the following statements about adenocarcinoma of the small bowel is incorrect in this context?

   A. The ileum is the most common primary location for small bowel adenocarcinoma.
   B. Adenocarcinoma accounts for approximately 40% of all small bowel cancers.
   C. The median age of onset for small bowel adenocarcinoma is between 50 and 70 years.
   D. Small bowel adenocarcinoma can lead to obstruction of the common bile duct.
   E. Adenocarcinoma arises from the glandular epithelium of the small bowel.

   Answer: A

   Explanation: The most common primary location for small bowel adenocarcinoma is the duodenum, not the ileum. This question integrates clinical presentation with specific knowledge about the disease's epidemiology and pathology.

4. A 50-year-old patient with a history of familial adenomatous polyposis (FAP) undergoes an endoscopic evaluation for suspected small bowel lesions. Which of the following characteristics is incorrect regarding small bowel adenomas in this patient?

   A. Arise from the glandular epithelium.
   B. Most commonly located in the ileum; least common in the duodenum.
   C. Typically solitary, less than 2 cm in size, and asymptomatic.
   D. Possess a risk of malignant transformation.
   E. Frequently multiple in polyposis syndromes like FAP.

   Answer: B

Explanation: Small bowel adenomas are most common in the duodenum, not the ileum. This question requires specific knowledge about the distribution and characteristics of adenomas in polyposis syndromes.

5. In a discussion on the etiology of small bowel adenocarcinoma, a surgical oncologist lists various predisposing conditions. Which of the following is incorrect association with an increased risk of small intestine adenocarcinoma?

   A. FAP.
   B. HNPCC.
   C. PJS.
   D. Celiac disease.
   E. Crohn's disease.

Answer: D

Explanation: Celiac disease is more commonly associated with lymphoma rather than adenocarcinoma of the small intestine. This question assesses knowledge of the etiological factors associated with small bowel adenocarcinoma.

6. A radiologist reviews a series of small bowel imaging studies for suspected adenomas. Which of the following descriptions is incorrect for a typical small bowel adenoma as observed on imaging?

   A. Presents as a smoothly outlined intraluminal filling defect.
   B. Most adenomas are sessile in nature.
   C. Characterized by a broad base with a stalk.
   D. Generally, less than 2 cm in diameter.
   E. When multiple, usually confined to a single bowel segment, of varying sizes, and may be pedunculated.

Answer: C

Explanation: Small bowel adenomas are typically broad-based and not characteristically pedunculated (having a stalk). This question integrates radiological imaging characteristics with clinical knowledge about adenomas.

7. A 55-year-old patient with a history of intermittent abdominal pain and weight loss presents with a bowel obstruction. Imaging reveals a mass in the small bowel. Histopathological examination is most likely to reveal malignant lesions. The incorrect option of small bowel malignant lesions is:

   A. Adenocarcinomas.
   B. Neuroendocrine tumors (NETs).
   C. Lymphomas.
   D. Sarcomas.
   E. GISTs.

Answer: E

Explanation: GISTs, though a significant entity in small bowel neoplasms, are not as common as the other listed malignancies. This scenario integrates clinical presentation with histopathology, requiring in-depth knowledge.

8. A 48-year-old patient presents with nonspecific gastrointestinal symptoms, and an endoscopic examination reveals a polyp in the small bowel. The incorrect statement regarding the histopathological finding is that it is most likely malignant:

   A. Carcinoid tumor.
   B. Adenomas.
   C. Hamartomas.
   D. Leiomyomas.
   E. Lipomas.

Answer: A

Explanation: Carcinoid tumors, although initially presenting as small and benign-looking lesions, are malignant NETs, contrasting with the other benign entities listed.

9. A 60-year-old patient with a history of hereditary nonpolyposis colorectal cancer (HNPCC) and long-standing irritable bowel syndrome (IBS) presents with signs of intestinal obstruction. Which of the following is incorrect recognized risk factor for small bowel tumors in this patient's profile?

   A. Consumption of a diet high in refined sugars and fats.
   B. Human immunodeficiency virus (HIV) infection.
   C. History of HNPCC.
   D. Long-standing IBS.
   E. Familial history of Peutz-Jeghers syndrome (PJS).

Answer: D

Explanation: IBS is not a risk factor for small bowel tumors. This question integrates a clinical scenario with differential risk factor identification, challenging the candidate to distinguish between IBS and conditions like IBD which are risk factors.

10. A 45-year-old patient with a history of intermittent intestinal obstruction undergoes endoscopy, revealing multiple small bowel polyps. Biopsy indicates hamartoma. Which of the following characteristics is incorrect for these hamartomas?

   A. Composed of smooth muscle covered by normal mucosa.
   B. Most commonly found in the jejunum, followed by the ileum and duodenum.
   C. Frequently multiple in FAP.
   D. Associated with an increased risk of intestinal adenocarcinoma and non-gastrointestinal or gynecologic tumors.
   E. Occasionally lobulated in appearance.

Answer: C

Explanation: Hamartomas of the small bowel are often multiple in PJS, not FAP. This question integrates clinical presentation with specific syndromic associations.

11. During a laparoscopic surgery for suspected small bowel obstruction, a surgeon encounters a well-defined mass. Pathology confirms a lipoma. Which of the following statements is incorrect regarding small bowel lipomas?

    A. Composed of mature adipose tissue encased in a thin capsule.
    B. Originate from the submucosal layer.
    C. Typically sessile but can occasionally be pedunculated.
    D. Possess malignant potential.
    E. May cause intermittent obstruction or bleeding.

Answer: D

Explanation: Lipomas are benign tumors and do not have malignant potential. This question challenges the examinee to differentiate between benign and malignant characteristics of small bowel tumors.

12. A radiologist reviewing imaging for a patient with suspected small bowel lipoma notes various features. Which of the following descriptions is incorrect for a typical small bowel lipoma as observed on imaging studies?

    A. Sharply marginated on barium studies.
    B. Presents as a solitary, sessile intraluminal filling defect on barium studies.
    C. Appears as a smooth, homogeneous, ovoid mass with fat attenuation on a CT scan.
    D. Exhibits signal intensity consistent with macroscopic fat on all magnetic resonance imaging (MRI) sequences.
    E. Typically shows enhancement on MRI.

Answer: E

Explanation: Lipomas do not typically show enhancement on MRI, as they are composed of fat tissue. This question requires specific knowledge of radiological imaging characteristics of small bowel lipomas.

13. A 58-year-old patient presents with an incidental finding of a small bowel mass during a CT scan for unrelated abdominal pain. Biopsy suggests a benign GIST. Which of the following statements about benign GISTs is incorrect?

    A. Originate from interstitial cells of Cajal.
    B. Characterized by the expression of KIT (CD117), a tyrosine kinase growth factor receptor.
    C. Approximately 40% arise in the small bowel, predominantly in the duodenum or jejunum.
    D. Typically show significant enhancement on imaging studies.
    E. Frequently exhibit exophytic growth.

Answer: D

Explanation: Benign GISTs show variable but generally poor enhancement on imaging. This question requires knowledge of both the biological nature and imaging characteristics of GISTs.

14. During a routine endoscopic examination, a submucosal mass in the small bowel is noted and biopsied, revealing a leiomyoma. Which of the following statements about leiomyomas of the small bowel is incorrect?

    A. A rare benign mesenchymal tumor.
    B. More commonly found in the ileum.
    C. CT and MRI typically reveal a well-circumscribed soft-tissue mass with enhancement.
    D. Larger tumors may exhibit calcification or ulceration.
    E. Imaging features can overlap with those of GISTs.

Answer: B

Explanation: Leiomyomas are more frequently found in the jejunum. This question challenges the examinee's knowledge of the epidemiology and radiological features of small bowel leiomyomas.

15. During a multidisciplinary team discussion, a case of a 60-year-old patient with a suspected carcinoid tumor is reviewed. Which of the following statements about carcinoid tumors is incorrect?

    A. Originate from chromaffin cells at the base of crypts of Lieberkühn.
    B. 90% arise in the proximal ileum.
    C. May be associated with mesenteric metastasis.
    D. Can be multifocal in nature.
    E. Can originate in a Meckel's diverticulum or the appendix.

Answer: B

Explanation: 90% of carcinoid tumors arise in the distal ileum, not the proximal ileum. This question tests specific anatomical knowledge about the origin of carcinoid tumors.

16. A radiologist is reviewing the imaging of a patient suspected to have a carcinoid tumor. Which of the following is an incorrect description of carcinoid tumor characteristics on imaging?

    A. The primary lesion appears as a small intraluminal filling defect on small bowel follow-through (SBFT) imaging.
    B. The primary lesion is usually visible on CT and MRI.
    C. Metastatic disease to the mesentery is more often identified on CT or MRI.
    D. May contain calcifications.
    E. Presents as a spiculated mesenteric mass, often with a desmoplastic or fibrotic reaction.

Answer: B

Explanation: Primary carcinoid tumors are often not visible on CT or MRI but can be identified on SBFT imaging. This question assesses knowledge of the imaging characteristics of carcinoid tumors.

17. A 65-year-old male patient presents with abdominal pain and weight loss. Imaging and biopsy suggest lymphoma of the small bowel. Which of the following statements about small bowel lymphoma is incorrect?

    A. The small bowel can be a primary site or involved as part of widespread systemic disease.
    B. Primary gastrointestinal lymphoma is the most common extranodal lymphoma.
    C. Peak prevalence occurs in the seventh decade of life.
    D. More commonly diagnosed in males.
    E. Most frequently located in the duodenum.

    Answer: E

    Explanation: Small bowel lymphoma is most frequently found in the ileum, not the duodenum, due to the abundant lymphoid tissue. This question assesses knowledge of the epidemiology and anatomical distribution of small bowel lymphoma.

18. In a case study of intestinal lymphoma, a variety of forms are discussed. Which of the following descriptions is incorrect regarding the forms of lymphoma in the intestine?

    A. Polypoid type is the most common form of intestinal lymphoma.
    B. Pseudoaneurysmal type manifests as mass-like wall thickening with preservation or dilation of the lumen.
    C. The endoexoenteric form appears cavitary.
    D. Mesenteric form is rare and more common in the distal duodenum, associated with celiac disease.
    E. Mesenteric type involves tumor extension into surrounding mesentery.

    Answer: D

    Explanation: The stenosing type, not the mesenteric form, is more common in the distal duodenum and associated with celiac disease. This question challenges the understanding of different morphological types of intestinal lymphoma.

19. A radiologist reviews imaging of a patient with suspected metastasis to the small bowel. Which of the following statements is incorrect regarding metastasis to the small bowel?

    A. Metastasis occurs via hematogenous spread or direct invasion.
    B. The most common sources of hematogenous metastases are from renal cell carcinoma.
    C. Common tumors that directly invade the small bowel include ovarian and colon cancer.
    D. CT and MRI often show single or multiple polypoid intraluminal lesions or focal wall thickening.
    E. Frequently results in luminal narrowing.

    Answer: B

Explanation: The most common sources of hematogenous metastases to the small bowel are lung cancer, breast cancer, and melanoma, not renal cell carcinoma. This question tests the knowledge of metastatic patterns to the small bowel.

20. A 62-year-old patient presents with gastrointestinal bleeding. Imaging and biopsy confirm a malignant GIST. Which of the following statements about malignant GISTs is incorrect?

    A. Tend to grow exophytically.
    B. Surgical resection is recommended regardless of size.
    C. Often exhibit areas of necrosis.
    D. Can cavitate and communicate with the bowel lumen.
    E. Can be easily distinguished from benign GIST based on imaging and microscopic features.

Answer: E

Explanation: Distinguishing between malignant and benign GISTs can be challenging due to overlapping imaging and microscopic features. This question assesses understanding of the complexities involved in diagnosing and managing GISTs.

21. A 55-year-old patient undergoes abdominal imaging following an episode of gastrointestinal bleeding, revealing a suspicious mass in the small bowel. Imaging characteristics suggest a malignant GIST. Which of the following imaging features has incorrect association with malignant GISTs?

    A. Presents as a large, bulky, predominantly exophytic mass.
    B. Often has lobulated margins.
    C. Shows heterogeneous enhancement.
    D. Frequently accompanied by bulky adenopathy.
    E. May exhibit necrosis, ulceration, cavitation, or hemorrhage.

Answer: D

Explanation: Bulky adenopathy is rare in malignant GIST. This question requires knowledge of specific imaging characteristics of malignant GISTs.

22. A 45-year-old patient undergoes an appendectomy, and the pathology report reveals a carcinoid tumor. Considering the treatment protocols for appendiceal carcinoid tumors, which of the following statements is incorrect?

    A. Tumors up to 1 cm are typically treated with appendectomy alone.
    B. Tumors measuring 1–2 cm require right hemicolectomy if located at the tip or mid-appendix.
    C. Tumors measuring 1–2 cm necessitate right hemicolectomy if located at the base, invading the mesoappendix, or with LN involvement.
    D. Right hemicolectomy is indicated for tumors larger than 2 cm.
    E. Appendectomy alone is often sufficient treatment for small tumors without adverse features.

Answer: B

Explanation: For 1–2 cm tumors located at the tip or mid-appendix, appendectomy alone is often sufficient, not right hemicolectomy. This question assesses knowledge of treatment guidelines based on tumor size and location in appendiceal carcinoids.

23. During a routine abdominal CT scan, a mucocele of the appendix is discovered in a patient. Which of the following statements about appendiceal mucoceles is incorrect?

    A. Mucocele is an obstructive dilatation caused by the accumulation of mucoid material.
    B. Can be caused by retention cysts, mucosal hyperplasia, cystadenomas, and cystadenocarcinomas.
    C. Intact mucoceles smaller than 5 cm are almost always benign.
    D. Larger mucoceles are more likely to be neoplastic.
    E. Clinical presentation is often nonspecific and can be an incidental finding during surgery.

   Answer: C

   Explanation: Intact mucoceles smaller than 2 cm, not 5 cm, are almost always benign. This question tests understanding of the pathology and prognosis of mucoceles based on their size.

24. A 60-year-old patient presents with appendicitis symptoms, and subsequent surgery reveals appendiceal adenocarcinoma. Which of the following statements is incorrect regarding appendiceal adenocarcinomas?

    A. Found in less than 1% of appendectomy specimens.
    B. Most are discovered incidentally.
    C. Typically affect older patients, with a longer duration of symptoms.
    D. Appendectomy is the recommended treatment.
    E. Mucinous adenocarcinoma is the most common cell type.

   Answer: D

   Explanation: Right hemicolectomy, not just appendectomy, is recommended for appendiceal adenocarcinoma. This question challenges the examinee's knowledge of the appropriate surgical treatment for appendiceal adenocarcinoma.

25. A 67-year-old patient presents with abdominal pain and weight loss. Imaging reveals a mass in the small bowel, suggestive of a sarcoma. Which of the following statements about sarcoma of the small bowel is incorrect?

    A. The most common sarcoma occurring in the small bowel is leiomyosarcoma.
    B. Sarcomas of the small bowel are most frequently found in the duodenum.
    C. CT and MRI typically show a large, heterogeneously enhancing mass with central necrosis.
    D. Can cavitate and communicate with the bowel lumen.
    E. Imaging features often overlap with those of malignant GIST.

Answer: B

Explanation: The most frequent location for small bowel sarcomas is the jejunum, followed by the ileum and then the duodenum. This question tests the knowledge of the anatomical distribution of small bowel sarcomas.

26. During a surgical procedure, a mass in the appendix is noted and biopsied, revealing a carcinoid tumor. Which of the following statements about appendiceal tumors is incorrect?

    A. Carcinoid tumors are the most common tumor type in the appendix.
    B. Typically appear as firm, yellow, bulbar masses in the appendix.
    C. The majority of appendiceal carcinoids are located at the tip of the appendix.
    D. The mean size of appendiceal carcinoids is approximately 2.5 cm.
    E. Appendiceal carcinoid tumors usually present with systemic disease.

Answer: E

Explanation: Appendiceal carcinoid tumors typically present with localized disease, not systemic disease. This question assesses the understanding of the presentation and characteristics of appendiceal carcinoids.

27. A patient presents with right lower quadrant pain, and a subsequent appendectomy reveals a carcinoid tumor. Which of the following statements about the clinical features of carcinoid tumors is incorrect?

    A. Carcinoid syndrome is commonly associated with appendiceal carcinoid.
    B. Symptoms directly attributable to the carcinoid tumor are rare.
    C. The tumor can obstruct the appendiceal lumen, leading to acute appendicitis.
    D. The malignant potential of carcinoid tumors is related to their size.
    E. Patients with carcinoid tumors generally have a high 5-year survival rate (83%).

Answer: A

Explanation: Carcinoid syndrome is rarely associated with appendiceal carcinoids unless there are widespread metastases. This question challenges the examinee to differentiate between typical and atypical presentations of appendiceal carcinoid tumors.

Bibliography

1. Brandi ML, Agarwal SK, Perrier ND, Lines KE, Valk GD, Thakker RV. Multiple endocrine neoplasia type 1: latest insights. Endocr Rev. 2021;42(2):133–70. PMID: 33249439; PMCID: PMC7958143. https://doi.org/10.1210/endrev/bnaa031.
2. Buckley JA, Fishman EK. CT evaluation of small bowel neoplasms: spectrum of disease. Radiographics. 1998;18(2):379–92.
3. Bilimoria KY, Bentrem DJ, Wayne JD, et al. Small bowel cancer in the United States: changes in epidemiology, treatment, and survival over the last 20 years. Ann Surg. 2009;249:63–71.

4. Jasti R, Carucci LR. Small bowel neoplasms: a pictorial review. Radiographics. 2020;40(4):1020–38.
5. Marafini I, Monteleone G, Stolfi C. Association between celiac disease and cancer. Int J Mol Sci. 2020;21(11):4155.
6. Quinones GA, Suheb MZ, Woolf A. Small bowel cancer. In: StatPearls. Treasure Island, FL: StatPearls; 2022.
7. Reynolds I, Healy P, Mcnamara DA. Malignant tumours of the small intestine. Surgeon. 2014;12(5):263–70. Epub 2014 Mar 14. PMID: 24637026. https://doi.org/10.1016/j.surge.2014.02.003.
8. Chung CS, Tai CM, Huang TY, Chang CW, Chen KC, Tseng CM, Wang HY, Chu CH, Wu JM, Chen Y, Wang HP. Small bowel tumors: a digestive endoscopy society of Taiwan (DEST) multicenter enteroscopy-based epidemiologic study. J Formos Med Assoc. 2018;117(8):705–10. PMID: 28988888. https://doi.org/10.1016/j.jfma.2017.09.003.
9. Canavan C, Abrams KR, Mayberry JF. Meta-analysis: mortality in Crohn's disease. Aliment Pharmacol Ther. 2007;25(8):861–70.
10. Boland CR, Idos GE, Durno C, Giardiello FM, Anderson JC, Burke CA, Dominitz JA, Gross S, Gupta S, Jacobson BC, Patel SG. Diagnosis and management of cancer risk in the gastrointestinal hamartomatous polyposis syndromes: recommendations from the US Multi-Society Task Force on colorectal cancer. Gastroenterology. 2022;162(7):2063–85.
11. Farkas N, Wong J, Bethel J, Monib S, Frampton A, Thomson S. A systematic review of symptomatic small bowel lipomas of the jejunum and ileum. Ann Med Surg. 2020;58:52–67.
12. Williams EA, Bowman AW. Multimodality imaging of small bowel neoplasms. Abdom Radiol. 2019;44:2089–103.
13. Yoo J, Kim SH, Han JK. Multiparametric MRI and 18 F-FDG PET features for differentiating gastrointestinal stromal tumors from benign gastric subepithelial lesions. Eur Radiol. 2020;30:1634–43.
14. Vinik A, Hughes MS, Feliberti E, Perry RR, Casellini C, Sinesi M, Vingan H, Johnson L. Carcinoid tumors. In: Endotext [Internet]; 2018.
15. Abou Saleh M, Mansoor E, Anindo M, Isenberg G. Prevalence of small intestine carcinoid tumors: a US population-based study 2012–2017. Dig Dis Sci. 2019;64:1328–34.
16. Thomas AS, Schwartz M, Quigley E. Gastrointestinal lymphoma: the new mimic. BMJ Open Gastroenterol. 2019;6(1):e000320.
17. Lo Re G, Federica V, Midiri F, Picone D, La Tona G, Galia M, Lo Casto A, Lagalla R, Midiri M. Radiological features of gastrointestinal lymphoma. Gastroenterol Res Pract. 2016;2016:1–9.
18. Miller HC, Frampton AE, Malczewska A, Ottaviani S, Stronach EA, Flora R, Kaemmerer D, Schwach G, Pfragner R, Faiz O, Kos-Kudła B. MicroRNAs associated with small bowel neuroendocrine tumours and their metastases. Endocr Relat Cancer. 2016;23(9):711–26.
19. Ohshima K, Fujiya K, Nagashima T, Ohnami S, Hatakeyama K, Urakami K, Naruoka A, Watanabe Y, Moromizato S, Shimoda Y, Ohnami S. Driver gene alterations and activated signaling pathways toward malignant progression of gastrointestinal stromal tumors. Cancer Sci. 2019;110(12):3821–33.
20. Rajravelu RK, Ginsberg GG. Management of gastric GI stromal tumors: getting the GIST of it. Gastrointest Endosc. 2020;91(4):823–5.
21. Galanopoulos M, Toumpanakis C. The problem of appendiceal carcinoids. Endocrinol Metab Clin. 2018;47(3):661–9.
22. Singh MP. A general overview of mucocele of appendix. J Fam Med Prim Care. 2020;9(12):5867–71.
23. Ito H, Osteen RT, Bleday R, Zinner MJ, Ashley SW, Whang EE. Appendiceal adenocarcinoma: long-term outcomes after surgical therapy. Dis Colon Rectum. 2004;47:474–80.

24. Shenoy S. Small bowel sarcoma: tumor biology and advances in therapeutics. Surg Oncol. 2015;24(3):136–44.
25. Njere I, Smith LL, Thurairasa D, Malik R, Jeffrey I, Okoye B, Sinha C. Systematic review and meta-analysis of appendiceal carcinoid tumors in children. Pediatr Blood Cancer. 2018;65(8):e27069.
26. Tsang ES, McConnell YJ, Schaeffer DF, Lee L, Yin Y, Zerhouni S, Schaff K, Speers C, Kennecke HF. Outcomes of surgical and chemotherapeutic treatments of goblet cell carcinoid tumors of the appendix. Ann Surg Oncol. 2018;25:2391–9.

Chapter 4
Colorectal Cancers

Munthir A. Alobaidi, Haider A. H. Ahmed, Sabah Noori Abdulraheem, Saleh Abdulkareem Saleh, and Aqeel Shakir Mahmood

1. A 55-year-old male patient presents with a 6-month history of altered bowel habits and rectal bleeding. He has a family history of colorectal cancer (CRC). Colonoscopy reveals a mass in the sigmoid colon, and biopsy confirms adenocarcinoma. Based on the epidemiology of CRC, identify the incorrect statement:

    A. CRC is the third most common cancer worldwide, with a higher incidence in developed countries.
    B. The incidence of CRC is higher in men than in women, attributed to lifestyle and dietary differences.
    C. Mortality rates of CRC are higher in women than in men, despite the higher incidence in males.
    D. A shift in CRC localization has been observed, with proximal colon cancers becoming more prevalent than distal colon cancers.
    E. There has been an increasing trend in CRC incidence among individuals under the age of 50, leading to revised screening guidelines.

   Answer: C

M. A. Alobaidi
Department of Surgery, College of Medicine, University of Baghdad, Baghdad, Iraq

H. A. H. Ahmed
Medical City Complex, Baghdad, Iraq

S. N. Abdulraheem
Baghdad Teaching Hospital, Baghdad, Iraq

S. A. Saleh
College of Medicine University of Baghdad, Baghdad, Iraq

A. S. Mahmood (✉)
Department of General Surgery, University of Baghdad, Baghdad, Iraq

A. S. Mahmood, A. Koulouris (eds.), *MCQs in General Surgical Oncology*,
https://doi.org/10.1007/978-3-031-65738-2_4

Explanation: Rates of both incidence and mortality are substantially higher in males than in females. This can probably be attributed due to lifestyle and dietary differences between males and females.

2. A 62-year-old male with a history of chronic smoking presents with weight loss, rectal bleeding, and a change in bowel habits. Colonoscopy reveals a mass in the descending colon, and subsequent biopsy confirms adenocarcinoma. Based on the epidemiology of colorectal cancer (CRC), identify the incorrect statement:

   A. CRC ranks as the third most common cancer worldwide, with significant variations in incidence across different regions.
   B. CRC is second only to lung cancer in terms of mortality, highlighting the importance of early detection and treatment.
   C. The majority of newly diagnosed CRC cases are classified as metastatic at presentation, emphasizing the need for advanced therapeutic strategies.
   D. There is a higher incidence of CRC in males compared to females, which may be influenced by genetic and environmental factors.
   E. The overall 5-year survival rate for CRC exceeds 50%, with early-stage diagnosis being a critical factor for favorable outcomes.

Answer: C

Explanation: Metastatic CRC accounts for 35% of newly diagnosed cases.

3. A 45-year-old female with a family history of colorectal cancer (CRC) presents for a routine checkup. She has a sedentary lifestyle, consumes a high-fat diet, and has a history of heavy alcohol use. Based on the risk factors for early-onset CRC, identify the incorrect statement:

   A. Hyperlipidemia is recognized as a contributing factor to the development of early-onset CRC, possibly due to its association with metabolic syndrome.
   B. Individuals with low socioeconomic status are at a higher risk for early-onset CRC, which may be attributed to limited access to healthcare and preventive screenings.
   C. Heavy alcohol use is a well-established risk factor for early-onset CRC, with a dose-response relationship observed in epidemiological studies.
   D. A deficiency in vitamin D is implicated in the increased risk of early-onset CRC, highlighting the importance of adequate sun exposure and dietary intake.
   E. The use of nonsteroidal anti-inflammatory drugs (NSAIDs) is associated with a decreased risk of colonic adenomas and CRC, making it an incorrect risk factor for early-onset CRC.

Answer: E

Explanation: Aspirin and other NSAIDs are associated with a 20 to 40% reduction in the risk of colonic adenomas and CRC in individuals at average risk. These potential benefits of long-term therapy must be weighed against the potential adverse effects (gastroduodenal toxicity and, with nonaspirin NSAIDs, increased cardiovascular risk).

4. A 40-year-old female with a family history of CRC seeks advice on lifestyle modifications to reduce her risk of developing the disease. She is a nonsmoker, consumes a balanced diet, and exercises regularly. Based on the protective factors against CRC, identify the incorrect statement:

   A. Regular consumption of dairy products has been associated with a reduced risk of CRC, possibly due to their calcium content.
   B. While antioxidants are generally considered beneficial for overall health, there is no convincing evidence that antioxidant supplements significantly prevent colorectal adenomas or CRC.
   C. Coffee consumption has been linked to a decreased risk of CRC, with studies suggesting a protective effect of certain compounds found in coffee.
   D. Higher intake of magnesium, found in foods like nuts and leafy green vegetables, has been associated with a lower risk of CRC.
   E. The use of oral contraceptives has been shown to have a protective effect against CRC, likely due to hormonal modulation.

Answer: B

Explanation: No convincing evidence that antioxidant supplements had a significant beneficial effect on primary or secondary prevention of colorectal adenomas.

5. A 35-year-old patient with a family history of CRC presents with multiple colonic polyps detected during a screening colonoscopy. Genetic testing confirms a diagnosis of FAP. Based on the characteristics of FAP, identify the incorrect statement:

   A. FAP accounts for less than 1% of all CRC cases in the United States, making it a rare but significant hereditary condition.
   B. Less than 5% of FAP cases are due to new or de novo adenomatous polyposis coli (APC) mutations, with the majority being inherited from an affected parent.
   C. Patients with FAP have a 5% lifetime risk of developing duodenal cancer, necessitating regular surveillance of the upper gastrointestinal tract.
   D. Individuals with FAP are at an increased risk for developing thyroid cancer, particularly the follicular or papillary subtypes.
   E. Attenuated FAP is typically characterized by oligopolyposis, with patients developing 10 to 99 adenomas, fewer than in classic FAP.

Answer: B

Explanation: FAP follows an autosomal dominant pattern of inheritance with nearly complete penetrance of colonic polyposis but variable penetrance of the extracolonic manifestations of the disease. Up to 25% of FAP cases are due to new or de novo APC mutations. Such patients do not have a family history of FAP but are at risk of passing the mutation on to offspring.

6. A 40-year-old patient with a family history of CRC undergoes genetic testing due to multiple polyps found during a colonoscopy. The results reveal a mutation

associated with a hereditary CRC syndrome. Based on the hereditary CRC syndromes and associated genes, identify the incorrect statement:

A. Lynch syndrome, characterized by an increased risk of CRC and other cancers, is commonly due to a mutation in the MLH1 gene.
B. Peutz-Jeghers syndrome, marked by the presence of hamartomatous polyps and mucocutaneous pigmentation, is caused by a mutation in the STK11 gene.
C. Juvenile polyposis, which presents with hamartomatous polyps in the gastrointestinal tract, is associated with a mutation in the SMAD4 gene.
D. Attenuated familial adenomatous polyposis (FAP), a milder form of FAP with fewer polyps, is caused by a mutation in the PMS2 gene.
E. MUTYH-associated polyposis, an autosomal recessive condition leading to multiple adenomatous polyps and CRC, is due to a mutation in the MUTYH gene.

Answer: D

Explanation: Attenuated FAP is typically associated with mutations in the APC gene, not the PMS2 gene. The PMS2 gene is more commonly associated with Lynch syndrome. This makes option D the incorrect statement in the context of hereditary CRC syndromes and their associated genes.

7. A 68-year-old male presents with a 6-month history of progressive fatigue, unintentional weight loss, and a recent onset of hematochezia. He has a history of smoking and a family history of CRC. Colonoscopy reveals a mass in the descending colon. Based on the clinical presentation of CRC, identify the incorrect statement:

A. A change in bowel habits, such as increased frequency or constipation, is more commonly associated with left-sided CRCs due to the smaller lumen and firmer stool consistency in the distal colon.
B. Dyspnea may be a presenting symptom of CRC metastasis, particularly when the cancer has spread to the lungs, leading to respiratory complications.
C. Hematochezia, or bright red blood in the stool, is more often indicative of rectosigmoid cancer than right-sided colon cancer, due to the proximity to the anal canal.
D. Iron-deficiency anemia resulting from unrecognized chronic blood loss is more frequently observed in patients with right-sided CRCs, as the blood has time to oxidize and may not be visibly apparent in the stool.
E. The specificity of dark-red rectal bleeding and the presence of a palpable abdominal mass for the diagnosis of CRC are high, but it is not as definitive as 95% for confirming the disease.

Answer: A

Explanation: A change in bowel habits is a more common presenting symptom for left-sided than right-sided CRCs. Fecal contents are liquid in the proximal colon, and the lumen caliber is larger, and CRCs are therefore less likely to be associated with obstructive symptoms, including colicky pain.

8. A 55-year-old patient presents with a history of altered bowel habits, intermittent rectal bleeding, and a palpable mass in the left lower quadrant. A colonoscopy reveals a tumor in the sigmoid colon. Based on the symptomatology of CRC, identify the incorrect statement:

   A. Obstruction is more prevalent in proximal colonic lesions, often presenting with symptoms such as constipation or distention.
   B. Altered bowel habits, such as changes in stool consistency or frequency, are usually observed with malignancies in the distal colon.
   C. The main presentation of colonic cancer is bleeding per rectum, which can range from bright red blood to dark, tarry stools depending on the tumor's location.
   D. Perforation of colonic cancer is most evident in the cecum, where the wall is thinner and the intraluminal pressure is higher.
   E. It is rare for CRC to be presented with a palpable abdominal mass, as this typically indicates advanced disease.

Answer: A

Explanation: Obstruction is more commonly observed with distal colonic tumors, such as those in the sigmoid colon, due to the narrower lumen and more solid consistency of the stool. Proximal lesions are less likely to cause obstruction and may present with symptoms related to anemia or occult bleeding. This makes option A the incorrect statement in the context of CRC symptomatology.

9. A 60-year-old male with a family history of CRC undergoes a screening colonoscopy. The procedure reveals several polyps, one of which appears suspicious for malignancy. Based on colonoscopy findings, identify the incorrect statement:

   A. Colonoscopy miss rates for CRC are estimated to be between 2% and 6%, emphasizing the importance of thorough examination and technique.
   B. The vast majority of colon and rectal cancers present as endoluminal masses, which can be detected during colonoscopy.
   C. Endoscopic criteria suggesting malignancy of a polyp include ulceration, soft consistency, adherence, and friability, which are indicative of potential invasive neoplasm.
   D. Tattooing adjacent to a suspicious lesion is important for subsequent localization, especially if an invasive neoplasm is found and surgical intervention is required.
   E. Colonoscopy has superior sensitivity compared to CT colonography in the diagnosis of nonpolypoid adenomas, which are flat or slightly raised lesions that may be more challenging to detect.

Answer: C

Explanation: Endoscopic criteria suggesting malignancy of a polyp include ulceration, firm consistency, adherence, and friability.

10. A 58-year-old female with a history of rectal bleeding and a family history of CRC undergoes diagnostic evaluation. An incomplete colonoscopy due to technical difficulties leads to further testing. Based on the diagnostic tests for CRC, identify the incorrect statement:

    A. The use of PillCam 2, a capsule endoscopy device, is beneficial in patients who have had incomplete colonoscopy to visualize the remainder of the colon.
    B. CA 19-9 serum markers, while used in the management of pancreatic cancer, are not recommended for the screening of CRC due to limited specificity and sensitivity.
    C. Liver function tests, though nonspecific, can provide clues but cannot be reliably used alone to detect liver metastasis in CRC patients.
    D. CT colonography, also known as virtual colonoscopy, aids in tumor staging by providing detailed images of the colon and surrounding structures.
    E. The absence of iron-deficiency anemia does not exclude the diagnosis of CRC as not all tumors cause significant bleeding to result in anemia.

Answer: B

Explanation: The specificity and sensitivity of serum tumor markers such as carcinoembryonic antigen (CEA) and CA 19-9 are limited.

11. A 50-year-old patient with a history of weight loss and rectal bleeding undergoes a colonoscopy, and a biopsy is taken from a suspicious mass in the ascending colon. The histopathology report reveals a mucinous adenocarcinoma. Based on the histology of CRC, identify the incorrect statement:

    A. Signet ring cell carcinomas, characterized by the presence of cells with intracellular mucin displacing the nucleus, carry a poor prognosis due to their aggressive behavior.
    B. Medullary adenocarcinoma, often associated with deficient mismatch repair proteins, presents as a distinct subtype with a better prognosis compared to other CRCs.
    C. Mucinous carcinomas, which contain a significant amount of extracellular mucin, have a predilection for the right side of the colon and are often associated with microsatellite instability.
    D. In signet ring cell carcinoma, the diagnosis requires that at least 75% of the tumor cells have displaced nuclei due to intracellular mucin, which is a hallmark of this aggressive variant.
    E. Appendiceal adenocarcinomas, while relatively rare, commonly spread intraperitoneally, leading to peritoneal carcinomatosis.

Answer: D

Explanation: In some non-gland-forming carcinomas, intracellular mucin may be a dominant feature that displaces tumor cell nuclei to the side. When ≥50% of the tumor is made up of cells of this type, it is classified as a signet ring cell carcinoma. It accounts for only 1–2% of all CRCs, but signet ring cell carcinoma is an aggressive variant with a propensity for extensive intramural spread and peritoneal carcinomatosis.

12. A 65-year-old patient undergoes a screening colonoscopy. The procedure is completed successfully, with adequate bowel preparation and cecal intubation. The endoscopist reports a withdrawal time of 6 min from the cecum. Based on the quality indicators of colonoscopy, identify the incorrect statement:

    A. A cecal intubation rate of greater than 90% is considered a key quality indicator, reflecting the thoroughness of the examination.
    B. Adequate bowel preparation is crucial for a high-quality colonoscopy, as it allows for clear visualization of the colonic mucosa and detection of lesions.
    C. A post-polypectomy bleeding rate of less than 0.5% is a benchmark for safety in colonoscopy procedures.
    D. A post-polypectomy perforation rate of less than 0.1% is another important measure of safety during colonoscopic interventions.
    E. A withdrawal time from the cecum of 6 min is considered a standard for improving the quality of endoscopy and enhancing adenoma detection.

Answer: E

Explanation: There is insufficient evidence to suggest a minimum withdrawal time from the cecum of 6 min improves quality of endoscopy or improves the adenoma detection rate.

13. A 55-year-old female presents with a 4-month history of weight loss, abdominal pain, and occasional rectal bleeding. She has no prior history of CRC screening. A colonoscopy reveals a mass in the sigmoid colon, and biopsy confirms adenocarcinoma. Based on the prognosis of CRC, identify the incorrect statement:

    A. Patients who are not diagnosed through screening programs have a higher risk of death and recurrence due to the potential for later-stage detection.
    B. The development of obstruction in CRC is considered a poor prognostic factor, as it often indicates advanced disease.
    C. Approximately 20% of CRC patients in the United States present with distant metastatic disease at the time of diagnosis, impacting their overall prognosis.
    D. Tumors presenting with rectal bleeding, particularly those in the distal colon and rectum, tend to have a better prognosis as they are often detected at an earlier stage.
    E. The involvement of regional lymph nodes is the second strongest predictor of prognosis in CRC, following the depth of tumor invasion.

Answer: D

Explanation: Tumors presenting with rectal bleeding (more commonly those involving the distal colon and rectum and at an earlier stage than proximal tumors) have a better prognosis. However, bleeding is not an independent predictor of outcome.

14. A 50-year-old patient with no family history of CRC comes to your clinic for a routine health checkup and inquires about CRC screening. Based on the general screening guidelines for CRC, identify the incorrect statement:

    A. Colonoscopy should be performed every 10 years starting at the age of 45 until the age of 75, as recommended by the US Preventive Services Task Force (USPSTF).
    B. High-sensitivity guaiac fecal occult blood test (HSgFOBT) or fecal immunochemical test (FIT) should be performed annually for noninvasive CRC screening.
    C. CT colonography, also known as virtual colonoscopy, should be performed every 5 years as an alternative to traditional colonoscopy for individuals at average risk.
    D. Flexible sigmoidoscopy, which examines the lower part of the colon, should be performed every 5 years as a less invasive screening option.
    E. A combination of flexible sigmoidoscopy every 10 years and an annual fecal immunochemical test is an acceptable screening strategy.

    Answer: A

    Explanation: The US Preventive Services Task Force (USPSTF) recommends offering CRC screening starting at age 45 years, not 50, for individuals at average risk. This makes option A the incorrect statement in the context of general screening guidelines for CRC.

15. A 55-year-old patient with rectal cancer undergoes a low anterior resection. The pathology report indicates a close circumferential resection margin (CRM). Based on the significance of CRM, identify the incorrect statement:

    A. CRM refers to the distance in millimeters between the tumor's deepest point of invasion and the resection margin from the retroperitoneal or mesenteric side, and it is a critical factor in surgical oncology.
    B. Positive CRM, defined as a margin less than 1 mm, is associated with an increased risk of local recurrence and poorer prognosis in rectal cancer.
    C. Tumor spread to the CRM can be established through various pathways, including continuous spread, discontinuous foci, and vascular or lymphatic invasion.
    D. CRM has a more important role in colon cancer than in rectal cancer, as it directly influences the likelihood of achieving a complete resection and the need for adjuvant therapy.
    E. The TNM staging system for CRC takes into account the status of the CRM, as it is an important prognostic factor.

    Answer: D

    Explanation: CRM has a more important role in rectal cancer than in colon cancer due to the anatomical constraints and the higher risk of local recurrence in rectal cancer. This makes option D the incorrect statement in the context of the significance of CRM.

16. A 70-year-old patient with a CRC diagnosis undergoes surgical resection. The pathology report indicates that the tumor has invaded through the muscularis propria into pericolorectal tissues and three regional lymph nodes are found to be positive. Based on the TNM staging of CRC, identify the incorrect statement:

    A. T3: Tumor invades through the muscularis propria into pericolorectal tissues, indicating an advanced local invasion.
    B. M1c: Metastasis to the peritoneal surface is identified alone or with other site or organ metastases, representing distant spread of the disease.
    C. N2a: Four to six regional lymph nodes are positive, indicating a higher nodal involvement.
    D. N1c: Two or three regional lymph nodes are positive, suggesting a misclassification of the nodal stage.
    E. T4b: Tumor directly invades or adheres to adjacent organs or structures, indicating extensive local spread.

    Answer: D

    Explanation: N1b is the correct classification for two or three regional lymph nodes being positive, not N1c. N1c refers to the presence of tumor deposits in the subserosa, mesentery, or non-peritonealized pericolic or perirectal tissues without regional nodal metastasis. This makes option D the incorrect statement in the context of the TNM staging of CRC.
17. A 25-year-old patient with a confirmed diagnosis of FAP presents to your clinic for a consultation. The patient has a family history of CRC and is seeking advice on management. Based on the characteristics of FAP, identify the incorrect statement:

    A. FAP is inherited in an autosomal dominant pattern, with affected individuals having a 50% chance of passing the condition to their offspring.
    B. The condition results from a germline mutation in the adenomatous polyposis coli (APC) gene, which plays a crucial role in regulating cell growth and apoptosis.
    C. Individuals with FAP have a nearly 100% lifetime risk of developing CRC if prophylactic surgery is not performed.
    D. Desmoid tumors, which are benign fibrous growths, have a significant association with FAP and can cause complications.
    E. Regular surveillance with colonoscopy is usually advised for patients with FAP to monitor for polyp development and malignancy.

    Answer: E

    Explanation: While regular surveillance is important in the early detection of polyps in FAP patients, the nearly 100% risk of developing CRC necessitates a more definitive intervention, such as total proctocolectomy, rather than surveillance alone. This makes option E the incorrect statement in the context of FAP management.
18. A 35-year-old patient with a diagnosis of Gardner syndrome presents with a newly diagnosed desmoid tumor. The patient has a family history of FAP and is

concerned about the management of the condition. Based on the characteristics of Gardner syndrome, identify the incorrect statement:

A. Surgery is the treatment of choice for intra-abdominal desmoid tumors, while nonsurgical therapies such as sulindac and/or tamoxifen are used for extra-abdominal tumors.
B. Most adrenal masses in Gardner syndrome are found incidentally during imaging studies and are typically nonfunctioning, posing minimal risk.
C. Nasal angiofibromas, although histologically benign, are locally aggressive vascular tumors that can cause significant morbidity.
D. Screening for thyroid cancer in patients with Gardner syndrome should include physical examination and ultrasound annually, starting at age 10 to 20 years, due to an increased risk of malignancy.
E. Surveillance for hepatoblastoma in children with Gardner syndrome should be conducted every 6 months using liver palpation, liver function tests, abdominal ultrasound, and alpha-fetoprotein (AFP) test.

Answer: A

Explanation: Surgery is the treatment for extra-abdominal desmoids, while sulindac and/or increasing doses of tamoxifen are the treatment for intra-abdominal tumors.

19. A 28-year-old patient with FAP undergoes a total colectomy with ileal pouch-anal anastomosis due to the presence of numerous colonic polyps and rectal adenomas. The patient inquires about postoperative surveillance and management. Based on the management of FAP, identify the incorrect statement:

A. Post-colectomy surveillance of the rectum or ileal pouch should be performed annually, not every 5 years, to monitor for polyp development and potential malignancy.
B. In patients with profuse polyposis and more than ten rectal adenomas, proctocolectomy with ileal pouch-anal anastomosis is indicated to reduce the risk of CRC.
C. The presence of adenomas with high-grade dysplasia or multiple adenomas larger than 6 mm is an indication for colectomy in FAP to prevent the progression to cancer.
D. Elective colectomy can be deferred to the early 20 s in teenagers with classic FAP who only have sparse (fewer than 10) or small (less than 5 mm) adenomas, allowing for normal growth and development.
E. Aspirin has not been demonstrated to prevent adenoma progression in FAP, and its use for chemoprevention remains under investigation.

Answer: A

Explanation: Endoscopic evaluation of the rectum or ileal pouch should be performed every 6 to 12 months (or every year for end ileostomies).

20. A 45-year-old patient with a family history of CRC and endometrial cancer is referred for genetic counseling. The patient is concerned about the risk of

developing cancer due to a potential hereditary condition. Based on the characteristics of HNPCC, identify the incorrect statement:

A. HNPCC accounts for approximately 3% of all CRC cases, making it one of the most common hereditary colorectal cancer syndromes.
B. Individuals with mutations in the related genes have a 100% lifetime risk of developing CRC, which necessitates aggressive surveillance and management strategies.
C. The syndrome is inherited in an autosomal dominant pattern, meaning that having just one copy of the mutated gene can increase the risk of cancer.
D. Females who carry mutations associated with HNPCC have an increased risk of developing endometrial carcinoma, in addition to colorectal cancer.
E. HNPCC results from germline mutations in DNA mismatch repair genes, which lead to microsatellite instability and an increased risk of certain cancers.

Answer: B

Explanation: Lifetime risk is 70–80%. Not all individuals with related gene mutation will develop CRC.

21. A 60-year-old patient with a newly diagnosed localized colon cancer undergoes surgical consultation for treatment planning. The tumor is located in the ascending colon, and the patient has no history of synchronous colon cancers. Based on the treatment of CRC, identify the incorrect statement:

A. Surgical resection is the only curative treatment modality for localized colon cancer, with the goal of completely removing the tumor and associated lymph nodes.
B. Synchronous colon cancer, defined as the presence of more than one primary tumor at the time of diagnosis, has been reported to be present in approximately 4% of patients with sporadic colon cancer.
C. Proximal and distal resection margins should be at least 3 cm from the tumor to ensure complete removal of the cancer and prevent local recurrence.
D. For patients undergoing right hemicolectomy for colon cancer, the length of ileum resected does not influence local recurrence rates, as long as adequate margins are achieved.
E. Radial margin positivity, which indicates tumor involvement at the outermost edge of the resected specimen, is rare with colon cancer resections, but it is an important factor in rectal cancer surgery.

Answer: C

Explanation: Proximal and distal resection margins should be at least 5 to 7 cm from the tumor. These margins should allow for an adequate resection of the appropriate segment of the bowel with its vascular supply and associated lymphatics.

22. A 55-year-old patient with colon cancer undergoes a surgical resection with lymphadenectomy. The pathology report indicates that ten lymph nodes were

examined, and two of them show metastatic involvement. Based on the principles of lymphadenectomy in CRC, identify the incorrect statement:

A. Complete mesocolic excision includes an extended lymphadenectomy beyond the primary feeding vessel and associated central lymph node basin to ensure thorough removal of potential metastatic sites.
B. At least eight lymph nodes should be assessed for adequate staging, as this number is sufficient to accurately determine the nodal status of the patient.
C. Complete mesocolic excision is analogous to D3 lymphadenectomy in the Japanese Society for Cancer of the Colon and Rectum classification, which aims for a more extensive lymph node dissection.
D. Complete mesocolic excision may lead to improved oncologic outcomes for patients with colon cancer by reducing the risk of local recurrence and improving survival rates.
E. Metastasis to central lymph nodes occurs in up to 8% of patients with CRC, highlighting the importance of thorough lymph node evaluation.

Answer: B

Explanation: There is a direct correlation between the number of lymph nodes evaluated per patient after surgical resection and survival. Examination of fewer than 12 lymph nodes is a high-risk feature for stage II colon cancer, which increases the risk of recurrence to that of stage IIIA disease. As such, consensus guidelines recommend that at least 12 lymph nodes be assessed for adequate staging. Adjuvant chemotherapy may be offered to those who have fewer than 12 lymph nodes examined, even if they have no demonstrable metastatic disease in the examined nodes.

23. A 65-year-old patient with a tumor located at the hepatic flexure of the colon undergoes surgical resection. The pathology report indicates no lymphatic spread. Based on the principles of vascular ligation in hepatic flexure tumor resection, identify the incorrect statement:

A. The ileocolic artery is ligated to ensure adequate blood supply is cut off from the tumor site and to facilitate lymphadenectomy.
B. The right colic artery is ligated to remove the blood supply to the tumor and to address potential lymphatic drainage routes.
C. The right branch of the middle colic artery is ligated to ensure the removal of the tumor along with its feeding vessels.
D. The left branch of the middle colic artery is not typically ligated in a hepatic flexure tumor resection with no lymphatic spread, as it supplies the transverse colon.
E. The right gastroepiploic artery is routinely ligated in hepatic flexure tumor resections to ensure complete removal of potential lymphatic spread.

Answer: E

Explanation: Right gastroepiploic artery is not routinely ligated unless there is evidence of nodal disease along its distribution.

24. A 55-year-old patient undergoes a colonoscopy, and a large polyp is found and removed. The pathology report indicates the presence of cancerous cells within the polyp. The patient is referred to a surgical oncologist for further evaluation. Based on the indications for radical surgery in the presence of polyps, identify the incorrect statement:

    A. Poorly differentiated histology within the polyp is an indication for radical surgery due to the aggressive nature of the tumor and increased risk of metastasis.
    B. Lymphovascular invasion detected in the polyp suggests a higher risk of systemic spread, warranting consideration for radical surgery.
    C. Tumor budding, which is the presence of isolated tumor cells at the invasive front, is a poor prognostic factor and may indicate the need for radical surgery.
    D. Cancer at the resection margin or submucosal invasion depth ≥1 cm is an indication for radical surgery to ensure complete removal of the tumor and prevent recurrence.
    E. Perineural invasion within the polyp is associated with a higher risk of local recurrence and distant metastasis, justifying radical surgical intervention.

    Answer: D

    Explanation: The correct threshold for submucosal invasion depth that typically warrants radical surgery is ≥1 mm, not ≥1 cm. This is because even a small depth of invasion can significantly increase the risk of lymph node metastasis. This makes option D the incorrect statement in the context of indications for radical surgery in the presence of polyps.

25. A 60-year-old patient undergoes a CRC resection with primary anastomosis. The surgical team discusses postoperative care to minimize the risk of anastomotic leaks. Based on factors that decrease leaks from anastomosis after CRC resection, identify the incorrect statement:

    A. The use of an ileostomy over a colostomy is considered a factor that decreases the risk of anastomotic leaks, although both have their own set of complications that need to be managed carefully.
    B. Maintaining normovolemia intraoperatively and postoperatively is important to ensure adequate tissue perfusion and healing of the anastomosis.
    C. The use of vasopressors intraoperatively should be minimized, as they can decrease blood flow to the anastomosis and increase the risk of leaks.
    D. Maintaining oxygen saturations of more than 97% can help ensure adequate tissue oxygenation, which is crucial for the healing process.
    E. Ensuring that there is no torsion or tension on the bowel loops at the site of the anastomosis is essential to prevent ischemia and promote proper healing.

    Answer: A

    Explanation: There is no proof of superiority of an ileostomy over a colostomy: both have their complications which need to be considered in conjunction with the wishes of the patient. Ileostomies are known for their high fluid outputs and risk of dehydration, which may ultimately lead to renal failure if not correctly managed, while colostomies are known to lead to prolapse and wound closure infections.

26. A 55-year-old patient with CRC is found to have isolated liver metastasis on imaging. The patient is being evaluated for potential curative resection. Based on the management of metastasis in CRC, identify the incorrect statement:

    A. Curative resection is indicated in cases of isolated lung or liver metastasis, as it can significantly improve survival outcomes for patients with CRC.
    B. Bilateral oophorectomy is not indicated if only one ovary is involved in metastasis, as removal of both ovaries may not be necessary.
    C. Cytoreductive surgery (CRS) is not recommended for high-risk patients in the absence of overt disseminated peritoneal metastases, as the risks may outweigh the benefits.
    D. Cancers located in the hepatic flexure or sigmoid colon are associated with a high recurrence rate, necessitating careful surveillance and management.
    E. PET scan is indicated if staging CT scans are negative, but there is a high suspicion of metastatic disease, as it can provide additional information for accurate staging.

Answer: B

Explanation: Complete resection of isolated ovarian metastases may improve survival. If one ovary is involved with disease, a bilateral oophorectomy should be performed because of the potential for microscopic disease in the other ovary as well as of the development of metachronous metastases. However it is generally acknowledged that ovarian metastases (particularly if synchronous and bilateral) represent a poor prognostic factor.

27. A 70-year-old patient with stage IV CRC presents with rectal bleeding and is being evaluated for palliative care options. The patient has received chemotherapy with a regimen that includes bevacizumab. Based on the principles of palliative care in CRC, identify the incorrect statement:

    A. Bevacizumab leads to an increased risk of obstruction, which is a common complication in patients receiving this antiangiogenic agent.
    B. Laser ablation can be used as a palliative measure to control rectal bleeding in patients with advanced CRC, providing symptomatic relief.
    C. The 5-year survival rates for CRC at stage IV are less than 10%, reflecting the poor prognosis associated with advanced disease.
    D. Chemotherapy regimens that incorporate fluorouracil (FU) or capecitabine are typically used in the palliative treatment of CRC to prolong survival and improve quality of life.
    E. The most important prognostic factor in the palliative care setting is the ability to achieve microscopic negative margins, which can significantly impact survival.

Answer: A

Explanation: Accumulating data suggest a significantly increased risk of perforation in patients treated with the antiangiogenic agent bevacizumab. Thus, colonic stenting should not be performed in patients who are receiving bevacizumab.

28. A 60-year-old patient with a rectal tumor located 5 cm from the anal verge is being evaluated for surgical options. The surgical team is considering various approaches, including transanal total mesorectal excision (TaTME) and laparoscopic surgery. Based on the principles of surgery in CRC, identify the incorrect statement:

    A. Transanal total mesorectal excision (TaTME) is an effective and safe technique for the resection of rectal tumors, offering good visualization and precision.
    B. Traditional open surgery has inferior outcomes and increased complication rates compared to robotic-assisted surgery, which provides better dexterity and visualization.
    C. Laparoscopic surgery for CRC has similar long-term outcomes to open surgery, including equivalent rates of survival and recurrence.
    D. Intraoperative fluorescence imaging using indocyanine green has no role in sentinel lymph nodes mapping during CRC surgery, as its utility is limited to assessing perfusion.
    E. Sphincter-preserving resection is not possible for tumors of the lower rectum, as these tumors often require more radical surgery to ensure complete removal.

Answer: E

Explanation: Sphincter-preserving surgical resection of rectal tumors (even those found in the lower rectum), as it has better prognosis and quality of life for the patients.

29. A 55-year-old patient with CRC and liver metastasis is being evaluated for surgical resection. The primary tumor is located in the right colon, and the liver metastasis is deemed resectable. The surgical team discusses the optimal approach for resection. Based on the management of liver metastasis in CRC, identify the incorrect statement:

    A. The classic approach to resection involves removing the primary colorectal tumor first, followed by a separate procedure to resect the liver metastasis.
    B. In simultaneous resection, the primary tumor is removed before the liver metastasis, ensuring that the primary source of cancer is addressed first.
    C. Simultaneous resection is preferred in right-sided colon tumors, as it allows for a more efficient surgical approach and potentially reduces the overall treatment time.
    D. Approximately 80% of patients with metastatic CRC are not candidates for resection at diagnosis, highlighting the importance of careful patient selection for surgery.

E. Achieving a negative margin at resection is associated with better survival outcomes, underscoring the importance of complete tumor removal.

Answer: B

Explanation: When simultaneous resection is performed, the liver resection is performed first. If the hepatic resection is more extensive than anticipated, or there is greater blood loss than anticipated, and/or the patient is not tolerating the procedure, the colorectal portion should be postponed and a staged approach utilized.

30. A 65-year-old patient with rectal cancer is being evaluated for treatment options. The tumor is clinically staged as T3, with positive lymph nodes, and is located close to the mesorectal fascia. The surgical team is discussing the indication for neoadjuvant CRT. Based on the indications for neoadjuvant CRT in rectal cancer, identify the incorrect statement:

A. Neoadjuvant CRT is indicated for clinically staged T3 or T4 tumors to downstage the tumor and improve resectability.
B. Node-positive tumors are candidates for neoadjuvant CRT to address micrometastatic disease and reduce the risk of local recurrence.
C. Tumors with invasion of the mesorectal fascia are indicated for neoadjuvant CRT to increase the likelihood of achieving clear resection margins.
D. Tumor size, such as being less than 3 cm in diameter, is a criterion for neoadjuvant CRT to reduce the tumor burden before surgery.
E. Tumors with a threatened circumferential resection margin (CRM) are indicated for neoadjuvant CRT to improve the chances of a complete resection.

Answer: D

Explanation: Tumor size has no impact on the decision to initiate CRT. In the United States, neoadjuvant CRT is generally administered over 5.5 weeks (1.8 Gy per day, five fractions per week) with concurrent infusional fluorouracil or daily oral capecitabine. The benefits of neoadjuvant, as compared with adjuvant, CRT include a superior sphincter preservation rate, a lower rate of anastomotic stenosis as a long-term complication of pelvic RT, and better local control while providing similar long-term survival.

31. A 55-year-old patient with stage III CRC has completed treatment and is now in the posttreatment surveillance phase. The patient inquires about the recommended surveillance schedule. Based on the American Cancer Society guidelines for posttreatment surveillance for resected CRC, identify the incorrect statement:

A. History and physical examination should be performed every 3 months for the first 2 years, and then every 6 months up to 5 years, to monitor for any signs of recurrence.
B. Carcinoembryonic antigen (CEA) levels should be checked every 3 months for the first 2 years, and then every 6 months up to 5 years, as a marker for potential recurrence.

C. CT scans of the abdomen, pelvis, and chest should be performed every 12 months for 5 years for stage III patients to detect any metastatic disease early.
D. Colonoscopy should be done 1 year after the initial surgery, and if normal, it should be repeated every 5 years to monitor for new polyps or cancer.
E. The purpose of surveillance is the early identification of recurrent disease, which can improve the chances of successful treatment if recurrence occurs.

Answer: D

Explanation: Colonoscopy should be performed 1 year after the initial surgery, and if normal, it should be repeated every 3 years, not every 5 years. This is to ensure early detection of any new polyps or cancer that may develop. This makes option D the incorrect statement in the context of posttreatment surveillance for resected CRC.

32. A 60-year-old patient with a low-lying rectal cancer is being evaluated for surgical options. The surgical team discusses the possibility of an abdominoperineal resection (APR). Based on the principles of APR, identify the incorrect statement:

A. APR involves the removal of the sigmoid colon, rectum, and anus, making it a radical procedure for low-lying rectal cancers.
B. The type of colostomy created in APR is a permanent end colostomy, as the anal sphincter complex is removed during the procedure.
C. All rectal cancers, regardless of their location, are amenable to be operated on by this technique, providing a one-size-fits-all solution.
D. Benign causes such as Crohn's proctitis can be managed by this technique when other treatments have failed and the disease is localized to the rectum.
E. The procedure is usually performed in the prone position to facilitate the mobilization of the rectum and ensure complete removal of the cancer.

Answer: C

Explanation: Not all rectal cancers are amenable to be managed by APR. This technique is specifically indicated for low-lying rectal cancers where sphincter preservation is not feasible. For higher rectal cancers, sphincter-preserving surgeries are often preferred. This makes option C the incorrect statement in the context of abdominoperineal resection.

33. A 50-year-old male with a history of chronic inflammatory bowel disease presents for a CRC screening consultation. He has a family history of Lynch syndrome and has undergone abdominopelvic radiation for a previous malignancy. Based on the risk factors that currently influence CRC screening guidelines, identify the incorrect statement:

A. Lynch syndrome, a hereditary nonpolyposis colorectal cancer, significantly increases the risk of CRC and influences early screening recommendations.
B. Crohn's disease, as part of inflammatory bowel disease, is associated with an increased risk of CRC, warranting more frequent screening intervals.

C. Previous abdominopelvic radiation for other malignancies is a known risk factor for CRC, necessitating earlier and more frequent screening.
D. Cholecystectomy, while associated with an increased risk of right-sided colon cancer, does not currently influence CRC screening guidelines.
E. Cystic fibrosis, due to the associated gastrointestinal complications, is considered a risk factor for CRC, impacting screening recommendations.

Answer: D

Explanation: Although there is a described relationship between cholecystectomy and an increased risk of right-sided colon cancer, this factor does not currently influence CRC screening guidelines. The other options are recognized risk factors that directly impact screening recommendations.

34. A 60-year-old patient with an average risk of CRC undergoes a screening colonoscopy, and several polyps are detected and removed. The histopathology report reveals a mix of hyperplastic polyps, tubular adenomas, and a sessile serrated polyp with dysplasia. Based on the recommendations for post-colonoscopy follow-up in average-risk adults, identify the incorrect statement:

A. The finding of 20 or fewer hyperplastic polyps in the rectum or sigmoid colon, each smaller than 10 mm, indicates a 10-year surveillance colonoscopy interval.
B. An adenoma with tubulovillous or villous histology warrants a 3-year surveillance colonoscopy to monitor for potential malignant transformation.
C. The presence of five to ten tubular adenomas, each smaller than 10 mm, suggests a 5-year surveillance colonoscopy interval, despite their relatively low risk of progression.
D. Piecemeal resection of an adenoma 20 mm or larger necessitates a 6-month surveillance colonoscopy to ensure complete removal and assess for recurrence.
E. A sessile serrated polyp with dysplasia requires a 3-year surveillance colonoscopy due to its increased risk of progression to CRC.

Answer: C

Explanation: The presence of five to ten tubular adenomas, each smaller than 10 mm, actually indicates a 3-year surveillance colonoscopy interval, not 5 years, due to the increased risk associated with multiple adenomas. This makes option C the incorrect statement in the context of post-colonoscopy follow-up recommendations.

35. A 35-year-old patient with a 10-year history of ulcerative colitis presents for a follow-up consultation. The patient has pancolitis and is concerned about the risk of developing CRC. Based on the association between CRC and ulcerative colitis, identify the incorrect statement:

A. The risk of CRC in patients with ulcerative colitis is related to both the duration of the disease and the extent of colonic involvement, with pancolitis posing the highest risk.

B. The risk of CRC for any patient with ulcerative colitis is estimated to be 2%, with the risk increasing significantly after 10 years of disease duration.
C. Adenocarcinomas found in patients with ulcerative colitis are typically flatter and have fewer overhanging margins compared to sporadic CRC, making them more challenging to detect.
D. In cases of toxic megacolon, complete proctocolectomy with Brook's ileostomy is considered the best surgical approach to prevent the risk of CRC and manage the acute condition.
E. Colonoscopy is indicated every 5 years for patients with ulcerative colitis beginning 8 years after the time of diagnosis with pancolitis, to monitor for dysplasia and early signs of CRC.

Answer: E

Explanation: Patients with ulcerative colitis should get surveillance colonoscopy starting at least 8 years after they are diagnosed with IBD. Follow-up colonoscopies should be done every 1 to 3 years, depending on the person's risk factors for CRC and the findings on the previous colonoscopy.

36. A 45-year-old patient with a family history suggestive of Lynch syndrome undergoes genetic counseling and testing. The patient's father had CRC at age 52, and an aunt had endometrial cancer at age 48. Based on the characteristics of Lynch syndrome, identify the incorrect statement:

A. Lynch syndrome is the most common inherited CRC susceptibility syndrome, accounting for about 3% of all CRC cases.
B. CRCs in Lynch syndrome are predominantly left-sided in location, contrasting with the typical right-sided location seen in sporadic cases.
C. The most common extracolonic tumor in Lynch syndrome is endometrial cancer, with a lifetime risk of up to 60% in affected women.
D. Lynch syndrome-associated cancers often involve at least two generations, reflecting the autosomal dominant inheritance pattern of the syndrome.
E. Tumor-based genetic screening for Lynch syndrome with microsatellite instability (MSI) or immunohistochemistry (IHC) testing is indicated in individuals with CRC or endometrial cancer at age 50 years or older, especially when there is a family history suggestive of the syndrome.

Answer: B

Explanation: CRCs in Lynch syndrome are predominantly right-sided in location, not left-sided. This is a key distinguishing feature from sporadic CRC cases, making option B the incorrect statement in the context of Lynch syndrome.

37. A 65-year-old patient with a newly diagnosed CRC is being evaluated for surgical resection. The tumor is located at the rectosigmoid junction. The surgical team discusses the anatomy relevant to the planned procedure. Based on the surgical anatomy of CRC, identify the incorrect statement:

A. The most common location of CRC is the descending colon, accounting for the majority of cases.

B. The lymphatic drainage of the mesorectal fat is mainly directed to the preaortic lymph nodes, which is important for staging and surgical planning.
C. Not all surgeries for CRC require an open approach; minimally invasive techniques such as laparoscopic or robotic-assisted surgery are increasingly used.
D. Carcinoma of the rectosigmoid junction requires ligation of the inferior mesenteric artery at its origin to ensure adequate lymph node removal and reduce the risk of recurrence.
E. The superior mesenteric vein lies to the right of the superior mesenteric artery (SMA), which is a key anatomical relationship in the mesentery.

Answer: A

Explanation: The most common location of CRC is the rectosigmoid junction, not the descending colon. This is an important consideration for surgical planning and understanding the presentation of the disease. This makes option A the incorrect statement in the context of CRC surgical anatomy.

38. During a surgical planning session for a patient with colon cancer, the surgical team discusses the blood supply to various segments of the colon. Based on the anatomy of the colon's blood supply, identify the incorrect statement:

A. The middle colic artery, a branch of the superior mesenteric artery, supplies the hepatic flexure, transverse colon, and splenic flexure.
B. The cecum is supplied by cecal branches originating from the ileocolic artery, which is a branch of the superior mesenteric artery.
C. The descending colon is mainly supplied by branches of the inferior mesenteric artery, including the left colic artery.
D. The inferior mesenteric artery provides blood supply to the sigmoid colon and upper part of the rectum, while the lower rectum is supplied by branches of the internal iliac artery.
E. The watershed area of the colon is the hepatic flexure, which is where the blood supply from the superior and the blood supply from the inferior mesenteric arteries meet.

Answer: E

Explanation: Splenic flexure is the watershed area of the colon and hence the most susceptible to ischemia (ischemic colitis).

39. A 50-year-old patient is scheduled for a lower gastrointestinal (GIT) endoscopy to investigate symptoms of rectal bleeding and altered bowel habits. The patient inquires about the procedure and its specifics. Based on the principles of lower GIT endoscopy, identify the incorrect statement:

A. Flexible sigmoidoscopy can visualize up to 70 cm of the colon, allowing for examination of the distal part of the large intestine.
B. Rigid sigmoidoscopy has a more limited reach of up to 40 cm of the colon, primarily used for examining the rectum and sigmoid colon.
C. A complete and successful colonoscopy requires reaching the cecum, with ileal intubation considered an additional measure of thoroughness.

D. The failure rate for reaching the cecum in colonoscopy can be up to 10%, influenced by factors such as patient anatomy and bowel preparation.
E. Prophylactic antibiotics are required for all patients undergoing lower GIT endoscopy to prevent post-procedure infections.

Answer: E

Explanation: Prophylactic antibiotics are not routinely recommended for lower GIT endoscopy procedures, except in specific circumstances such as patients with certain cardiac conditions or those at high risk for endocarditis. This makes option E the incorrect statement in the context of lower GIT endoscopy.

Bibliography

1. Global Cancer Observatory. International Agency for Research on Cancer. World Health Organization. [Internet]. https://gco.iarc.fr/. Accessed 23 Jan 2023.
2. Schwartz SI, Charles Brunicardi F, Andersen DK, Billiar TR, Dunn DL, Hunter JG, et al. Schwartz's principles of surgery. New York: McGraw-Hill Education; 2014.
3. Archambault AN, Lin Y, Jeon J, et al. JNCI Cancer Spectr. 2021;5(4):pkab064.
4. Moreno CC, Mittal PK, Sullivan PS, Rutherford R, Staley CA, Cardona K, Hawk NN, Dixon WT, Kitajima HD, Kang J, Small WC, Oshinski J, Votaw JR. Colorectal cancer initial diagnosis: screening colonoscopy, diagnostic colonoscopy, or emergent surgery, and tumor stage and size at initial presentation. Clin Colorectal Cancer. 2016;15(1):67–73. https://doi.org/10.1016/j.clcc.2015.07.004.
5. Bisgaard ML, Fenger K, Bülow S, Niebuhr E, Mohr J. Familial adenomatous polyposis (FAP): frequency, penetrance, and mutation rate. Hum Mutat. 1994;3(2):121–5. https://doi.org/10.1002/humu.1380030206.
6. Markowitz SD, Bertagnolli MM. Molecular origins of cancer: molecular basis of colorectal cancer. N Engl J Med. 2009;361(25):2449–60. PMID: 20018966; PMCID: PMC2843693. https://doi.org/10.1056/NEJMra0804588.
7. Stapley S, Peters TJ, Sharp D, Hamilton W. The mortality of colorectal cancer in relation to the initial symptom at presentation to primary care and to the duration of symptoms: a cohort study using medical records. Br J Cancer. 2006;95(10):1321–5. PMID: 17060933; PMCID: PMC2360591. https://doi.org/10.1038/sj.bjc.6603439.
8. Calanzani N, Chang A, Van Melle M, Pannebakker MM, Funston G, Walter FM. Recognising colorectal cancer in primary care. Adv Ther. 2021;38:2732–46.
9. Konishi T, Shimada Y, Hsu M, Tufts L, Jimenez-Rodriguez R, Cercek A, Yaeger R, Saltz L, Smith JJ, Nash GM, Guillem JG, Paty PB, Garcia-Aguilar J, Gonen M, Weiser MR. Association of preoperative and postoperative serum carcinoembryonic antigen and colon cancer outcome. JAMA Oncol. 2018;4(3):309–15. PMID: 29270608; PMCID: PMC5885834. https://doi.org/10.1001/jamaoncol.2017.4420.
10. SEER*Stat Database: Incidence—SEER 9 Regs Research Data with Delay-Adjustment, Malignant Only, Nov 2018 Sub (1975–2016) <Katrina/Rita population adjustment>—linked to county attributes—Total US, 1969–2017 counties. National Cancer Institute.
11. Sullivan BA, Noujaim M, Roper J. Cause, epidemiology, and histology of polyps and pathways to colorectal cancer. Gastrointest Endosc Clin N Am. 2022;32(2):177–94.

12. Tinmouth J, Kennedy EB, Baron D, Burke M, Feinberg S, Gould M, et al. Colonoscopy quality assurance in Ontario: systematic review and clinical practice guideline. Can J Gastroenterol Hepatol. 2014;28(5):251–74.
13. Shaukat A, Kaltenbach T, Dominitz JA, Robertson DJ, Anderson JC, Cruise M, Burke CA, Gupta S, Lieberman D, Syngal S, Rex DK. Endoscopic recognition and management strategies for malignant colorectal polyps: recommendations of the US multi-society task force on colorectal cancer. Am J Gastroenterol. 2020;115(11):1751–67. https://doi.org/10.14309/ajg.0000000000001013.
14. Gupta S, Lieberman D, Anderson JC, et al. Recommendations for follow-up after colonoscopy and polypectomy: a consensus update by the US multi-society task force on colorectal cancer. Am J Gastroenterol. 2020;115:415–34. https://doi.org/10.14309/ajg.0000000000000544.
15. Ihnát P, Martínek L, Ihnát Rudinská L, Mitták M, Vávra P, Zonča P. Cirkumferenčný resekčný okraj v modernej liečbe karcinómu rekta [Circumferential resection margin in the modern treatment of rectal cancer]. Rozhl Chir. 2013;92(6):297–303. Czech.
16. AJCC Cancer Staging Manual. Eighth Edition (2017) published by Springer International Publishing. Corrected at 4th printing, 2018.
17. Dinarvand P, Davaro EP, Doan JV, Ising ME, Evans NR, Phillips NJ, et al. Familial adenomatous polyposis syndrome: an update and review of extraintestinal manifestations. Arch Pathol Lab Med. 2019;143(11):1382–98.
18. Sobczuk P, Agnieszczak IM, Grycuk W, Czarnecka AM, Świtaj T, Koseła-Paterczyk H, Morysiński T, Zdzienicki M, Rutkowski P. What is the best front-line approach in patients with desmoid fibromatosis?—a retrospective analysis from a reference center. Eur J Surg Oncol. 2021;47(10):2602–8. https://doi.org/10.1016/j.ejso.2021.05.002.
19. Syngal S, Brand RE, Church JM, Giardiello FM, Hampel HL, Burt RW, American College of Gastroenterology. ACG clinical guideline: genetic testing and management of hereditary gastrointestinal cancer syndromes. Am J Gastroenterol. 2015;110(2):223–62; quiz 263. PMID: 25645574; PMCID: PMC4695986. https://doi.org/10.1038/ajg.2014.435.
20. Pellat A, Netter J, Perkins G, Cohen R, Coulet F, Parc Y, et al. Lynch syndrome: what is new? Bull Cancer. 2019;106(7–8):647–55. Accessed 24 Dec 2021.
21. Hashiguchi Y, Hase K, Ueno H, Mochizuki H, Shinto E, Yamamoto J. Optimal margins and lymphadenectomy in colonic cancer surgery. Br J Surg. 2011;98(8):1171–8. https://doi.org/10.1002/bjs.7518.
22. McGory ML, Shekelle PG, Ko CY. Development of quality indicators for patients undergoing colorectal cancer surgery. J Natl Cancer Inst. 2006;98(22):1623–33. https://doi.org/10.1093/jnci/djj438.
23. Chaouch MA, Kellil T, Jeddi C, Saidani A, Chebbi F, Zouari K. How to prevent anastomotic leak in colorectal surgery? A systematic review. Ann Coloproctol. 2020;36(4):213–22. Epub 2020 Aug 31. PMID: 32919437; PMCID: PMC7508486. https://doi.org/10.3393/ac.2020.05.14.2.
24. Vogel JD, Felder SI, Bhama AR, Hawkins AT, Langenfeld SJ, Shaffer VO, Thorsen AJ, Weiser MR, Chang GJ, Lightner AL, Feingold DL, Paquette IM. The American Society of Colon and Rectal Surgeons clinical practice guidelines for the management of colon cancer. Dis Colon Rectum. 2022;65(2):148–77. https://doi.org/10.1097/DCR.0000000000002323.
25. Chen J, Wang DR, Zhang JR, Li P, Niu G, Lu Q. Metaanalysis of temporary ileostomy versus colostomy for colorectal anastomoses. Acta Chir Belg. 2013;113(5):330–9.
26. Erroi F, Scarpa M, Angriman I, Cecchetto A, Pasetto L, Mollica E, Bettiol M, Ruffolo C, Polese L, Cillo U, D'Amico DF. Ovarian metastasis from colorectal cancer: prognostic value of radical oophorectomy. J Surg Oncol. 2007;96(2):113–7. https://doi.org/10.1002/jso.20803.
27. Ganapathi AM, Westmoreland T, Tyler D, Mantyh CR. Bevacizumab-associated fistula formation in postoperative colorectal cancer patients. J Am Coll Surg. 2012;214(4):582–8; discussion 588-90. Epub 2012 Feb 8. https://doi.org/10.1016/j.jamcollsurg.2011.12.030.
28. Marks JH Frenkel JL, D'Andrea AP, Greenleaf CE. Maximizing rectal cancer results: TEM and TATA techniques to expand sphincter preservation. Surg Oncol Clin N Am. 2011;20(3):501–20, viii–ix. https://doi.org/10.1016/j.soc.2011.01.008.

29. Reddy SK, Pawlik TM, Zorzi D, Gleisner AL, Ribero D, Assumpcao L, Barbas AS, Abdalla EK, Choti MA, Vauthey JN, Ludwig KA, Mantyh CR, Morse MA, Clary BM. Simultaneous resections of colorectal cancer and synchronous liver metastases: a multi-institutional analysis. Ann Surg Oncol. 2007;14(12):3481–91. Epub 2007 Sep 1. https://doi.org/10.1245/s10434-007-9522-5.
30. Fokas E, Liersch T, Fietkau R, Hohenberger W, Beissbarth T, Hess C, Becker H, Ghadimi M, Mrak K, Merkel S, Raab HR, Sauer R, Wittekind C, Rödel C. Tumor regression grading after preoperative chemoradiotherapy for locally advanced rectal carcinoma revisited: updated results of the CAO/ARO/AIO-94 trial. J Clin Oncol. 2014;32(15):1554–62. Epub 2014 Apr 21. https://doi.org/10.1200/JCO.2013.54.3769.
31. American Cancer Society Colorectal Cancer Survivorship Care Guidelines. American Cancer Society Colorectal Cancer Survivorship Care Guidelines. CA Cancer J Clin. 2015;65:427–55.
32. Hawkins AT, Albutt K, Wise PE, Alavi K, Sudan R, Kaiser AM, Bordeianou L, Continuing Education Committee of the SSAT. Abdominoperineal resection for rectal cancer in the twenty-first century: indications, techniques, and outcomes. J Gastrointest Surg. 2018;22:1477–87.
33. Bjelakovic G, Nagorni A, Nikolova D, Simonetti RG, Bjelakovic M, Gluud C. Meta-analysis: antioxidant supplements for primary and secondary prevention of colorectal adenoma. Aliment Pharmacol Ther. 2006;24(2):281–91.
34. Nissan A, Guillem JG, Paty PB, Wong WD, Cohen AM. Signet-ring cell carcinoma of the colon and rectum: a matched control study. Dis Colon Rectum. 1999;42(9):1176–80. https://doi.org/10.1007/BF02238570.
35. Vogel JD, Eskicioglu C, Weiser MR, Feingold DL, Steele SR. The American Society of Colon and Rectal Surgeons clinical practice guidelines for the treatment of colon cancer. Dis Colon Rectum. 2017;60(10):999–1017. https://doi.org/10.1097/DCR.0000000000000926.
36. Ahadova A, Gallon R, Gebert J, Ballhausen A, Endris V, Kirchner M, Stenzinger A, Burn J, von Knebel DM, Bläker H, Kloor M. Three molecular pathways model colorectal carcinogenesis in lynch syndrome. Int J Cancer. 2018;143(1):139–50. https://doi.org/10.1002/ijc.31300.
37. Dekker E, Tanis PJ, Vleugels JL, Kasi PM, Wallace M. Colorectal cancer. Lancet. 2019;394:1467–80.
38. Mayo CW. Blood supply of the colon: surgical considerations. Surg Clin N Am. 1955;35(4):1117–22.
39. Deb A, Perisetti A, Goyal H, Aloysius MM, Sachdeva S, Dahiya D, Sharma N, Thosani N. Gastrointestinal endoscopy-associated infections: update on an emerging issue. Dig Dis Sci. 2022;67(5):1718–32.

Chapter 5
Pre- and Nonmalignant Colorectal Conditions

Aqeel Shakir Mahmood, Haider A. H. Ahmed, Waseem M. Al Hamidy, Abdulazeez S. Al-Janabi, and Mustafa Ismail

1. A 55-year-old patient presents for a routine colonoscopy. Multiple polyps are identified during the procedure. Considering the nature of intestinal polyps, identify the incorrect statement:

    A. Polyps are any projection from the intestinal mucosa regardless of histology.
    B. A significant proportion of colorectal carcinomas (CRC) arise from adenomatous polyps.
    C. Polyps can be classified into neoplastic, hyperplastic, inflammatory, and hamartomatous types.
    D. Approximately 25% of individuals older than 50 years have adenomatous polyps.
    E. All types of polyps, including hyperplastic and inflammatory, have a significant risk of malignant transformation.

Answer: E

Explanation: Nonneoplastic polyps such as inflammatory and hyperplastic polyps are generally not associated with an increased risk of malignant transformation.

A. S. Mahmood
Department of General Surgery, University of Baghdad, Baghdad, Iraq

H. A. H. Ahmed
Medical City Complex, Baghdad, Iraq

W. M. Al Hamidy
Gastroenterology and Hepatology Teaching Hospital, Medical City, Baghdad, Iraq

A. S. Al-Janabi
College of Medicine University of Baghdad, Baghdad, Iraq

M. Ismail (✉)
Department of Surgery, College of Medicine, University of Baghdad, Baghdad, Iraq

A. S. Mahmood, A. Koulouris (eds.), *MCQs in General Surgical Oncology*,
https://doi.org/10.1007/978-3-031-65738-2_5

2. During a health screening, a 60-year-old patient is found to have a large bowel polyp. Biopsy results are pending. Which of the following statements about large bowel polyps is incorrect?

   A. They are classified into neoplastic and nonneoplastic types.
   B. Hyperplastic polyps, frequently observed in adults, are a high-risk factor for developing malignancy.
   C. In children, juvenile polyps are the most common type and are generally nonneoplastic.
   D. Tubular adenoma is the predominant type among neoplastic polyps.
   E. Villous adenoma carries the greatest risk for malignant transformation due to its morphology.

Answer: B

Explanation: Hyperplastic polyps are a type of nonneoplastic polyp and are generally not associated with a high risk of malignancy.

3. A 45-year-old patient presents with a history of recurrent rectal bleeding. Colonoscopy reveals several polyps, predominantly in the sigmoid colon. Concerning hyperplastic polyps, which of the following statements is incorrect?

   A. They pose a significant risk of malignant transformation.
   B. These are the most common polyp type in adults.
   C. They are predominantly located in the sigmoid colon.
   D. Hyperplastic polyps fall under the category of hamartomatous polyps.
   E. Histologically, they exhibit a characteristic sawtooth pattern.

Answer: A

Explanation: Hyperplastic polyps, while common, are generally considered nonmalignant and do not carry a significant risk of malignant transformation.

4. A 50-year-old patient undergoes a colonoscopy where several small polyps are found. Regarding the characteristics of hyperplastic polyps, which of the following statements is incorrect?

   A. They represent the most prevalent type of polyps.
   B. Typically, these polyps are smaller than 5 mm in diameter.
   C. Routine removal is not necessary for these types of polyps.
   D. Larger hyperplastic polyps (>2 cm) may have a heightened risk of malignancy.
   E. They are not considered premalignant and exhibit hyperplasia without dysplasia.

Answer: C

Explanation: Even though hyperplastic polyps are nonneoplastic, they cannot be distinguished from neoplastic polyps macroscopically, necessitating removal of suspicious polyps.

5. A patient with a history of inflammatory bowel disease (IBD) presents with multiple colonic polyps on imaging. Concerning inflammatory polyps, identify the incorrect statement:

   A. They are most commonly encountered in cases of IBD.
   B. These polyps are not considered to be premalignant.
   C. Removal of these polyps is generally not required.
   D. Histologically, they exhibit normal regenerating mucosa.
   E. Extensive polyposis can be observed, particularly in patients with severe colitis.

Answer: C

Explanation: Despite being nonneoplastic, inflammatory polyps should be removed as they cannot be reliably distinguished from adenomatous polyps microscopically.

6. A child presents with rectal bleeding and a protruding rectal mass. A colonoscopy reveals several polyps. Regarding juvenile polyps, which statement is incorrect?

   A. They are the most common type of polyps in children.
   B. They are most frequently found in the sigmoid colon.
   C. There is an association with polyposis syndromes.
   D. These polyps can carry a risk of malignant transformation.
   E. They can prolapse out of the rectum and cause bleeding.

Answer: B

Explanation: Juvenile polyps are most commonly located in the rectum.

7. A 60-year-old patient undergoes a screening colonoscopy. Several colorectal polyps are identified. Regarding neoplastic colorectal polyps, which of the following statements is incorrect?

   A. Their incidence increases with age.
   B. They are more frequently encountered in males than in females.
   C. The majority are tubular adenomas.
   D. The most common site for these polyps is the sigmoid colon.
   E. They can present as solitary or multiple and can be either sessile or pedunculated.

Answer: B

Explanation: Unlike colorectal carcinoma, which is more common in males, neoplastic polyps occur with equal frequency in both sexes.

8. A 55-year-old patient with a family history of colorectal cancer presents for evaluation. A colonoscopy reveals multiple polyps. Which of the following is incorrect risk factor for malignant transformation of polyps?

   A. Size greater than 2 cm.
   B. Increased tubular component.
   C. Presence of juvenile polyps.
   D. Having multiple polyps.
   E. Advanced age.

Answer: B

Explanation: An increased villous component, not tubular component, is a significant factor associated with a higher risk of malignant transformation in polyps.

9. A 68-year-old patient undergoes a colonoscopy, and a polyp is biopsied in the sigmoid colon. Concerning tubular adenomas, which statement is incorrect?

   A. They account for approximately 20% of neoplastic polyps.
   B. These are considered premalignant polyps.
   C. The sigmoid colon is their most common location.
   D. Typically, they present as stalked polyps.
   E. Morphologically, they resemble a mushroom and histologically show complex branching of glands.

Answer: A

Explanation: Tubular adenomas actually account for about 60% of neoplastic polyps, not 20%.

10. During a surveillance colonoscopy in a patient with a history of polyps, a new lesion is identified and biopsied. In the context of villous adenomas, which of the following statements is incorrect?

   A. They have the highest risk of malignant transformation.
   B. These polyps are usually sessile.
   C. They constitute about 10% of neoplastic polyps.
   D. They secrete protein- and potassium-rich mucous.
   E. Can lead to hypoalbuminemia and hypokalemia due to their secretions.

Answer: C

Explanation: Villous adenomas, associated with a 40% malignancy risk, are not as common as implied by the statement that they make up 10% of neoplastic polyps.

11. A 45-year-old patient undergoes a colonoscopy due to a family history of CRC. Several serrated polyps are identified. Regarding serrated polyps, which of the following statements is incorrect?

    A. They are distinct from adenomatous polyps.
    B. They are considered nonneoplastic polyps.
    C. Familial serrated polyposis syndrome has been identified.
    D. They can present as either sessile serrated adenomas or traditional serrated adenomas.
    E. Endoscopically, they appear as flat lesions and are challenging to visualize.

Answer: B

Explanation: Serrated polyps are neoplastic and can contribute to colorectal carcinogenesis.

12. A pediatric patient presents with a gastrointestinal bleed, and a colonoscopy reveals multiple polyps. Concerning hamartomatous polyps, which statement is incorrect?

    A. They are also referred to as juvenile polyps.
    B. PJS is characterized by the presence of hamartomatous polyps.
    C. They carry an increased risk of malignancy.
    D. They can occur at any age but are most commonly found in childhood.
    E. Polypectomy is the recommended treatment for all types of hamartomatous polyps.

Answer: C

Explanation: Hamartomatous polyps, while part of certain syndromes like PJS, are generally not associated with a significant increase in malignancy risk.

13. A 30-year-old patient with a known diagnosis of PJS presents for a routine checkup. Regarding PJS, which statement is incorrect?

    A. It involves polyposis of the small intestine and, to a lesser extent, the colon and rectum.
    B. The polyps are considered hamartomatous and are not generally at significant risk of malignant transformation.
    C. Screening includes baseline colonoscopy and upper endoscopy at 20 years, followed by annual flexible sigmoidoscopy.
    D. Melanin spots may be noted on the buccal mucosa.
    E. Carcinoma can never develop in this condition.

Answer: E

Explanation: Despite low malignant potential, carcinoma can develop in patients with PJS.

14. During a routine colonoscopy for a 70-year-old patient, multiple neoplastic polyps are found. Identify the incorrect statement about neoplastic polyps:

    A. They are characterized by dysplasia.
    B. Tubular adenomas are associated with malignancy in 30% of cases.
    C. Villous adenomas have a 40% association with malignancy.
    D. The risk of invasive carcinoma is rare in polyps smaller than 1 cm.
    E. Most neoplastic polyps do not progress to cancer.

Answer: B

Explanation: Tubular adenomas are associated with a malignancy risk of about 5%, not 30%.

15. A 70-year-old patient with a history of large, sessile colorectal polyps is referred for treatment. Regarding the management of neoplastic polyps, which of the following statements is incorrect?

    A. Sessile polyps pose more challenges in removal than pedunculated polyps.
    B. Colonoscopic/proctoscopic polypectomy is typically the preferred treatment modality.
    C. Colectomy might be indicated if the polyp is large or flat or if invasive cancer is confirmed in the specimen.
    D. Potential complications of polypectomy include perforation and bleeding.
    E. Transanal operative excision is less effective than proctoscopic intervention for rectal sessile polyps.

Answer: E

Explanation: Transanal operative excision, rather than being inferior, is actually considered the gold standard for managing rectal sessile polyps.

16. A 55-year-old male with a history of colonic polyps undergoes a colonoscopy, revealing a 2 cm adenomatous polyp with high-grade dysplasia and invasion into the submucosa. The multidisciplinary team discusses the management strategy considering the patient's overall health status and preferences. Which of the following statements is incorrect regarding the management of malignant adenomas?

    A. Surgical resection is recommended for high-risk adenomas when therapeutic polypectomy is deemed insufficient.
    B. The decision-making process should involve a multidisciplinary team including a surgeon, pathologist, and endoscopist.
    C. Patient preference should not significantly influence the management strategy of malignant adenomas.
    D. High-risk features of adenomas include completeness and margin of excision, degree of differentiation, and Haggitt level of invasion.
    E. Therapeutic polypectomy alone may be sufficient for patients with low-risk adenomas after a comprehensive evaluation.

Answer: C

Explanation: Patient preference should not significantly influence the management strategy of malignant adenomas.

17. A 30-year-old female with a family history of FAP is evaluated for her risk of developing colorectal cancer. She has no symptoms but is concerned about her risk and future management. Which of the following statements is incorrect about the management of FAP?

    A. Prophylactic colectomy is considered necessary for all diagnosed patients with FAP.
    B. Regular endoscopic surveillance of the upper gastrointestinal tract is crucial for detecting malignant transformation.
    C. Surgical management of complex desmoid tumors is preferred over medical management in FAP patients.
    D. FAP patients are at risk for both colonic and extracolonic cancers.
    E. HNPCC involves regular colonoscopic or gynecologic examinations as preventive measures.

Answer: C

Explanation: Surgical management of complex desmoid tumors is preferred over medical management in FAP patients.

18. A 45-year-old patient undergoes a screening colonoscopy, and multiple adenomatous polyps are identified and removed. The endoscopist plans the patient's follow-up and surveillance strategy. Which of the following statements is incorrect on the endoscopic management of colorectal polyps?

    A. Endoscopic polypectomy is not an effective strategy for preventing colorectal cancer morbidity.
    B. Techniques for endoscopic resection of polyps continue to evolve, requiring endoscopists to update their skills.
    C. The evaluation and classification of polyps are crucial for determining the optimal treatment strategy.
    D. Innovative methods and concepts in polypectomy are being discussed to improve patient outcomes.
    E. Regular surveillance is essential for patients after polypectomy to monitor for new polyp development or recurrence.

Answer: A

Explanation: Endoscopic polypectomy is not an effective strategy for preventing colorectal cancer morbidity.

19. A 60-year-old patient is diagnosed with early-stage CRC. The surgical team is considering the most appropriate surgical approach, taking into account the patient's condition and the characteristics of the tumor. Which of the following statements is incorrect regarding minimally invasive surgery for CRC?

    A. Minimally invasive surgery has not shown any benefits over conventional surgical approaches in the treatment of CRC.
    B. Advancements in video and robotic technologies have significantly contributed to the field of minimally invasive surgery.
    C. Laparoscopic and robotic surgeries offer reduced operative trauma and potentially better outcomes for patients.
    D. The treatment of benign colorectal pathology via the endoscopic route has been widely accepted due to technological advancements.
    E. The selection of minimally invasive techniques must adhere to state-of-the-art oncological principles.

Answer: A

Explanation: Minimally invasive surgery has not shown any benefits over conventional surgical approaches in the treatment of CRC.

20. A 35-year-old patient with a 10-year history of ulcerative colitis undergoes a surveillance colonoscopy. The gastroenterologist is focused on detecting any dysplasia or early signs of CRC. Which of the following statements is incorrect regarding CRC screening in patients with inflammatory bowel disease?

    A. Chromoendoscopy with targeted biopsies of visible lesions is the preferred method over traditional random biopsies.
    B. All dysplastic lesions in IBD patients are invisible and cannot be detected through current endoscopic techniques.
    C. Surveillance colonoscopy is recommended for patients with long-standing ulcerative colitis or Crohn's colitis.
    D. Newer colonoscopic techniques are shifting the focus from random to targeted biopsies.
    E. Efforts are being made to endoscopically remove resectable visible dysplasia, reserving surgery for when it's not possible.

Answer: B

Explanation: All dysplastic lesions in IBD patients are invisible and cannot be detected through current endoscopic techniques.

Bibliography

1. Aust DE, Rüschoff J. Polypen im Kolorektum: Nichtneoplastisch und nichthamartomatös [Polyps of the colorectum: non-neoplastic and non-hamartomatous]. Pathologe. 2011;32(4):297–302. German. https://doi.org/10.1007/s00292-011-1435-1.

2. Jass J. Hyperplastic polyps and colorectal cancer: is there a link? Clin Gastroenterol Hepatol. 2004;2(1):1–8.
3. Loffeld RJ, Dekkers PE, Flens M. What is the consequence of hyperplastic polyps? Do adenomas and colorectal cancer develop in these patients? A clinical study. Acta Gastroenterol Belg. 2010;73(4):441–4.
4. Loscalzo J, Fauci AS, Kasper DL, Hauser SL, Longo DL, Larry J, Jameson. Harrison's principles of internal medicine. 21st ed. New York: McGraw Hill; 2022.
5. Soyer T. Polypoid disease of colon in children. Pediatr Surg Int. 2020;36(4):447–55.
6. Sullivan BA, Noujaim M, Roper J. Cause, epidemiology, and histology of polyps and pathways to colorectal cancer. Gastrointest Endosc Clin N Am. 2022;32(2):177–94.
7. Ponz de Leon M, Di Gregorio C. Pathology of colorectal cancer. Dig Liver Dis. 2001;33(4):372–88.
8. Ma MX, Bourke MJ. Sessile serrated adenomas: how to detect, characterize and resect. Gut Liver. 2017;11(6):747–60.
9. Yoo TW, Park DI, Kim YH, Kim HS, Kim WH, Kim TI, Kim HJ, Yang SK, Byeon JS, Lee MS, Jung IK, Chung MK, Jung SA, Jeen YT, Choi JH, Choi H, Han DS, Song JS. Clinical significance of small colorectal adenoma less than 10 mm: the KASID study. Hepatogastroenterology. 2007;54(74):418–21.
10. Šachlová M. Premalignancies of colon. Klin Onkol. 2013;26(Suppl):S38–43.
11. Schwartz SI, Charles Brunicardi F, Andersen DK, Billiar TR, Dunn DL, Hunter JG, et al. Schwartz's principles of surgery. New York: McGraw-Hill Education; 2014.
12. Tacheci I, Kopacova M, Bures J. Peutz-Jeghers syndrome. Curr Opin Gastroenterol. 2021;37(3):245–54.
13. Murakami T, Sakamoto N, Nagahara A. Endoscopic diagnosis of sessile serrated adenoma/polyp with and without dysplasia/carcinoma. World J Gastroenterol. 2018;24(29):3250–9.
14. Monreal-Robles R, Jaquez-Quintana JO, Benavides-Salgado D, González-González JA. Serrated polyps of the colon and rectum: a concise review. Rev Gastroenterol Mex. 2021;86(3):276–86.
15. Crockett SD, Nagtegaal ID. Terminology, molecular features, epidemiology, and management of serrated colorectal neoplasia. Gastroenterology. 2019;157(4):949–966.e4.
16. Mitchell P, Haboubi N. The malignant adenoma: when to operate and when to watch. Surg Endosc. 2008;22:1563–9.
17. Soravia C, Bapat B, Cohen Z. Familial adenomatous polyposis (FAP) and hereditary non-polyposis colorectal cancer (HNPCC): a review of clinical, genetic and therapeutic aspects. Schweiz Med Wochenschr. 1997;127(16):682–90.
18. Gao P, Zhou K, Su W, Yu J, Zhou P. Endoscopic management of colorectal polyps. Gastroenterol Rep. 2022;11:goad027.
19. Karcz WK, von Braun W. Minimally invasive surgery for the treatment of colorectal cancer. Visc Med. 2016;32:192–8.
20. Clarke W, Feuerstein J. Updates in colorectal cancer screening in inflammatory bowel disease. Curr Opin Gastroenterol. 2018;34:208–16.

Chapter 6
Peritoneal Malignancies

Salih Ahmed Aljiburi, Talib A. Majeed, Samer Sabri, and Aqeel Shakir Mahmood

1. A 60-year-old man with a history of asbestos exposure presents with abdominal pain and weight loss. Imaging reveals diffuse peritoneal thickening. Biopsy confirms malignant peritoneal mesothelioma (MPM). Regarding the epidemiology of MPM, identify the incorrect statement:

   A. MPM shows a stronger male predominance compared to pleural mesothelioma, with a male to female ratio of approximately four to one.
   B. The association between asbestos exposure and MPM is less robust than that for pleural mesothelioma.
   C. The median age at presentation for MPM is typically younger than for pleural mesothelioma, ranging between 51 and 59 years.
   D. Among workers exposed to asbestos, the lifetime risk of developing mesothelioma is estimated to be up to 10%.
   E. Patients who have received direct peritoneal external beam radiation for other cancers have a slightly elevated risk of developing MPM.

Answer: A

Explanation: MPM does not show a stronger male predominance compared to pleural mesothelioma; in fact, the male to female ratio is less pronounced in MPM.

S. A. Aljiburi
Baghdad Teaching Hospital, Baghdad, Iraq

T. A. Majeed
GIT and Liver Hospital, Medical City Baghdad, Baghdad, Iraq

S. Sabri
Department of Surgery, Baghdad Teaching Hospital, Medical City Complex, Baghdad, Iraq

A. S. Mahmood (✉)
Department of General Surgery, University of Baghdad, Baghdad, Iraq

A. S. Mahmood, A. Koulouris (eds.), *MCQs in General Surgical Oncology*,
https://doi.org/10.1007/978-3-031-65738-2_6

2. A 55-year-old female presents with a 6-month history of increasing abdominal girth and discomfort. CT imaging reveals ascites and diffuse peritoneal lesions. Biopsy findings are consistent with MPM. Which of the following statements about the clinical features of MPM is incorrect?

   A. Symptoms are primarily due to diffuse peritoneal involvement rather than localized, focal disease.
   B. The clinical presentation of MPM often includes ascites or tumor progression within the abdominal cavity.
   C. Abdominal distention, the most common initial symptom, is present in 30 to 80% of patients.
   D. Pain, often the second symptom to manifest, is a common presenting feature in MPM.
   E. Distant metastases are exceedingly rare in MPM.

   Answer: E

   Explanation: Distant metastases, while uncommon, are not as rare in MPM as the option suggests.

3. A 58-year-old female with a history of occupational asbestos exposure presents with abdominal pain and weight loss. Abdominal CT reveals diffuse peritoneal thickening and omental caking. Considering the use of radiographic imaging in the diagnosis of MPM, identify the incorrect statement:

   A. CT scan is the primary initial diagnostic tool due to its widespread availability and detailed visualization of abdominal structures.
   B. PET scanning, while useful for staging, does not reliably assess the full extent of MPM due to its unique spread patterns.
   C. Calcified pleural plaques, a common finding in pleural mesothelioma, are less frequently observed in MPM.
   D. MRI and CT are equally effective in delineating the imaging patterns and features characteristic of MPM.
   E. CT scans often underrepresent the actual disease burden in MPM, as they may not capture microscopic peritoneal spread.

   Answer: B

   Explanation: PET scanning has limitations in accurately assessing the extent of MPM due to the disease's diffuse peritoneal spread.

4. A 63-year-old man with unexplained ascites and a history of asbestos exposure undergoes diagnostic evaluation for suspected MPM. Which of the following statements regarding the diagnosis of MPM is incorrect?

   A. In any patient with signs of a diffuse malignant process in the abdomen, MPM should be a differential diagnosis, especially with a history of asbestos exposure.
   B. Ultrasonography, while useful for evaluating ascites, is not the most informative initial study for diagnosing MPM.

   C. Serum chemistries and tumor markers have limited utility in establishing a diagnosis of MPM.
   D. Fluid cytology from ascitic fluid, despite being a minimally invasive option, often yields inconclusive results and has a low diagnostic rate for MPM.
   E. Both CT-guided core needle biopsy and laparoscopic biopsy can provide adequate tissue for histopathological diagnosis of MPM.

Answer: B

Explanation: CT, not ultrasonography, is the most useful initial diagnostic study for MPM.

5. A 52-year-old woman presents with abdominal bloating and pain. Imaging and biopsy confirm MPM. In discussing the staging and prognosis of MPM, which of the following statements is incorrect?

   A. Currently, there is no universally accepted staging system for MPM, making the assessment of disease extent challenging.
   B. Patients diagnosed with localized MPM often have a favorable prognosis following complete surgical excision.
   C. MPM variants containing a sarcomatoid component typically exhibit a poorer prognosis compared to other histological types.
   D. Routine staging for distant metastases is a critical component of MPM evaluation, due to the frequent occurrence of extraperitoneal spread.
   E. The spread of MPM beyond the peritoneum is infrequent, and hence, distant metastases are relatively rare.

Answer: D

Explanation: Because MPM rarely spreads beyond the peritoneum, routine distant metastasis staging is generally unnecessary unless symptoms of distant organ involvement are present.

6. A 60-year-old male with abdominal distension and pain is diagnosed with MPM without evidence of extraperitoneal metastases. He has a good performance status. Regarding the treatment of MPM, identify the incorrect statement:

   A. Patients with no extraperitoneal metastases and good performance status are considered good candidates for surgical intervention.
   B. CRS combined with hyperthermic intraoperative peritoneal perfusion with chemotherapy (HIPEC) has shown superior outcomes compared to initial systemic chemotherapy or debulking surgery alone.
   C. The efficacy of adjunctive systemic chemotherapy, either before or after CRS plus HIPEC, remains unclear and is the subject of ongoing investigation.
   D. For patients ineligible for CRS/HIPEC, systemic chemotherapy is generally the treatment of choice.
   E. Administering systemic chemotherapy as consolidation after CRS/HIPEC in patients with high-risk features is unnecessary.

Answer: E

Explanation: Systemic chemotherapy as consolidation is recommended for MPM patients with high-risk features following CRS/HIPEC, contrary to the implication of option E.

7. A 48-year-old female with advanced ovarian cancer presents for surgical evaluation. Imaging shows extensive peritoneal involvement. In considering CRS for her, which of the following statements is incorrect?

   A. CRS typically involves only peritonectomy procedures without the need for visceral resections.
   B. The primary objective of CRS is to achieve complete cytoreduction, removing as much tumor as possible.
   C. CRS is particularly effective for patients with large volume but low-grade tumors.
   D. The presence of liver metastases is a contraindication for CRS.
   E. Achieving complete cytoreduction is less likely in cases with aggressive, large volume disease.

Answer: A

Explanation: CRS often includes both peritonectomy procedures and visceral resections, not just peritonectomy alone.

8. A 55-year-old man with a history of gastric cancer now presents with symptoms suggestive of peritoneal carcinomatosis (PC). CT scan shows peritoneal nodules and omental caking. Regarding the resectability of PC, which of the following statements is incorrect?

   A. CT scans provide the most detailed radiological assessment of PC, crucial for surgical planning.
   B. The extent of disease observed during surgical exploration often exceeds that predicted by CT imaging.
   C. Peripheral liver metastases are considered a contraindication for CRS.
   D. The administration of intraperitoneal chemotherapy at the time of surgery is an essential component of the treatment strategy.
   E. The decision for CRS is primarily based on the extent and distribution of peritoneal lesions.

Answer: C

Explanation: Peripheral liver metastases are not an absolute contraindication for CRS; decisions are often based on the overall extent of disease and surgical feasibility.

9. A 50-year-old female with ovarian cancer develops peritoneal carcinomatosis. The treatment team considers cytoreductive surgery followed by HIPEC. Which of the following statements is incorrect regarding the management of peritoneal carcinomatosis?

   A. HIPEC combined with cytoreductive surgery is considered ineffective for peritoneal carcinomatosis.

B. Advances in diagnostic techniques have enhanced the early detection of peritoneal disease.
C. Laparoscopic techniques have contributed to less morbid cytoreductive procedures.
D. Proper patient selection based on prognostic scores is crucial for the success of treatment.
E. The treatment has shown significant survival gains in patients with peritoneal disease.

Answer: A

Explanation: HIPEC combined with cytoreductive surgery is considered ineffective for peritoneal carcinomatosis.

10. A 45-year-old male is diagnosed with diffuse malignant peritoneal mesothelioma. The multidisciplinary team discusses an intensive local-regional treatment strategy. Which of the following statements is incorrect about the treatment of diffuse malignant peritoneal mesothelioma?

A. Treatment involves cytoreductive surgery with peritonectomy and hyperthermic intraoperative intraperitoneal chemotherapy.
B. Early postoperative intraperitoneal chemotherapy is never used in treating diffuse malignant peritoneal mesothelioma.
C. Identifiable clinical features can help select patients most likely to benefit from treatment.
D. Experience in management has led to a reduction in morbidity and mortality associated with the treatment.
E. Approximately half of the treated patients are alive at 5 years.

Answer: B

Explanation; Early postoperative intraperitoneal chemotherapy is never used in treating diffuse malignant peritoneal mesothelioma.

11. A surgical team prepares for a HIPEC procedure for a patient with colorectal peritoneal carcinomatosis. Which of the following statements is incorrect regarding safety during HIPEC procedures?

A. Perioperative personnel face no risk of exposure to cytotoxic agents during HIPEC.
B. High-voltage electrocautery is used, generating surgical smoke that may pose a risk to healthcare workers.
C. Delivering chemotherapy directly into the peritoneal cavity maximizes dose intensity while minimizing systemic toxicity.
D. Proper precautions and policies are necessary to avoid occupational exposure to cytotoxic agents.
E. Inhalation of surgical smoke generated during the procedure may pose a risk to healthcare workers.

Answer: A

Explanation: Perioperative personnel face no risk of exposure to cytotoxic agents during HIPEC.

12. A 60-year-old patient with peritoneal carcinomatosis from gastric cancer is evaluated for potential treatment with CRS and HIPEC. Which of the following statements is incorrect regarding CRS and HIPEC for peritoneal carcinomatosis?

    A. CRS and HIPEC can only improve the quality of life without extending patient survival.
    B. The completeness of cytoreduction is a leading predictor of postoperative patient outcome.
    C. Consistent preoperative diagnostics and patient selection are critical for achieving complete macroscopic cytoreduction.
    D. Selected patients with peritoneal carcinomatosis can experience improved survival and quality of life with CRS and HIPEC.
    E. The volume of intraperitoneal tumor dissemination is a significant factor in patient selection for this treatment.

Answer: A

Explanation: CRS and HIPEC can only improve the quality of life without extending patient survival.

13. A 55-year-old female with gastric cancer develops peritoneal carcinomatosis. The team considers perioperative intraperitoneal chemotherapy plus CRS. Which of the following statements is incorrect regarding surgical treatments for gastric cancer peritoneal carcinomatosis?

    A. Systemic chemotherapy is the most effective treatment for peritoneal carcinomatosis from gastric cancer.
    B. Perioperative intraperitoneal chemotherapy targets the peritoneal dissemination directly, resulting in high locoregional intensity of drugs.
    C. Neoadjuvant intraperitoneal/systemic chemotherapy has been developed as a new bidirectional chemotherapy.
    D. Complete cytoreduction, low peritoneal carcinomatosis index, and negative peritoneal free cancer cells are significant favorable prognostic factors.
    E. HIPEC after CRS is associated with improved survival with an acceptable postoperative morbidity and mortality.

Answer: A

Explanation: Systemic chemotherapy is the most effective treatment for peritoneal carcinomatosis from gastric cancer.

14. A 54-year-old woman presents with abdominal distension and ascites. Imaging and biopsy are suggestive of peritoneal carcinomatosis, but no primary tumor is identified. In the context of peritoneal carcinomatosis in females, which statement is incorrect?

    A. PC can be a manifestation of cancers of unknown primary origin.

B. PC typically originates from colonic or extracolonic tissues with similar histological characteristics.
C. The clinical presentation of primary peritoneal carcinoma often mimics that of advanced ovarian cancer.
D. Women at increased risk for ovarian cancer are also at risk for developing primary peritoneal carcinoma.
E. Management options for women with peritoneal carcinomatosis of unknown primary origin may include surgical debulking followed by systemic chemotherapy.

Answer: B

Explanation: In females, PC usually originates from the ovary or extraovarian tissues similar to the ovary, not colonic or extracolonic tissues.

15. A 50-year-old male with a history of CRC treated with surgery and adjuvant chemotherapy presents with abdominal pain and weight loss. CT scan reveals peritoneal thickening and nodules, suggestive of peritoneal carcinomatosis. Regarding the diagnosis, staging, and prevention of PC, identify the incorrect statement:

A. PC is classified as stage IV disease irrespective of the primary tumor's stage.
B. CT scan is the preferred initial imaging modality for the evaluation of suspected PC.
C. Effective early treatment of primary tumors does not completely eliminate the risk of subsequent development of PC.
D. The main surgical approach for primary tumors to prevent PC is extensive local excision.
E. Administering adjuvant therapy after primary tumor treatment significantly reduces the risk of PC recurrence.

Answer: E

Explanation: While early treatment and adjuvant therapy reduce recurrence risk, they do not necessarily prevent the development of peritoneal carcinomatosis.

Bibliography

1. Boffetta P. Epidemiology of peritoneal mesothelioma: a review. Ann Oncol. 2007;18(6):985–90. Epub 2006 Oct 9. https://doi.org/10.1093/annonc/mdl345.
2. Eltabbakh GH, Piver MS, Hempling RE, Recio FO, Intengen ME. Clinical picture, response to therapy, and survival of women with diffuse malignant peritoneal mesothelioma. J Surg Oncol. 1999;70(1):6–12. https://doi.org/10.1002/(sici)1096-9098(199901)70:1<6::aid-jso2>3.0.co;2-x.
3. Levy AD, Arnáiz J, Shaw JC, Sobin LH. From the archives of the AFIP: primary peritoneal tumors: imaging features with pathologic correlation. Radiographics. 2008;28(2):583–607; quiz 621-2. https://doi.org/10.1148/rg.282075175.

4. Guest PJ, Reznek RH, Selleslag D, Geraghty R, Slevin M. Peritoneal mesothelioma: the role of computed tomography in diagnosis and follow up. Clin Radiol. 1992;45(2):79–84. https://doi.org/10.1016/s0009-9260(05)80059-5.
5. Jacquet P, Sugarbaker PH. Clinical research methodologies in diagnosis and staging of patients with peritoneal carcinomatosis. Cancer Treat Res. 1996;82:359–74. https://doi.org/10.1007/978-1-4613-1247-5_23.
6. Hesdorffer ME, Chabot JA, Keohan ML, Fountain K, Talbot S, Gabay M, Valentin C, Lee SM, Taub RN. Combined resection, intraperitoneal chemotherapy, and whole abdominal radiation for the treatment of malignant peritoneal mesothelioma. Am J Clin Oncol. 2008;31(1):49–54. https://doi.org/10.1097/COC.0b013e3180684181.
7. Yan TD, Deraco M, Baratti D, Kusamura S, Elias D, Glehen O, Gilly FN, Levine EA, Shen P, Mohamed F, Moran BJ, Morris DL, Chua TC, Piso P, Sugarbaker PH. Cytoreductive surgery and hyperthermic intraperitoneal chemotherapy for malignant peritoneal mesothelioma: multi-institutional experience. J Clin Oncol. 2009;27(36):6237–42. Epub 2009 Nov 16. https://doi.org/10.1200/JCO.2009.23.9640.
8. Feldman AL, Libutti SK, Pingpank JF, Bartlett DL, Beresnev TH, Mavroukakis SM, Steinberg SM, Liewehr DJ, Kleiner DE, Alexander HR. Analysis of factors associated with outcome in patients with malignant peritoneal mesothelioma undergoing surgical debulking and intraperitoneal chemotherapy. J Clin Oncol. 2003;21(24):4560–7. https://doi.org/10.1200/JCO.2003.04.150.
9. Rajeev R, Turaga K. Hyperthermic intraperitoneal chemotherapy and cytoreductive surgery in the management of peritoneal carcinomatosis. Cancer Control. 2016;23(1):36–46.
10. Sugarbaker P, Yan T, Stuart O, Yoo D. Comprehensive management of diffuse malignant peritoneal mesothelioma. Eur J Surg Oncol. 2006;32(6):686–91.
11. Gonzalez-Bayón L, González-Moreno S, Ortega-Pérez G. Safety considerations for operating room personnel during hyperthermic intraoperative intraperitoneal chemotherapy perfusion. Eur J Surg Oncol. 2006;32(6):619–24.
12. Glockzin G, Schlitt H, Piso P. Peritoneal carcinomatosis: patients selection, perioperative complications and quality of life related to cytoreductive surgery and hyperthermic intraperitoneal chemotherapy. World J Surg Oncol. 2009;7:5.
13. Yonemura Y, Endou Y, Sasaki T, Hirano M, Mizumoto A, Matsuda T, Takao N, Ichinose M, Miura M, Li Y. Surgical treatment for peritoneal carcinomatosis from gastric cancer. Eur J Surg Oncol. 2010;36(12):1131–8.
14. Comin CE, Saieva C, Messerini L. H-caldesmon, calretinin, estrogen receptor, and Ber-EP4: a useful combination of immunohistochemical markers for differentiating epithelioid peritoneal mesothelioma from serous papillary carcinoma of the ovary. Am J Surg Pathol. 2007;31(8):1139–48. https://doi.org/10.1097/PAS.0b013e318033e7a8.
15. Magge D, Zenati MS, Austin F, Mavanur A, Sathaiah M, Ramalingam L, Jones H, Zureikat AH, Holtzman M, Ahrendt S, Pingpank J, Zeh HJ, Bartlett DL, Choudry HA. Malignant peritoneal mesothelioma: prognostic factors and oncologic outcome analysis. Ann Surg Oncol. 2014;21(4):1159–65. Epub 2013 Dec 10. PMID: 24322529; PMCID: PMC4100549. https://doi.org/10.1245/s10434-013-3358-y.

Chapter 7
Hepatocellular Carcinoma

Raafat Raoof Alturfi, Talib A. Majeed, Sajjad G. Al-Badri, Saleh Abdulkareem Saleh, and Aqeel Shakir Mahmood

1. A 58-year-old male with a history of chronic alcoholism and hepatitis C presents with an abdominal mass and weight loss. CT scan reveals a liver lesion. Biopsy confirms hepatocellular carcinoma (HCC). Which of the following statements about HCC is incorrect?

   A. HCC is the fifth most common cancer and the third leading cause of cancer mortality worldwide.
   B. It is the leading cause of cancer mortality in Southeast Asia and sub-Saharan Africa.
   C. The incidence of HCC is higher in men than in women.
   D. Chronic hepatitis A is a recognized major risk factor for the development of HCC.
   E. Dietary exposure to aflatoxin is correlated with an increased risk of HCC.

   Answer: D

   Explanation: Hepatitis A, being an acute self-limiting infection, rarely causes chronic liver disease or HCC.

2. A 45-year-old female with a 10-year history of nonalcoholic steatohepatitis (NASH) is diagnosed with a liver tumor. Her family history is significant for

R. R. Alturfi
Department of Digestive Surgery, Gastroenterology and Hepatology Teaching Hospital, Baghdad, Iraq

T. A. Majeed
GIT and Liver Hospital, Medical City Baghdad, Baghdad, Iraq

S. G. Al-Badri · S. A. Saleh
College of Medicine University of Baghdad, Baghdad, Iraq

A. S. Mahmood (✉)
Department of General Surgery, University of Baghdad, Baghdad, Iraq

A. S. Mahmood, A. Koulouris (eds.), *MCQs in General Surgical Oncology*,
https://doi.org/10.1007/978-3-031-65738-2_7

liver cancer. On further evaluation, HCC is diagnosed. Identify the incorrect statement regarding risk factors for HCC:

A. More than half of global HCC cases are attributed to chronic hepatitis C virus infection.
B. Integration of hepatitis B virus (HBV) DNA into hepatocyte genomes is a precursor in HCC development.
C. Implementation of HBV vaccination programs has reduced HCC incidence in high-risk regions.
D. Metabolic syndromes, including conditions impairing glucose metabolism, are implicated in HCC pathogenesis.
E. The risk of HCC is elevated in patients with hepatic nonalcoholic fatty liver disease (NAFLD).

Answer: A

Explanation: Worldwide, HBV infection, not hepatitis C virus, accounts for the majority of HCC cases.

3. In assessing a 55-year-old cirrhotic patient with decompensated liver disease, the Child-Pugh classification is being used. Which of the following factors is incorrect in the Child-Pugh classification?

A. The presence and severity of ascites.
B. Levels of serum bilirubin.
C. Serum albumin concentrations.
D. Evidence of portal vein invasion.
E. Presence and severity of hepatic encephalopathy.

Answer: D

Explanation: Child-Pugh classification includes ascites, bilirubin, albumin levels, and hepatic encephalopathy, but not portal vein invasion.

4. A 48-year-old woman with a long history of diabetes and heavy alcohol use is being evaluated for a liver mass. In discussing potential risk factors for HCC with her medical team, which of the following is incorrect risk factor for HCC?

A. Chronic infection with hepatitis C virus.
B. Chronic infection with HBV.
C. Prolonged heavy alcohol consumption.
D. Long-standing diabetes.
E. History of IBS.

Answer: E

Explanation: IBS is not a known risk factor for HCC, whereas the other options are well-documented risk factors.

5. A 70-year-old male with a history of liver cirrhosis due to chronic hepatitis B infection presents with abdominal discomfort and weight loss. Imaging suggests a liver lesion consistent with HCC. Which of the following statements about HCC is incorrect?

A. HCC is the most common primary liver malignancy in adults.
B. HCC predominantly affects patients with preexisting liver disease, such as liver cirrhosis or chronic hepatitis.
C. Early-stage HCC is usually asymptomatic.
D. Advanced HCC typically presents without symptoms.
E. Hepatoblastoma is the most common primary liver malignancy in children.

Answer: D

Explanation: While early-stage HCC can be asymptomatic, advanced HCC often presents with nonspecific symptoms like abdominal pain, weight loss, and anorexia.

6. A 54-year-old male with chronic hepatitis C undergoes imaging for a suspected liver lesion. The radiologist is evaluating the characteristics of the lesion for HCC. Which statement about the imaging features of HCC is incorrect?

A. On CT, HCC lesions typically appear hyperdense.
B. MRI often shows the lesion as hyperintense or isointense on T2-weighted images.
C. Arterial phase hyperenhancement is a common feature in HCC.
D. An enhancing capsule may be visible around the lesion.
E. HCC lesions can present with irregular borders and potential signs of local invasion.

Answer: A

Explanation: On CT, HCC lesions usually appear hypodense or isodense, not hyperdense.

7. During a case review, a patient with HCC exhibits erythrocytosis. The medical team is discussing paraneoplastic syndromes in HCC. Which statement about paraneoplastic syndromes in HCC is incorrect?

A. Hypoglycemia typically occurs in early-stage HCC.
B. Erythrocytosis in HCC may be due to tumor secretion of erythropoietin.
C. Anemia at diagnosis is common in HCC patients due to various tumor effects.
D. Hypercalcemia in HCC may occur in association with osteolytic metastases.
E. Less than 5% of HCC tumors secrete insulin-like growth factor-II.

Answer: A

Explanation: Hypoglycemia is more commonly a feature of advanced HCC, thought to result from the tumor's high metabolic demands.

8. A multidisciplinary team is discussing the long-term outcomes of HCC in different patient populations. Which of the following statements about HCC is incorrect?

A. Patients with HBV-related HCC often have more preserved liver function than those with hepatitis C virus.
B. NASH patients are more likely to develop HCC within non-cirrhotic liver parenchyma.

C. Recurrence rates following resection for HCC are low, about 10% at 5 years.
D. The benefit of resection may be greater in patients with NASH-related HCC.
E. There is a significant risk of disease recurrence following partial hepatectomy.

Answer: C

Explanation: Recurrence rates following resection for HCC are high, with 50–75% recurrence at 5 years, not low as previously stated.

9. In a discussion about liver transplantation for a patient with end-stage liver disease, the Model for End-Stage Liver Disease (MELD) score is being calculated. Which parameter is incorrect in the MELD score calculation?

A. Severity and prognosis assessment of liver disease in candidates for transplantation.
B. Serum bilirubin levels.
C. Serum creatinine levels.
D. International normalized ratio (INR) for prothrombin time.
E. White blood cell (WBC) count.

Answer: E

Explanation: The MELD score includes serum bilirubin, serum creatinine, and INR, but it does not factor in the WBC count.

10. During a liver cancer conference, the use of tumor markers in the diagnosis of HCC is discussed. Which of the following is *not* a recognized tumor marker for HCC?

A. AFP.
B. Des-gamma-carboxy prothrombin (DCP).
C. CEA.
D. Lens culinaris agglutinin-reactive AFP (AFP-L3).
E. Methylated DNA markers (MDMs).

Answer: C

Explanation: CEA is not a marker for HCC; it is more commonly associated with CRC and other tumors.

11. A 65-year-old woman with a large liver mass is being staged for HCC. The team is considering various staging systems, including the Okuda staging system. Which of the following is incorrect in the Okuda staging system for HCC?

A. Tumor size.
B. Presence of ascites.
C. Serum albumin levels.
D. Serum bilirubin levels.
E. Presence of hepatic encephalopathy.

Answer: E

Explanation: The Okuda staging system includes tumor size, ascites, albumin, and bilirubin, but it does not include hepatic encephalopathy.

12. In a tumor board meeting, a 55-year-old patient with HCC is being staged using the Okuda staging system. Which of the following statements about the Okuda staging system for HCC is incorrect?

    A. Stage I is characterized by having no positive criteria.
    B. A bilirubin level of less than 3 mg/dL is considered positive.
    C. Stage III is defined by the presence of three or four positive criteria.
    D. A positive criterion is met if the tumor occupies more than 25% of the liver's largest cross-sectional area.
    E. A bilirubin level of more than 3 mg/dL is a positive criterion.

 Answer: D

 Explanation: In the Okuda staging system, a positive criterion is met if the tumor size exceeds 50% of the liver's largest cross-sectional area, not 25%.

13. A 62-year-old male with advanced liver cirrhosis is being evaluated for potential liver resection due to HCC. The surgical team is discussing risk factors for postoperative liver failure. Which of the following is *not* a risk factor for postoperative liver failure following resection for HCC?

    A. Significant portal hypertension.
    B. Presence of splenomegaly.
    C. Presence of varices.
    D. Low preoperative platelet count.
    E. Young age at onset.

 Answer: E

 Explanation: Younger age is not a recognized risk factor for postoperative liver failure. Factors such as portal hypertension, splenomegaly, varices, and a low preoperative platelet count are more pertinent risks.

14. During a surgical planning session for a 48-year-old female undergoing resection for HCC, techniques to minimize intraoperative blood loss are being discussed. Which of the following techniques is incorrect to minimize blood loss during HCC resection?

    A. Employing low central venous pressure anesthesia
    B. Utilizing intermittent vascular exclusion, such as Pringle's maneuver
    C. Implementing total vascular exclusion
    D. Performing laparoscopic resection

 Answer: D

 Explanation: While low CVP anesthesia, Pringle's maneuver, and total vascular exclusion are techniques to minimize intraoperative blood loss, laparoscopic resection is not specifically aimed at reducing blood loss during HCC resection.

15. In a surgical oncology conference, a case of a 56-year-old patient with HCC is being discussed for potential surgical resection. Which of the following statements about surgical resection in HCC is incorrect?

A. Only 20–40% of patients with HCC are eligible for surgical resection.
B. According to BCLC guidelines, resection is not recommended for patients with >3 nodules or 2–3 nodules with one >3 cm.
C. A large tumor without microvascular invasion may have a prognosis similar to a small tumor with microvascular invasion.
D. Surgical resection is typically reserved for patients with a single lesion or three lesions <3 cm and good liver function.
E. Large tumor size, vascular invasion, and multifocal disease are absolute contraindications to surgical resection.

Answer: E

Explanation: While large tumor size, vascular invasion, and multifocal disease are poor prognostic factors, they are not absolute contraindications for surgical intervention in HCC.

16. During a transplant evaluation for a 55-year-old patient with HCC, the suitability for transplantation is being assessed using the Milan criteria. Which of the following statements about the Milan criteria for HCC transplantation is incorrect?

A. Eligibility includes one lesion smaller than 5 cm.
B. Up to three lesions, each smaller than 3 cm, are acceptable.
C. There should be no extrahepatic manifestations of HCC.
D. There must be no evidence of gross vascular invasion.
E. The patient must be below the age of 60.

Answer: E

Explanation: The Milan criteria do not include an age limit; they focus on tumor size, number, absence of extrahepatic disease, and lack of gross vascular invasion.

17. In a recent liver cancer conference, the use of the Barcelona Clinic Liver Cancer (BCLC) staging system was discussed. A 65-year-old patient with a single liver lesion and preserved liver function (Child-Pugh A) is being considered for treatment. Which statement about the BCLC staging system is incorrect?

A. It employs the Child-Pugh system for assessing underlying liver function.
B. The system is particularly prognostic for patients with early-stage liver cancer.
C. Its conservative approach toward surgical resection in certain stages has faced criticism.
D. BCLC staging is primarily utilized for pathological staging post-resection or transplantation.
E. It evaluates tumor characteristics, liver function, and patient performance status.

Answer: D

Explanation: The BCLC staging system is used for clinical staging of liver cancer, not pathological staging.

18. A 60-year-old male with hepatitis B-related HCC is being staged using the American Joint Committee on Cancer/International Union Against Cancer (AJCC/UICC) system. His liver resection specimen is being reviewed. Which of the following statements about the AJCC/UICC staging system for HCC is incorrect?

    A. The system is based on a retrospective central histology review of surgically resected patients.
    B. It takes into account tumor size and the presence or absence of vascular invasion.
    C. Emphasizes the significance of macroscopic vascular invasion in staging.
    D. Validation of the system has been limited to patients with HCV-related HCC.
    E. Tumor size is considered the most crucial histopathological prognostic factor in HCC.

    Answer: E

    Explanation: Vascular invasion, not tumor size, is the key histopathological prognostic indicator in HCC according to AJCC/UICC.

19. During a liver cancer symposium, various etiologies of HCC are discussed. A patient with HCC and a background of genetic hemochromatosis is being used as a case study. Which of the following is an incorrect cause of HCC?

    A. Hereditary hemochromatosis.
    B. Wilson's disease.
    C. Alpha-1 antitrypsin deficiency.
    D. Schistosomiasis.
    E. Liver cirrhosis which accounts for only 25% of HCC cases.

    Answer: E

    Explanation: Liver cirrhosis is a major risk factor for HCC, contributing to about 80% of cases, not 25%.

20. A 60-year-old woman with chronic liver disease is undergoing evaluation for a suspected liver tumor. The clinical team is discussing the diagnostic approach for HCC. Which of the following statements about the diagnosis of HCC is incorrect?

    A. Liver biopsy is always required to establish the diagnosis of HCC.
    B. Ultrasound is typically the initial imaging modality for suspected HCC.
    C. Screening for HCC is recommended in high-risk patient groups.
    D. Diagnosis often involves identifying a solid nodule, typically ≥10 mm in size.
    E. HCC nodules can appear heterogeneous with irregular borders on ultrasound.

    Answer: A

    Explanation: Liver biopsy is not routinely required for HCC diagnosis in patients with underlying liver disease and characteristic imaging findings.

21. A 55-year-old female with HCC is undergoing staging. The team is considering the possibility of extrahepatic metastases. Which statement about extrahepatic metastases in HCC is incorrect?

    A. They can be present at diagnosis, especially in patients with advanced-stage primary tumors.
    B. Approximately 10 to 15% of cases show large vessel vascular invasion with tumors larger than 5 cm.
    C. The brain is the most common site of extrahepatic metastases.
    D. Perihepatic lymphadenopathy should not be automatically interpreted as extrahepatic metastases.
    E. Extrahepatic metastases may occur as part of disease recurrence after locoregional therapy.

Answer: C

Explanation: The most frequent sites of extrahepatic metastases in HCC are the lung, intra-abdominal lymph nodes, and bone, while brain metastases are rare.

22. In a multidisciplinary team meeting, a 58-year-old male with chronic liver disease is being evaluated for HCC. The team discusses the role of AFP in HCC. Which statement about AFP is incorrect?

    A. Serum AFP concentration is the most commonly used serum marker for HCC.
    B. A threshold of 8 ng/mL AFP is standard in clinical practice for initiating an HCC evaluation.
    C. Elevated AFP levels in patients with chronic liver disease indicate an increased risk for HCC.
    D. AFP is not the primary test used for HCC surveillance.
    E. AFP levels do not consistently correlate with the clinical characteristics of the tumor.

Answer: B

Explanation: The threshold AFP level commonly used to trigger evaluation for HCC is 20 ng/mL, not 8 ng/mL.

23. During a clinical review of a patient with HCC, the team discusses tumor characteristics associated with increased recurrence and poorer survival. Which of the following tumor features is incorrectly associated with increased recurrence and worse survival in HCC?

    A. Vascular invasion.
    B. Infiltrative growth pattern.
    C. Positive margin status.
    D. LN involvement.
    E. Unifocal tumor.

Answer: E

Explanation: Features associated with increased recurrence and worse survival in HCC include vascular invasion, infiltrative growth pattern, positive margin status, and LN involvement. A unifocal tumor is generally associated with a better prognosis.

24. In a case review of a 50-year-old patient with HCC, the NCCN guidelines for hepatic resection are being discussed. Which of the following is incorrect regarding absolute indications for hepatic resection according to NCCN guidelines?

    A. Child-Pugh Class A liver function without portal hypertension.
    B. Multifocal HCC with major vascular invasion.
    C. Remaining liver functionality of at least 20% in non-cirrhotic patients.
    D. Remaining liver functionality of 30%–40% with Child-Pugh Class A cirrhosis.
    E. Adequate vascular and biliary inflow/outflow for the remaining liver.

Answer: B

Explanation: According to NCCN guidelines, hepatic resection is not an absolute indication for multifocal HCC with major vascular invasion. Solitary lesions without major vascular invasion are more suitable for resection.

25. A 66-year-old patient with HCC is considered unsuitable for surgery, and ablation therapy is being discussed. Which statement about ablation therapy for HCC is incorrect?

    A. The tumor location must be accessible for the ablation approach.
    B. Ablation can be curative for tumors ≤3 cm in size.
    C. Inoperable lesions >5 cm should be considered for arterially directed therapy, systemic therapy, or radiotherapy (RT).
    D. Adjuvant therapy is routinely used to increase the success rate of ablation.
    E. Ablation of lesions 3 to 5 cm in size may be considered to improve survival rates.

Answer: D

Explanation: There is no evidence that adjuvant therapies post-ablation provide a benefit in the treatment of HCC.

26. A 50-year-old female with a recently diagnosed HCC is being discussed in a multidisciplinary tumor board for staging and treatment planning using the BCLC system. Which of the following statements about the BCLC staging system for HCC is incorrect?

    A. Stage 0–A HCC patients are considered for resection, transplantation, or local ablation.
    B. Stage B HCC patients are typically managed with transarterial chemoembolization (TACE).
    C. Stage C HCC is usually treated with systemic therapies like sorafenib.
    D. Stage D HCC management involves best supportive care.

E. Stage D HCC is typically managed with percutaneous ethanol injection or radiofrequency ablation (RFA).

Answer: E

Explanation: Percutaneous ethanol injection and RFA are treatments for early-stage HCC (Stage A), not for Stage D, which is managed with supportive care.

27. In a 63-year-old patient with HCC, a CT scan reveals multiple liver lesions and involvement of a major branch of the hepatic vein. How would this case be staged according to the AJCC/UICC HCC staging system? Identify the incorrect statement:

A. Stage I (T1) is characterized by a solitary tumor without vascular invasion.
B. Stage II (T2) includes either a solitary tumor with vascular invasion or multiple tumors, each ≤5 cm.
C. Stage IIIA (T3a) is defined by the presence of multiple tumors larger than 5 cm.
D. Stage IIIB (T3b) involves a single or multiple tumors of any size with involvement of a major portal or hepatic vein branch.
E. Stage IIIC includes any stage of HCC with distant metastases.

Answer: E

Explanation: Stage IIIC (T4) is defined by invasion of adjacent organs or perforation of the visceral peritoneum, not distant metastases.

28. A 55-year-old man with a history of chronic hepatitis B infection presents with elevated liver enzymes. Imaging suggests a liver lesion consistent with HCC. Which of the following statements about the diagnostic workup for HCC is incorrect?

A. Contrast-enhanced CT or MRI is essential for a definitive radiological diagnosis of HCC.
B. Serum AFP levels are specific for HCC.
C. Cross-sectional imaging is used to assess the morphological features characteristic of HCC.
D. Histological confirmation via core needle biopsy may be required in certain cases.
E. Ultrasound is often utilized in the initial assessment for HCC.

Answer: B

Explanation: AFP levels are not specific to HCC and may be elevated in various hepatic and non-hepatic conditions.

29. In a case conference discussing a 62-year-old patient with HCC, the BCLC staging system is being used to guide treatment decisions. Which of the following statements about the BCLC staging system is incorrect?

A. Stage 0 is characterized by a single tumor less than 2 cm.
B. Stage A can include a single tumor less than 3 cm or up to three tumors each less than 3 cm.

C. Stage B is defined by multiple tumors or a single tumor larger than 3 cm.
D. Stage C may involve vascular invasion.
E. Stage D is associated with distant metastasis.

Answer: E

Explanation: In the BCLC system, Stage C includes vascular invasion or metastasis, and Stage D is characterized by liver failure or tumor-related symptoms.

30. A 56-year-old patient with liver cirrhosis is being classified using the Child-Turcotte-Pugh (CTP) scoring system. Which of the following statements about the CTP classification is incorrect?

A. In class A, albumin levels are greater than 3.5 g/dL.
B. Class B is characterized by an INR between 1.7 and 2.3.
C. Class A includes bilirubin levels between 2.5 and 3.5 mg/dL.
D. Class A is associated with the absence of ascites.
E. Class B includes the absence of hepatic encephalopathy.

Answer: C

Explanation: In Class A of the CTP classification, bilirubin levels are less than 2.5 mg/dL, not between 2.5 and 3.5 mg/dL.

31. A 60-year-old male with advanced HCC presents with unusual laboratory findings. The oncology team is discussing potential paraneoplastic syndromes associated with HCC. Which of the following is *not* typically a paraneoplastic syndrome associated with HCC?

A. Hypoglycemia.
B. Erythrocytosis.
C. Diarrhea.
D. Hypercalcemia.
E. Syndrome of inappropriate antidiuretic hormone (SIADH).

Answer: E

Explanation: SIADH, characterized by excessive ADH production leading to hyponatremia, is more commonly associated with lung cancer than with HCC.

32. In a liver cancer seminar, the outcomes of partial hepatectomy in HCC patients are being discussed. A 58-year-old patient with a solitary HCC tumor is being considered for surgery. Which of the following statements about partial hepatectomy for HCC is incorrect?

A. It can be curative for patients with a solitary tumor without gross vascular invasion.
B. 5-year survival rates can exceed 50%.
C. Recurrence rates at 5 years are less than 30%.
D. The presence of comorbidities is an independent predictor of perioperative mortality.
E. CT imaging/MRI is crucial for determining the tumor's relation to vascular and biliary structures.

Answer: C

Explanation: Recurrence rates following partial hepatectomy for HCC often exceed 70% at 5 years, not less than 30%.

33. During a discussion on advanced HCC treatment options, external beam radiation therapy (EBRT) is considered for a 70-year-old patient. Which statement about the recommendation of EBRT in HCC is incorrect?

    A. It is recommended for confined multifocal or unresectable HCC.
    B. Suitable for patients with microvascular invasion.
    C. Can be sequenced with systemic or catheter-based therapies.
    D. Used as a bridge to transplantation or before surgery in selected cases.
    E. Employed as a salvage option for local recurrences.

Answer: B

Explanation: EBRT is recommended for patients with macrovascular invasion, not microvascular, as surgical options may not be feasible.

Bibliography

1. Iorio N, John S. Hepatitis A. In: StatPearls [Internet]. Treasure Island, FL: StatPearls; 2023. Accessed 14 Jul 2023.
2. Chen Y, Tian Z. HBV-induced immune imbalance in the development of HCC. Front Immunol. 2019;10:2048. https://doi.org/10.3389/fimmu.2019.02048.
3. Levy I, Sherman M. Staging of hepatocellular carcinoma: assessment of the CLIP, Okuda, and child-Pugh staging systems in a cohort of 257 patients in Toronto. Gut. 2002;50(6):881–5.
4. Yang JD, Hainaut P, Gores GJ, Amadou A, Plymoth A, Roberts LR. A global view of hepatocellular carcinoma: trends, risk, prevention and management. Nat Rev Gastroenterol Hepatol. 2019;16(10):589–604.
5. Bruix J, Sherman M. Hepatocellular carcinoma: clinical presentation, diagnosis, and staging. Hepatology. 2011;53(3):1020–2.
6. Chernyak V, Fowler KJ, Kamaya A, et al. Liver imaging reporting and data system (LI-RADS) version 2018: imaging of hepatocellular carcinoma in at-risk patients. Radiology. 2018;289(3):816–30. https://doi.org/10.1148/radiol.2018181494.
7. Ong Y, Huey CW, Shelat VG. Paraneoplastic syndromes in hepatocellular carcinoma: a review. Expert Rev Gastroenterol Hepatol. 2022;16(5):449–71.
8. Lang H, Sotiropoulos GC, Brokalaki EI, Schmitz KJ, Bertona C, Meyer G, et al. Survival and recurrence rates after resection for hepatocellular carcinoma in noncirrhotic livers. J Am Coll Surg. 2007;205(1):27–36. https://doi.org/10.1016/j.jamcollsurg.2007.03.002.
9. Kamath PS, Kim WR. The model for end-stage liver disease (MELD). Hepatology. 2007;45(3):797–805.
10. Debes JD, Romagnoli PA, Prieto J, Arrese M, Mattos AZ, Boonstra A, On Behalf Of The Escalon Consortium. Serum biomarkers for the prediction of hepatocellular carcinoma. Cancers (Basel). 2021;13(7):1681. PMID: 33918270; PMCID: PMC8038187. https://doi.org/10.3390/cancers13071681.
11. Leung TW, Tang AM, Zee B, Lau WY, Lai PB, Leung KL, Lau JT, Yu SC, Johnson PJ. Construction of the Chinese university prognostic index for hepatocellular carcinoma and

comparison with the TNM staging system, the Okuda staging system, and the cancer of the liver Italian program staging system: a study based on 926 patients. Cancer. 2002;94(6):1760–9.
12. Duseja A. Staging of hepatocellular carcinoma. J Clin Exp Hepatol. 2014;4:S74–9.
13. Maithel SK, Kneuertz PJ, Kooby DA, Scoggins CR, Weber SM, Martin RC 2nd, et al. Importance of low preoperative platelet count in selecting patients for resection of hepatocellular carcinoma: a multi-institutional analysis. J Am Coll Surg. 2011;212:638–48. discussion 648–50.
14. Johnson M, Mannar R, Wu AV. Correlation between blood loss and inferior vena caval pressure during liver resection. Br J Surg. 1998;85(2):188–90.
15. Pawlik TM, Poon RT, Abdalla EK, Zorzi D, Ikai I, Curley SA, et al. Critical appraisal of the clinical and pathologic predictors of survival after resection of large hepatocellular carcinoma. Arch Surg. 2005;140(5):450–7; discussion 457–8.
16. Mazzaferro V, Regalia E, Doci R, Andreola S, Pulvirenti A, Bozzetti F, Montalto F, Ammatuna M, Morabito A, Gennari L. Liver transplantation for the treatment of small hepatocellular carcinomas in patients with cirrhosis. N Engl J Med. 1996;334(11):693–9.
17. Llovet JM, Zucman-Rossi J, Pikarsky E, Sangro B, Schwartz M, Sherman M, et al. Hepatocellular carcinoma. Nat Rev Dis Primers. 2016;2:16018. https://www.ncbi.nlm.nih.gov/pmc/articles/PMC5440153/. Accessed 10 Jul 2023.
18. Kunutsor SK, Apekey TA, Van Hemelrijck M. Intrahepatic vascular invasion is the strongest predictor of mortality in hepatocellular carcinoma: a systematic review and meta-analysis. BMC Cancer. 2014;14:328. https://doi.org/10.1186/1471-2407-14-328.
19. El-Serag HB. Epidemiology of viral hepatitis and hepatocellular carcinoma. Gastroenterology. 2012;142(6):1264–73.
20. Bialecki ES, Di Bisceglie AM. Diagnosis of hepatocellular carcinoma. HPB. 2005;7(1):26–34.
21. Harding JJ, Abu-Zeinah G, Chou JF, Owen DH, Ly M, Lowery MA, Capanu M, Do R, Kemeny NE, O'Reilly EM, Saltz LB, Abou-Alfa GK. Frequency, morbidity, and mortality of bone metastases in advanced hepatocellular carcinoma. J Natl Compr Canc Netw. 2018;16(1):50–8. https://doi.org/10.6004/jnccn.2017.7024.
22. Kanwal F, Singal AG. Surveillance for hepatocellular carcinoma: current best practice and future direction. Gastroenterology. 2019;157(1):54–64. Epub 2019 Apr 12. PMID: 30986389; PMCID: PMC6636644. https://doi.org/10.1053/j.gastro.2019.02.049.
23. Schiffman SC, Woodall CE, Kooby DA, Martin RC, Staley CA, Egnatashvili V, et al. Factors associated with recurrence and survival following hepatectomy for large hepatocellular carcinoma: a multicenter analysis. J Surg Oncol. 2010;101:105–10.
24. Truty MJ, Vauthey JN. Surgical resection of high-risk hepatocellular carcinoma: patient selection, preoperative considerations, and operative technique. Ann Surg Oncol. 2010;17:1219–25.
25. Bruix J, Takayama T, Mazzaferro V, Chau GY, Yang J, Kudo M, Cai J, Poon RT, Han KH, Tak WY, Lee HC. Adjuvant sorafenib for hepatocellular carcinoma after resection or ablation (STORM): a phase 3, randomised, double-blind, placebo-controlled trial. Lancet Oncol. 2015;16(13):1344–54.
26. Minagawa M, Ikai I, Matsuyama Y, Yamaoka Y, Makuuchi M. Staging of hepatocellular carcinoma: assessment of the Japanese TNM and AJCC/UICC TNM systems in a cohort of 13,772 patients in Japan. Ann Surg. 2007;245(6):909–22.
27. Simpson JL, Snijders RJM, Sonek J, et al. The revised 2016 international standards for alphafetoprotein in maternal serum. Prenat Diagn. 2017;37(1):1–10.
28. Kaplan DE, Dai F, Aytaman A, Baytarian M, Fox R, Hunt K, Knott A, Pedrosa M, Pocha C, Mehta R, Duggal M. Development and performance of an algorithm to estimate the child-Turcotte-Pugh score from a national electronic healthcare database. Clin Gastroenterol Hepatol. 2015;13(13):2333–41.
29. Luo JC, Hwang SJ, Wu JC, Lai CR, Li CP, Chang FY, Chiang JH, Lui WY, Chu CW, Lee SD. Clinical characteristics and prognosis of hepatocellular carcinoma patients with paraneoplastic syndromes. Hepatogastroenterology. 2002;49(47):1315–9.

30. Kianmanesh R, Regimbeau JM, Belghiti J. Selective approach to major hepatic resection for hepatocellular carcinoma in chronic liver disease. Surg Oncol Clin. 2003;12(1):51–63.
31. Apisarnthanarax S, Barry A, Cao M, Czito B, DeMatteo R, Drinane M, Hallemeier CL, Koay EJ, Lasley F, Meyer J, Owen D. External beam radiation therapy for primary liver cancers: an ASTRO clinical practice guideline. Pract Radiat Oncol. 2022;12(1):28–51.

Chapter 8
Liver Metastases

Raafat Raoof Alturfi, Waseem M. Al Hamidy, Munthir A. Alobaidi, and Aqeel Shakir Mahmood

1. A 58-year-old man with a history of left-sided colon cancer presents with imaging studies showing multiple liver lesions suspicious for metastases. The multidisciplinary team is evaluating the patient for potential liver resection. Which of the following statements regarding colorectal liver metastases (CRLMs) is incorrect?

   A. Resectable CRC liver metastases simply as tumors that can be resected completely while leaving an adequate liver remnant.
   B. Of those patients with CRLMs, 20% will be candidate for curative liver resection.
   C. The perioperative risks may be prohibitive.
   D. Patients who develop rapidly progressive metastases beyond the liver during the trial of systemic chemotherapy will not benefit from surgery.
   E. There is an adverse impact of left- versus right-sided primary tumor location on liver resection.

   Answer: E

   Explanation: The embryonic origin of the primary colon cancer also appears to affect the prognosis of patients who develop liver metastases. The adverse impact of right- versus left-sided primary tumor location has been noted in

R. R. Alturfi
Department of Digestive Surgery, Gastroenterology and Hepatology Teaching Hospital, Baghdad, Iraq

W. M. Al Hamidy
Gastroenterology and Hepatology Teaching Hospital, Medical City, Baghdad, Iraq

M. A. Alobaidi
Department of Surgery, College of Medicine, University of Baghdad, Baghdad, Iraq

A. S. Mahmood (✉)
Department of General Surgery, University of Baghdad, Baghdad, Iraq

A. S. Mahmood, A. Koulouris (eds.), *MCQs in General Surgical Oncology*,
https://doi.org/10.1007/978-3-031-65738-2_8

other CRC populations, including those with unresectable metastatic disease and localized nonmetastatic disease.

2. Regarding preoperative evaluation for CRLMs, a 55-year-old patient with CRLMs is being evaluated for surgery. Which of the following is incorrect?

   A. Preoperative imaging is used to determine the number and extent of liver metastases.
   B. We prefer MRI over triphasic liver CT because it is most sensitive in detecting additional lesions that might preclude resection.
   C. CT is limited in the ability to identify lesions smaller than 1 cm and can have false negative rates as high as 10%.
   D. PET scans identify radiographically occult extrahepatic disease and optimize the selection of candidates for hepatic resection.
   E. Diagnostic laparoscopy is standard for evaluating patients with CRLMs.

Answer: E

Explanation: With improved sensitivity of cross-sectional imaging modalities, diagnostic laparoscopy is no longer standard for evaluating patients with CRLMs. Instead, we only use it in patients with a suspicion of small-volume carcinomatosis on radiographic imaging studies (i.e., CT, MRI, or PET) or who are at particularly high risk for harboring unresectable diseases (e.g., a metachronous presentation with several liver metastases that do not respond to chemotherapy).

3. A 62-year-old woman with a history of rectal cancer treated with neoadjuvant chemoradiation and surgical resection presents with isolated liver metastases. The multidisciplinary team is discussing the feasibility of local resection of these CRLMs. Which of the following statements regarding the anatomical factors for local resection of CRLMs is incorrect?

   A. Resectability of hepatic colorectal metastases should focus on the ability to obtain a complete resection (negative margins).
   B. Positive surgical margin is associated with a higher local recurrence.
   C. Anticipated margin of <1 cm should not be used as an exclusion criterion for resection.
   D. Presence of extrahepatic disease is considered an absolute contraindication for liver resection.
   E. Preservation of adequate future liver remnant (>20% in a healthy liver; >30% after chemotherapy) is crucial.

Answer: D

Explanation: The presence of extrahepatic disease should no longer be considered an absolute contraindication to hepatic resection provided the patient is carefully selected and a complete (margin-negative) resection of both intra- and extrahepatic disease is feasible.

4. A 55-year-old man with a history of sigmoid colon cancer, previously treated with surgery and adjuvant chemotherapy, presents with isolated liver metastases. The surgical team is evaluating various techniques for the upcoming

resection of CRLMs. During surgery for CRLMs, which of the following statements is incorrect?

A. Obtaining a negative resection margin remains an important determinant of survival.
B. We routinely perform an air cholangiogram at the time of surgery.
C. Intra-abdominal drains are routinely placed after hepatectomy.
D. Sixty to 70% of patients with CRLMs are candidates for minimally invasive resection.
E. The optimal extent of liver resection for CRLMs is subject to debate, but current trends are moving toward nonanatomic parenchymal-sparing resection.

Answer: C

Explanation: Routine placement of intra-abdominal drains after hepatectomy has no clear benefit. Thus, we do not recommend the use of drains.

5. A 60-year-old patient with CRLMs is being considered for surgical treatment. Which of the following is incorrect?

A. Surgical treatment of metachronous lesions is not different from surgery for any other liver lesions.
B. Resecting synchronous CRLMs is typically more complex than resecting metachronous CRLMs.
C. Curative resection cannot be performed in two stages.
D. Patients who present with symptoms from the primary CRC with synchronous CRLMs should undergo resection of the colorectal primary tumor first.
E. Asymptomatic patients from the primary CRC and synchronous CRLMs may undergo a simultaneous or staged resection, depending on the extent of their liver involvement.

Answer: C

Explanation: Although patients who have significant CRLMs in both lobes of the liver cannot be cured with a single operation, curative resection can still be performed in two stages. In the first stage, as many metastases are removed as possible. A second-stage operation is performed to remove the remaining CRLMs.

6. A patient with CRLMs is undergoing management considerations. Which of the following is incorrect?

A. Initial systemic chemotherapy is often undertaken as a means of assessing the natural history of metastatic disease.
B. Neoadjuvant systemic chemotherapy has the potential to convert initially unresectable liver metastases to resectable disease.
C. Patients whose disease progresses while on chemotherapy would not benefit from resection.
D. In disappearing liver metastases after neoadjuvant systemic chemotherapy, resection is not required.

E. Lesions at the greatest risk of disappearing after chemotherapy are those <2 cm in diameter and >1 cm deep in the liver parenchyma.

Answer: D

Explanation: Unfortunately, resection is still required because a true pathologic complete response or durable clinical response is rare (17%) after chemotherapy alone.

7. A 70-year-old patient with unresectable CRLMs is being evaluated for treatment options. Which of the following is incorrect?

A. Initial treatment options include chemotherapy and/or locoregional therapies such as ablation.
B. Initially unresectable hepatic metastases may have a sufficient objective response to permit a subsequent complete resection.
C. Forty percent of patients with metastatic CRC are not candidates for resection at diagnosis.
D. Ablation is a parenchymal-sparing strategy that is increasingly used for the management of small or unresectable tumors.
E. For patients with borderline resectable disease or inadequate future liver remnant for resection, a combined ablation/resection approach can be used.

Answer: C

Explanation: Approximately 80% of patients with metastatic CRC are not candidates for resection at diagnosis.

8. A patient with CRLMs that are unsuitable for resection is being considered for treatment options. Which of the following is incorrect?

A. Locoregional liver-directed treatment includes methods using RFA, microwave ablation, or stereotactic body radiotherapy (SBRT).
B. SBRT is an acceptable alternative to initial systemic chemotherapy.
C. TACE and radioembolization are not appropriate options if locoregional methods were not applicable.
D. Patients who are ineligible for locoregional therapy are treated with systemic chemotherapy.
E. A commonly employed strategy is to start with chemotherapy, and consolidate this, for appropriate candidates, with subsequent ablation.

Answer: C

Explanation: In most cases, the extent of disease will preclude tumor ablation or SBRT, and TACE and radioembolization are appropriate options. The choice is usually based on local expertise, patient preference, and patient/tumor characteristics.

9. A 58-year-old patient with recurrent CRLMs is being evaluated for treatment options. Which of the following is incorrect?

A. Recurrences following initial resection of CRLMs can occur in up to 57% of cases.
B. Liver is the most common site of recurrence.

C. Resection for recurrence of CRLM is a safe and feasible option in properly selected patients.
D. Recurrences at the margin are common.
E. Disease is thought to recur more frequently after two-stage hepatectomies than after single-stage liver resections.

Answer: D

Explanation: Interestingly, recurrences at the margin are uncommon.

10. A 55-year-old male with bilobar colorectal liver metastases is being evaluated for potential curative surgery. His oncologist is considering preoperative portal vein embolization to increase the future liver remnant volume. Which of the following statements regarding preoperative portal vein embolization is incorrect?

A. Portal vein embolization is utilized to induce hypertrophy of the future liver remnant, increasing the safety of resection.
B. Portal vein embolization can make patients, who were previously deemed inoperable due to insufficient future liver remnant, suitable candidates for surgery.
C. Portal vein embolization significantly increases the risk of postsurgical liver failure due to decreased liver volume.
D. Portal vein embolization is a well-established technique in the multidisciplinary management of colorectal liver metastases.
E. Combining portal vein embolization with staged liver resection allows potentially curative surgery in patients with extensive bilobar metastases.

Answer: C

Explanation: Portal vein embolization significantly increases the risk of postsurgical liver failure due to decreased liver volume. This statement is incorrect because PVE aims to prevent postsurgical liver failure by inducing hypertrophy of the future liver remnant, thereby increasing its volume and functional capacity.

11. A 48-year-old female with small, unresectable colorectal liver metastases is being evaluated for alternative treatment options. The treatment team is considering RFA. Which of the following statements about RFA is incorrect?

A. RFA is one of the least invasive techniques for treating unresectable hepatic malignancies.
B. RFA can be performed using percutaneous, laparoscopic, or open surgical techniques.
C. RFA is associated with high local tumor progression rates, making it an undesirable option for most patients.
D. RFA can provide effective palliation and potentially extend survival in selected patients.
E. The use of RFA is particularly considered for patients who are not appropriate candidates for surgical resection.

Answer: C

Explanation: RFA is associated with high local tumor progression rates, making it an undesirable option for most patients. This statement is incorrect as RFA, while having some risk of local tumor progression, is a valuable option for certain patients, offering effective palliation and potential survival benefits.

12. A 60-year-old patient with extensive synchronous bilobar liver metastases from colorectal cancer is evaluated for potential curative interventions. The surgical team proposes a two-stage hepatectomy. Which of the following statements about two-stage hepatectomy is incorrect?

    A. The two-stage hepatectomy approach is designed for patients with extensive bilobar liver metastases.
    B. The primary goal of the first stage is to resect metastases in one lobe and induce hypertrophy in the other.
    C. Two-stage hepatectomy typically results in shorter overall hospital stays compared to single-stage resections.
    D. This approach can convert patients from inoperable to operable status.
    E. The second stage involves resecting the remaining disease in the hypertrophied lobe after an interval of liver regeneration.

Answer: C

Explanation: Two-stage hepatectomy typically results in shorter overall hospital stays compared to single-stage resections. This statement is incorrect as the two-stage hepatectomy, while effective, involves multiple surgeries and recovery periods, potentially leading to longer cumulative hospital stays.

13. A 45-year-old patient with metastatic colorectal cancer confined to the liver is discussing treatment options. Liver transplantation is mentioned as a potential approach. Which of the following statements about liver transplantation for metastatic colorectal cancer is incorrect?

    A. Liver transplantation can offer a chance of cure for patients with metastatic colorectal cancer confined to the liver.
    B. Liver transplantation is a widely accepted standard treatment modality for all patients with liver-confined metastatic colorectal cancer.
    C. Candidates for liver transplantation should have no extrahepatic disease and limited hepatic tumor load.
    D. Liver transplantation is considered in highly selected patients due to the scarcity of donor organs and the risk of recurrence.
    E. The decision for liver transplantation involves a thorough evaluation by a multidisciplinary team.

Answer: B

Explanation: Liver transplantation is a widely accepted standard treatment modality for all patients with liver-confined metastatic colorectal cancer. This statement is incorrect as liver transplantation for metastatic colorectal cancer is considered in very highly selected patients and is not a standard treatment modality due to the reasons mentioned in option D.

14. A 50-year-old patient with resectable colorectal liver metastases is considering surgical options. The surgical oncology team discusses minimally invasive liver surgery. Which of the following statements about minimally invasive liver surgery is incorrect?

    A. Minimally invasive techniques, including laparoscopic surgery, are being increasingly used for liver metastases resection.
    B. Minimally invasive liver surgery is associated with significantly longer operative times than open surgery.
    C. These techniques can result in shorter hospital stays and less postoperative pain compared to open surgery.
    D. Major hepatectomies can be performed using minimally invasive techniques in selected patients.
    E. Minimally invasive liver surgery is limited to patients with single, small liver metastases.

   Answer: E

   Explanation: Minimally invasive liver surgery is limited to patients with single, small liver metastases. This statement is incorrect as minimally invasive techniques can be applied to a variety of cases, including those with multiple or larger metastases, depending on the patient's overall condition and the surgeon's expertise.

15. A patient with CRLMs is discussing potential outcomes with the medical team. Which of the following is incorrect?

    A. Perioperative mortality associated with colorectal liver metastasis (CRLM) resection is <25%.
    B. Resection offers the greatest likelihood of cure for patients with liver-isolated CRC.
    C. Having a RAS mutation is a risk factor for worse overall survival.
    D. Mutations in the BRAF gene have also been linked to poor prognosis after resection of CRLMs.
    E. Postoperative complications include bile leak, ascites, liver failure, and pulmonary and thrombotic complications.

   Answer: A

   Explanation: Perioperative mortality associated with colorectal liver metastasis (CRLM) resection is <5%.

Bibliography

1. Nordlinger B, Guiguet M, Vaillant JC, Balladur P, Boudjema K, Bachellier P, Jaeck D. Surgical resection of colorectal carcinoma metastases to the liver. A prognostic scoring system to improve case selection, based on 1568 patients. Association Française de Chirurgie. Cancer. 1996;77(7):1254–62.

2. Syn NL, Kabir T, Koh YX, Tan HL, Wang LZ, Chin BZ, Wee I, Teo JY, Tai BC, Goh BKP. Survival advantage of laparoscopic versus open resection for colorectal liver metastases: a meta-analysis of individual patient data from randomized trials and propensity-score matched studies. Ann Surg. 2020;272(2):253–65. https://doi.org/10.1097/SLA.0000000000003672.
3. Nagakura S, Shirai Y, Suda T, Hatakeyama K. Multiple repeat resections of intra- and extra-hepatic recurrences in patients undergoing initial hepatectomy for colorectal carcinoma metastases. World J Surg. 2002;26(2):141–7. Epub 2001 Dec 4. https://doi.org/10.1007/s00268-001-0196-z.
4. Squires MH 3rd, Lad NL, Fisher SB, Kooby DA, Weber SM, Brinkman A, Sarmiento JM, Scoggins CR, Egger ME, Cardona K, Cho CS, Martin RC, Russell MC, Winslow E, Staley CA 3rd, Maithel SK. Value of primary operative drain placement after major hepatectomy: a multi-institutional analysis of 1,041 patients. J Am Coll Surg. 2015;220(4):396–402. Epub 2015 Jan 2. https://doi.org/10.1016/j.jamcollsurg.2014.12.029.
5. Martin RC 2nd, Augenstein V, Reuter NP, Scoggins CR, McMasters KM. Simultaneous versus staged resection for synchronous colorectal cancer liver metastases. J Am Coll Surg. 2009;208(5):842–50; discussion 850–2. Epub 2009 Mar 26. https://doi.org/10.1016/j.jamcollsurg.2009.01.031.
6. Benoist S, Brouquet A, Penna C, Julié C, El Hajjam M, Chagnon S, Mitry E, Rougier P, Nordlinger B. Complete response of colorectal liver metastases after chemotherapy: does it mean cure? J Clin Oncol. 2006;24(24):3939–45. https://doi.org/10.1200/JCO.2006.05.8727.
7. Global Cancer Observatory. International Agency for Research on Cancer. World Health Organization. https://gco.iarc.fr
8. Benson AB 3rd, Geschwind JF, Mulcahy MF, Rilling W, Siskin G, Wiseman G, Cunningham J, Houghton B, Ross M, Memon K, Andrews J, Fleming CJ, Herman J, Nimeiri H, Lewandowski RJ, Salem R. Radioembolisation for liver metastases: results from a prospective 151 patient multi-institutional phase II study. Eur J Cancer. 2013;49(15):3122–30. Epub 2013 Jun 15. https://doi.org/10.1016/j.ejca.2013.05.012.
9. Pawlik TM, Scoggins CR, Zorzi D, Abdalla EK, Andres A, Eng C, Curley SA, Loyer EM, Muratore A, Mentha G, Capussotti L, Vauthey JN. Effect of surgical margin status on survival and site of recurrence after hepatic resection for colorectal metastases. Ann Surg. 2005;241(5):715–22, discussion 722–4. PMID: 15849507; PMCID: PMC1357126, 724. https://doi.org/10.1097/01.sla.0000160703.75808.7d.
10. Primrose J. Surgery for colorectal liver metastases. Br J Cancer. 2010;102(9):1313–8.
11. Wong J, Cooper A. Local ablation for solid tumor liver metastases: techniques and treatment efficacy. Cancer Control. 2016;23(1):30–7.
12. Mentha G, Terraz S, Andres A, Toso C, Rubbia-Brandt L, Majno P. Operative management of colorectal liver metastases. Semin Liver Dis. 2013;33(3):262–72.
13. Clavien P-A, Lesurtel M, Bossuyt PMM, Gores GJ, Langer B, Perrier A. Recommendations for liver transplantation for hepatocellular carcinoma: an international consensus conference report. Lancet Oncol. 2012;13(1):e11–22.
14. Reddy SK, Pawlik TM, Zorzi D, Gleisner AL, Ribero D, Assumpcao L, Barbas AS, Abdalla EK, Choti MA, Vauthey JN, Ludwig KA, Mantyh CR, Morse MA, Clary BM. Simultaneous resections of colorectal cancer and synchronous liver metastases: a multi-institutional analysis. Ann Surg Oncol. 2007;14(12):3481–91. Epub 2007 Sep 1. https://doi.org/10.1245/s10434-007-9522-5.

Chapter 9
Gallbladder Cancer

Waseem M. Al Hamidy, Haider A. H. Ahmed, Sabah Noori Abdulraheem, and Aqeel Shakir Mahmood

1. A 78-year-old male was recently diagnosed with GBC. Which of the following is an incorrect statement regarding the risk factors for gallbladder malignancy?
   A. Stones >3 cm carry a tenfold increased risk.
   B. Symptomatic stone disease carries a lower risk of developing malignancy than asymptomatic stones.
   C. GB polyps >10 mm carry a 25% risk of malignancy.
   D. Porcelain gallbladders are malignant in 10% of cases.
   E. It is advised to undergo prophylactic cholecystectomy when risk factors for gallbladder malignancy are present.

Answer: B

Explanation: Symptomatic gallstone disease carries a higher risk of developing malignancy than asymptomatic gallstones.

2. A 55-year-old woman presents to the clinic with complaints of upper abdominal pain and jaundice. She has a history of recurrent gallstone disease and was diagnosed with chronic cholecystitis two years ago. An ultrasound reveals gallbladder wall thickening, multiple gallstones, and calcification of the gallbladder wall. Which of the following is the incorrect statement regarding her risk factors for gallbladder carcinoma?

W. M. Al Hamidy
Gastroenterology and Hepatology Teaching Hospital, Medical City, Baghdad, Iraq

H. A. H. Ahmed
Medical City Complex, Baghdad, Iraq

S. N. Abdulraheem
Baghdad Teaching Hospital, Baghdad, Iraq

A. S. Mahmood (✉)
Department of General Surgery, University of Baghdad, Baghdad, Iraq

A. S. Mahmood, A. Koulouris (eds.), *MCQs in General Surgical Oncology*,
https://doi.org/10.1007/978-3-031-65738-2_9

A. Gallbladder stones are a risk factor for gallbladder carcinoma.
B. Chronic infection with Salmonella Typhi is a risk factor for gallbladder carcinoma.
C. Smoking is a significant risk factor for gallbladder carcinoma.
D. Obesity is associated with an increased risk of gallbladder carcinoma.
E. Gallbladder wall calcification is a risk factor for gallbladder carcinoma.

Answer: C

Explanation: While gallbladder stones, chronic infection with Salmonella Typhi, and obesity are established risk factors for gallbladder carcinoma, smoking is not typically associated with this type of cancer.

3. A 60-year-old male presents with intermittent right upper quadrant pain that has been ongoing for several years. He reports a history of gallstones and was advised to undergo a cholecystectomy, but he declined. During his current visit, an ultrasound reveals multiple gallstones, with the largest stone measuring 4 cm in diameter. The patient's symptoms and history prompt further evaluation for potential gallbladder carcinoma. Which of the following is the incorrect statement about gallstone disease as a risk factor for gallbladder carcinoma?

A. Gallstone disease is the strongest risk factor.
B. Having cholesterol gallstones is a risk factor for gallbladder carcinoma.
C. Patients who have stones larger than 3 cm have a higher risk of cancer.
D. Longer duration of gallstone presence is a risk factor.
E. Having a gallbladder stone less than 1 cm is a risk factor.

Answer: E

Explanation: Gallbladder stones less than 1 cm in size are generally not considered a significant risk factor for gallbladder carcinoma.

4. A 45-year-old woman presents with a calcified gallbladder wall, which was incidentally found during an abdominal CT scan. She has no history of GBC. In porcelain gallbladder, which of the following statements is incorrect?

A. It is a subtype of GBC.
B. It is more commonly diagnosed in men than women.
C. It involves complete or selective calcification of the gallbladder wall.
D. CT scan is the diagnostic imaging of choice.
E. Cholelithiasis is a risk factor for porcelain gallbladder.

Answer: B

Explanation: While porcelain gallbladder is associated with an increased risk of GBC, it is not a subtype of it and is more commonly diagnosed in women.

5. A 50-year-old man presents for a routine check-up and undergoes an abdominal ultrasound. The scan reveals a small polyp in the gallbladder, which measures 5 mm. The polyp appears to be benign, and there is no associated thickening of the gallbladder wall. Based on this finding, which of the following is the incorrect statement regarding benign gallbladder polyps?

A. Inflammatory polyps are typically benign with no malignant potential.
B. Cholesterol polyps are benign and common, with no risk of malignancy.
C. Adenomyomas polyps are benign and have no risk of malignant transformation.
D. Fibromas polyps are benign and typically do not undergo malignant transformation.
E. Adenoma polyps are benign with no risk of malignant transformation.

Answer: E

Explanation: While the other listed polyps can be benign, adenoma polyps are neoplastic and can increase the risk of GBC.

6. A 60-year-old African patient with a known history of primary sclerosing cholangitis (PSC) comes for a routine check-up. During the visit, an abdominal ultrasound is performed, revealing an 11 mm sessile polyp in the gallbladder. The patient is asymptomatic and has no family history of gallbladder cancer. Regarding the risk of malignancy in this case scenario, which of the following is the incorrect statement?

A. Age of the patient is a risk factor.
B. Size of the polyp is a risk factor.
C. Ethnicity of the patient is a significant risk factor.
D. History of PSC increases the risk.
E. The sessile nature of the polyp is a risk factor.

Answer: C

Explanation: While age, size of the polyp, history of PSC, and characteristics of the polyp are relevant factors, ethnicity, such as being Indian, increases the risk of gallbladder carcinoma in specific populations, but ethnicity alone in an African patient does not significantly influence the risk in this context.

7. A 55-year-old patient with a history of gallbladder polyps undergoes an abdominal ultrasound, which reveals a polyp. Regarding gallbladder polyps, the incorrect statement is:

A. Most of the polyps are benign.
B. Ultrasonography can differentiate between malignant and benign polyps.
C. Can be differentiated from gallstones on abdominal ultrasound by being fixed on the wall, showing no movement when the patient rolls from one side to another, and not causing acoustic shadow.
D. CT scan shows low sensitivity for small and cholesterol polyps.
E. Usually discovered incidentally on imaging and can be diagnosed by causing right upper quadrant abdominal pain.

Answer: B

Explanation: Ultrasonography alone cannot reliably differentiate between malignant and benign polyps.

8. A 65-year-old woman, who is asymptomatic, is found to have a gallbladder mass greater than 2 cm during a routine check-up. Regarding the clinical presentation of GBC, which of the following is the incorrect statement?

A. A 70-year-old patient who presented with obstructive jaundice.
B. Incidentally post-cholecystectomy due to symptomatic cholelithiasis.
C. Asymptomatic 65-year-old patient with a gallbladder mass > 2 cm.
D. A previously healthy 30-year-old patient who presented with fever, right abdominal pain, and jaundice.
E. Metastatic liver lesions with solitary sessile biliary mass.

Answer: D

Explanation: The features in a previously healthy young patient without mentioned risk factors are more indicative of cholangitis rather than gallbladder carcinoma.

9. In imaging of GBC, the incorrect statement is:

A. Ultrasound is the best initial test.
B. CT scan is an additional test for suspicious lesions and staging.
C. Magnetic resonance cholangiopancreatography (MRCP) is better than CT for differentiation between malignant and benign lesions.
D. Endoscopic retrograde pancreatocholangiography (ERCP) and percutaneous transhepatic cholangiopancreatography (PTCp) are diagnostic tests of choice for patients suspected of having GBC.
E. EUS is better than external ultrasound for the prediction of tumor histology.

Answer: D

Explanation: ERCP and PTCp are not the diagnostic tests of choice for diagnosing GBC.

10. In a 65-year-old patient with T4, N2 stage of biliary cancer, the incorrect statement is:

A. No invasion of vessels at this stage.
B. Invades the main portal vein or hepatic artery.
C. Can invade two or more extrahepatic structures.
D. Metastases to four or more regional lymph nodes.
E. Regular follow-up after management may not have an effect on survival outcome for this type of tumor.

Answer: A

Explanation: T4 stage of GBC invades the main portal vein/hepatic artery or invades two or more extrahepatic structures.

11. A 58-year-old patient with a history of GBC presents to the oncology clinic with symptoms of weight loss, abdominal pain, and shortness of breath. Imaging studies are performed to evaluate for potential metastases. The scans reveal lesions in multiple sites, suggesting metastatic spread. Regarding the sites for gallbladder carcinoma metastasis, the incorrect statement is:

A. Liver is a common site for metastasis.
B. Peritoneum is frequently involved in metastasis.
C. Lung is a known site for metastasis.
D. Brain is a common site for metastasis.
E. Abdominal wall can be involved in metastasis.

Answer: D

Explanation: The brain is not a common site for gallbladder carcinoma metastasis. Metastatic spread more commonly involves the liver, peritoneum, lungs, and abdominal wall.

12. A 62-year-old patient with advanced GBC is being evaluated for potential surgical resection. Regarding the absolute contraindications to surgical resection in this patient, the incorrect statement is:

    A. Liver metastasis is an absolute contraindication.
    B. T2 stage is an absolute contraindication.
    C. Lymph node involvement by tumor (para-aortic, paracaval, SMA, and/or celiac artery lymph nodes) is an absolute contraindication.
    D. Peritoneal metastases are an absolute contraindication.
    E. Encasement or occlusion of major vessels is an absolute contraindication.

Answer: B

Explanation: T2 stage of cancer, which penetrates perimuscular connective tissue but does not extend beyond the serosa or into the liver, does not represent an absolute contraindication for resection. Other factors like liver metastasis, peritoneal spread, and major vessel involvement are indeed contraindications.

13. A 55-year-old patient with T1a GBC is under evaluation for treatment options. The incorrect statement regarding T1a GBC is:

    A. Simple cholecystectomy is recommended.
    B. T1a GBC is limited to in situ or invades the lamina propria only.
    C. Radical cholecystectomy is the treatment of choice.
    D. LN metastases are rare.
    E. Radical cholecystectomy has no survival benefit.

Answer: C

Explanation: Simple cholecystectomy is often recommended for T1a GBC, as radical cholecystectomy may not provide a survival benefit in these cases.

14. A 60-year-old patient is diagnosed with T1b GBC; the incorrect statement regarding T1b GBC is:

    A. Simple cholecystectomy is the surgery of choice.
    B. Penetrates the muscular layer.
    C. Radical cholecystectomy with or without port site excision.
    D. Removal of the cystic duct margin with or without common bile duct resection if involved.
    E. LN resection includes porta hepatis, gastrohepatic ligament, and retroduodenal nodes.

Answer: A

Explanation: For T1b GBC, radical cholecystectomy is typically recommended as the treatment of choice.

15. A 56-year-old patient is diagnosed with T2 GBC. Regarding T2 tumor stage, the incorrect statement is:

    A. Penetrates peri-muscular connective tissue.
    B. No extension beyond the serosa or into the liver.
    C. Perforates serosa and/or directly invades the liver or other adjacent structures.
    D. Treatment includes radical cholecystectomy.
    E. Involves LN metastases.

   Answer: C

   Explanation: T2 GBC does not involve direct invasion into the liver or other adjacent structures, and radical cholecystectomy is often considered in its treatment.

16. A 65-year-old patient is diagnosed with T3 N1 GBC. As regards T3 N1, the incorrect statement is:

    A. Perforates serosa (visceral peritoneum).
    B. Metastases to one or three regional lymph nodes.
    C. Directly invades the liver.
    D. Invades adjacent organs like the stomach, duodenum, colon, pancreas, omentum, or extrahepatic bile ducts.
    E. Invades the main portal vein/hepatic artery.

   Answer: E

   Explanation: T4 GBC invades the main portal vein/hepatic artery, not T3.

17. A 50-year-old patient with incidentally found GBC is being considered for laparoscopic management. In laparoscopic management of GBC, the incorrect statement is:

    A. Laparoscopic cholecystectomy has the concern of port site metastasis after incidentally found GBC.
    B. Port site disease was seen only in patients with T2 or T3 disease.
    C. Port site disease correlated with the development of peritoneal metastases.
    D. Some have recommended port site excision at the time of re-exploration after laparoscopic cholecystectomy.
    E. Port site resection was associated with overall survival and recurrence-free survival.

   Answer: E

   Explanation: Port site resection was not associated with overall survival or recurrence-free survival in laparoscopic management of GBC.

18. A 58-year-old patient recently diagnosed with GBC with peritoneal metastasis presents with jaundice and upper abdominal pain. Which of the available management options is incorrect?

    A. Simple cholecystectomy.
    B. Endoscopic or percutaneous biliary drainage.

C. Endoscopic stenting or intestinal bypass.
D. Therapeutic radical cholecystectomy.
E. Biliary bypass.

Answer: D

Explanation: In the presence of peritoneal metastasis, a therapeutic radical cholecystectomy is not typically recommended; a palliative approach is more appropriate.

19. A 45-year-old patient inquires about the 5-year prognosis for GBC. The incorrect statement regarding the expected 5-year prognosis for GBC is:

A. Early stage nearly 60%.
B. Advanced resectable stages 4–13%.
C. Metastatic 2%.
D. Five-year survival for all patients with GBC is 20%.
E. Five-year survival for all patients with GBC is 60%.

Answer: E

Explanation: The 5-year survival for all patients with GBC is typically around 20%.

20. A 65-year-old patient with GBC is being considered for extended cholecystectomy. Regarding the management of GBC with extended cholecystectomy, the incorrect statement is:

A. An open procedure generally has been recommended.
B. A minimally invasive procedure generally has been recommended.
C. Intraoperative bile spillage should be avoided.
D. Lowering central venous pressure during liver dissection and the use of surgical hemostatic devices.
E. A sample of the cystic duct margin should be sent to the frozen section.

Answer: B

Explanation: An open procedure generally has been recommended for extended cholecystectomy, rather than a minimally invasive approach.

21. A 54-year-old patient with a history of GBC underwent routine follow-up imaging to assess for potential tumor recurrence after surgical resection. The incorrect statement regarding the location of a high recurrence rate in gallbladder carcinoma is:

A. Retroperitoneal lymph nodes are common sites of recurrence.
B. Intrahepatic recurrence is common in GBC.
C. Peritoneum is a frequent site of recurrence.
D. Locoregional recurrence is often observed.
E. Large bowel is a common site of recurrence.

Answer: E

Explanation: The large bowel is not a common location for recurrence in GBC compared to the other mentioned sites.

22. During a laparoscopic cholecystectomy for cholelithiasis, the surgeon suspects GBC. Regarding management, the incorrect statement is:

    A. If the surgeon is experienced in hepatobiliary surgery, the cholecystectomy can be done with a frozen section of the resected segment.
    B. For surgeons who do not have experience with hepatobiliary surgery, closing the incisions with simple cholecystectomy and referral to a more experienced center.
    C. For inexperienced surgeons with this type of surgery, closing the incisions without simple cholecystectomy and referral to a tertiary center.
    D. There is a difference in survival noticed between direct opening and referral.

Answer: D

Explanation: There is typically no difference in survival noticed between direct opening and referral for further management of suspected GBC.

23. A 67-year-old woman presents with right upper quadrant pain and jaundice. Imaging studies and biopsy confirm a diagnosis of gallbladder cancer. The surgical team is discussing the management plan, including staging and the potential need for re-resection. Regarding the management of gallbladder cancer, which of the following statements is incorrect?

    A. Staging with a CT scan must be done.
    B. Re-resection procedure must be done for those who have T1b, T2, or T3 stage.
    C. A high rate of residual disease patients, and those who undergo re-resection have better survival than those who do not.
    D. A staging laparoscopy may be performed to rule out peritoneal metastases, especially in those with T3 disease, poorly differentiated histology, or positive margins.
    E. No staging or re-resection needed.

Answer: E

Explanation: Staging of GBC must be done, and re-resection will be performed if needed according to the stage of the tumor.

24. A 54-year-old man undergoes cholecystectomy for presumed benign gallbladder disease. Postoperative histopathology reveals gallbladder cancer. The surgical oncology team is discussing the indications for re-resection. Regarding re-resection of the gallbladder, which of the following statements is incorrect?

    A. Re-resection for T1a tumors does not appear to provide an overall survival benefit.
    B. The optimal approach to incidental T1b disease is more controversial.
    C. An incidentally detected T2 tumor on histologic review of the cholecystectomy specimen, re-exploration and extended cholecystectomy are indicated.
    D. T3 GBC has very high rates of residual disease at re-exploration.
    E. Re-resection is recommended regardless of the stage.

Answer: E

Explanation: Re-resection is recommended depending on the stage of GBC, and for T1a tumors, it does not appear to provide an overall survival benefit.

25. A 56-year-old patient with incidentally found GBC is being evaluated for re-resection. Prior to re-resection for incidentally finding GBC, laparoscopy may be performed; the incorrect statement is regarding the purpose of staging laparoscopy is:

    A. To rule out peritoneal metastases.
    B. For staging with T3 disease.
    C. Staging poorly differentiated histology.
    D. Staging tumors with positive margins.
    E. CT scan alone is enough for staging GBC prior to resection in all cases.

Answer: E

Explanation: CT scan alone may not be sufficient for staging GBC, and other diagnostic tests may be necessary based on the patient's presentation.

26. A 60-year-old woman is undergoing surgery for GBC. The surgical team is discussing the extent of LN dissection required. Regarding lymph node dissection for GBC, which of the following statements is incorrect?

    A. If the stage of GBC is >T1a, LN removal is needed whether bile duct excision is planned or not.
    B. LNs that appear normal during surgery should not be removed.
    C. LN metastasis is found in 35–80% of patients with GBC that is ≥T2.
    D. LN involvement is a strong predictor of a poor outcome after surgery.
    E. At least six lymph nodes should be removed for dependable staging.

Answer: B

Explanation: LNs that appear normal during surgery should still be removed during LN dissection for GBC, as LN metastasis is not always clear during surgery.

27. A 70-year-old man with a diagnosis of GBC is scheduled for surgery. The surgical team is planning the extent of regional LN dissection. Regarding a proper regional lymph node dissection for GBC, which of the following statements is incorrect?

    A. Removing all lymph nodes in the porta hepatis.
    B. Removing all lymph nodes along the hepatoduodenal ligaments.
    C. Location of the metastatic LNs is more prognostic than the number of metastatic lymph nodes and the LN ratio.
    D. Removing all lymph nodes along the common bile duct.
    E. Removing all lymph along the hepatic artery and portal vein.

Answer: C

Explanation: The number of metastatic lymph nodes and the LN ratio are often more prognostic than the specific location of metastatic lymph nodes in GBC.

28. A 65-year-old woman with GBC is being evaluated for hepatic resection. The tumor is located at the gallbladder fundus and there is no evidence of distant

metastasis. The surgical team is discussing the extent of liver resection required. Regarding hepatic resection in GBC, which of the following statements is incorrect?

A. Minimal liver resection is needed to clear margins in most cases.
B. It may be necessary to remove additional segments of the liver beyond what is included in extended cholecystectomy.
C. Margin-negative liver resection with an at least 2 cm nonanatomic excision of the gallbladder fossa.
D. Excision of liver segments IVb and V is acceptable for gallbladder fundus tumor.
E. Nonanatomic liver excision decreases the risk for bleeding and bile leakage.

Answer: E

Explanation: Anatomic liver resection, not nonanatomic, reduces the risk for bleeding or bile leakage during hepatic resection for GBC.

29. A 62-year-old patient with GBC has undergone surgery, and prognostic factors are being evaluated. The incorrect statement regarding prognostic factors is:

A. Tumor staging (N) by location of lymph nodes affected.
B. Status of the surgical margins of the tumor.
C. Invasion depth of the tumor.
D. Presence of vascular and neural invasion.
E. Histologic grade of differentiation.

Answer: A

Explanation: The number of lymph nodes examined for staging assessment is often more important than the specific location of lymph nodes affected. At least six lymph nodes should be examined for proper postoperative staging of patients.

30. A 55-year-old patient with resected GBC is being considered for adjuvant therapy. The incorrect statement regarding adjuvant therapy is:

A. Adjuvant therapy is routinely recommended to patients with resected GBC at many institutions.
B. Adjuvant CRT has enhanced survival in patients with locally advanced disease.
C. Adjuvant therapy for patients with completely resected muscle-invasive (≥T1b), node-positive, or margin-positive GBC.
D. Therapy for a patient with a resected T1a, node-negative tumor, is strongly recommended.
E. Six months of postoperative chemotherapy alone with capecitabine monotherapy for most patients.

Answer: D

Explanation: Adjuvant therapy is typically not recommended for patients with a resected T1a, node-negative tumor, according to guidelines.

31. A 58-year-old patient with a history of GBC is being monitored for recurrence. The incorrect statement regarding the recurrence of GBC is:

    A. Majority of all recurrences occur in the first 12 months.
    B. One-third of cases recur within 2 years.
    C. Overall survival usually decreases over time, and the longer an individual has survived since treatment, the greater the chance of additional survival.
    D. Survival was greater among patients with cholangiocarcinoma (CC) compared with patients with GBC.
    E. Studies show that those with disease recurrence have the same prognosis as those without recurrence.

    Answer: E

    Explanation: Those with disease recurrence often have a worse prognosis than those without recurrence, making option E incorrect.

32. A 60-year-old patient with GBC is being considered for adjuvant therapy with capecitabine. The incorrect statement regarding adjuvant capecitabine therapy is:

    A. Postoperative chemotherapy may enhance overall survival in comparison with surgery alone.
    B. Postoperative chemotherapy alone with capecitabine monotherapy can be used.
    C. Capecitabine adverse effects include hand-foot syndrome, diarrhea, and fatigue.
    D. Regimen includes giving 1250 mg/m^2 twice daily on days 1–14 of a 3-week cycle, for eight cycles.
    E. Postoperative chemotherapy alone with capecitabine and cytarabine can be used.

    Answer: E

    Explanation: Postoperative chemotherapy alone with capecitabine monotherapy is the standard treatment for most patients with GBC.

33. A 58-year-old man with resected GBC is being discussed in a multidisciplinary tumor board meeting. The tumor was node-positive with clear margins. The team is considering the role of adjuvant therapy. Regarding the role of adjuvant therapy in resectable GBC, which of the following statements is incorrect?

    A. Survival benefit from adjuvant therapy was statistically significant.
    B. There is a survival benefit of chemotherapy and CRT.
    C. There is a survival benefit of radiation therapy alone.
    D. Patients with node-positive disease show great survival benefit from adjuvant therapy.
    E. Margin-positive disease shows survival benefits using adjuvant therapy.

    Answer: C

    Explanation: Radiation therapy alone has not shown a significant survival benefit in resectable GBC.

34. A 63-year-old woman with resectable GBC is undergoing a multidisciplinary treatment planning discussion. The surgical team is considering the role of adjuvant intraoperative RT. Regarding adjuvant intraoperative RT in resectable GBC, which of the following statements is incorrect?

    A. Preoperative external RT can increase complete resection and tolerance and is theoretically more effective (less hypoxia) than post-surgery external RT.
    B. Normal tissues surrounding the gallbladder have limitations for radiation, which is where intraoperative RT is mostly useful.
    C. Survival is better compared with patients having resection alone.
    D. Postsurgical external beam radiation is better than intraoperative radiation.
    E. Routine use of intraoperative radiation therapy can be considered a standard component of therapy for GBC.

    Answer: E

    Explanation: The lack of strong evidence for intraoperative radiation benefits, limited availability, and specific requirements for intraoperative treatment make routine use of this method of therapy not considered standard management for GBC.

35. A 56-year-old patient presents with jaundice and suspicious findings in the gallbladder on ultrasound. The incorrect statement regarding this scenario is:

    A. Preoperative jaundice is an absolute contraindication for radical resection.
    B. Many jaundiced patients are found to have disseminated disease.
    C. Neoadjuvant chemotherapy could be considered in this situation.
    D. Stenting via an endoscopic or percutaneous approach is usually needed.
    E. Patients presented with jaundice prior to surgery have a lower likelihood of curative resection.

    Answer: A

    Explanation: Preoperative jaundice is a relative contraindication for radical resection. Most patients with preoperative jaundice are found to have disseminated, unresectable disease, but curative resection can still be attempted in some cases.

36. A 66-year-old male presented with abdominal pain and jaundice; further evaluation showed unresectable GBC. The incorrect statement is:

    A. CRT and chemotherapy are acceptable choices for locoregional therapy of a locally advanced, unresectable GBC.
    B. Adjuvant therapies have shown to be effective with long-term outcomes in patients with advanced GBC, R1 disease, and LN metastasis.
    C. There is insufficient evidence to support the routine use of neoadjuvant therapy in advanced GBC.
    D. Most cases are managed by radiation therapy alone.
    E. Cisplatin plus gemcitabine is an adjuvant treatment option for patients with advanced GBC.

    Answer: D

Explanation: Tumor resection is seldom achieved with radiation alone, as it is often insufficient for effective tumor eradication due to proximity to dose-limiting normal tissues.

37. A 72-year-old female presented with abdominal pain and distension. Imaging studies exhibit unresectable GBC. Regarding chemotherapy in unresectable tumors, the incorrect statement is:

    A. Chemotherapy with gemcitabine alone in the treatment of unresectable GBC is an option.
    B. There is no survival benefit in unresectable cancer when comparing supportive care with chemotherapy treatment.
    C. Gemcitabine plus oxaliplatin (GEMOX) is better than fluorouracil and supportive care in improving overall survival.
    D. Transaminitis is a significant side effect, which was more prevalent in GEMOX.
    E. Median overall survival was 9.5 months in the GEMOX group.

Answer: B

Explanation: There is a survival benefit in unresectable cancer when comparing chemotherapy treatment with supportive care.

38. A 71-year-old male developed abdominal pain, jaundice, anorexia, and itching. Diagnostic studies revealed GBC. In terms of chemotherapy for gallbladder tumors, the incorrect statement is:

    A. Gemcitabine plus cisplatin is a chemotherapy option.
    B. Gemcitabine plus capecitabine is a chemotherapy option.
    C. Capecitabine alone is a chemotherapy option.
    D. Gemcitabine plus oxaliplatin is a chemotherapy option.
    E. Gemcitabine monotherapy is used rather than gemcitabine-based combinations for most patients with unresectable tumors.

Answer: E

Explanation: Gemcitabine combined with other chemotherapy agents is often preferred over gemcitabine monotherapy for most patients with unresectable tumors, provided they have good tolerance for chemotherapy and an acceptable bilirubin level.

39. A 54-year-old patient presented with resectable GBC. The incorrect statement regarding pre-surgical management is:

    A. The poorest prognosis was in the group of patients with elevation of both CA19-9 and CEA markers.
    B. There is no role for tumor markers in GBC.
    C. Preoperative CEA levels within the normal range are associated with a better prognosis.
    D. Preoperative CA19-9 levels within the normal limit are associated with a better prognosis.
    E. Surveillance is needed for resectable tumors.

Answer: B

Explanation: Tumor markers like CA19-9 and CEA can provide valuable prognostic information in GBC.

40. A 67-year-old female presents with right upper quadrant pain and jaundice. Imaging reveals a mass in the gallbladder with possible liver invasion. The patient's history includes chronic cholecystitis and gallstones. Laboratory findings indicate elevated CA19-9 levels. Based on the clinical and diagnostic findings, gallbladder cancer is suspected. Which of the following statements regarding GBC is incorrect?

    A. The prognosis of GBC significantly improves with early-stage diagnosis, where a 5-year survival rate can approach 80% in highly selected cases of stage I disease following surgical resection.
    B. GBC is often diagnosed incidentally during or after cholecystectomy for presumed benign conditions, reflecting its asymptomatic nature in early stages.
    C. Despite its overall rarity compared to other gastrointestinal cancers, GBC shows marked regional prevalence, correlating closely with areas of high gallstone disease incidence.
    D. The distribution of GBC demonstrates notable geographical variability, directly associated with the prevalence of recognized risk factors such as gallstones and chronic gallbladder inflammation.
    E. GBC incidence shows a clear gender predilection, being more frequently diagnosed in females, with hormonal and reproductive factors contributing to this disparity.

Answer: A

Explanation: Early-stage GBC (stage I) indeed has a better prognosis following surgical resection, but such cases are rare, and the overall 5-year survival rate across all stages remains low.

41. A 63-year-old male planned for GBC surgery. During cholecystectomy of advanced GBC, the incorrect statement is:

    A. LN dissection is indicated only if the cystic duct frozen section is positive.
    B. If the cystic duct margin is negative, there is no need for bile duct resection.
    C. If the cystic duct margin is positive, bile duct resection should be performed.
    D. Bile duct resection should be performed when the frozen section of cystic duct margins cannot be performed.
    E. LN dissection is indicated whether or not bile duct resection is performed if the GBC is >T1a.

Answer: A

Explanation: LN dissection is indicated in advanced GBC whether or not bile duct resection is performed if the GBC is >T1a.

42. A 66-year-old female, who has family history of GBC, presented with insidious onset jaundice. Regarding gallbladder malignancies, the incorrect statement is:

A. Most cases are adenocarcinoma.
B. The first LN draining the gallbladder is the hilar lymph node.
C. Tumor invasion is common to segments IVb and V of the liver because the draining gallbladder veins are to that area.
D. Lymphatics in the gallbladder are present in the subserosal area.
E. Carcinomas that do not breach the muscular layer have a higher risk of nodal involvement.

Answer: E

Explanation: Nodal involvement in gallbladder malignancies is higher when the carcinoma extends through the muscular layer because lymphatics are present in the subserosal area.

43. A 57-year-old patient with suspected gallbladder disease is scheduled for surgery. The incorrect statement regarding the surgical anatomy of the gallbladder is:

A. The cystic artery is a branch of the right hepatic artery.
B. The lateral border of the hepatocystic triangle is formed by the gallbladder and cystic duct.
C. The base of the hepatocystic duct is formed by liver parenchyma.
D. Calot's triangle has its base formed by the cystic duct.
E. The medial border of Calot's triangle is formed by the common hepatic duct.

Answer: C

Explanation: The base of Calot's triangle is formed by the cystic artery, and it is an important surgical landmark in the approach to the gallbladder.

44. A 47-year-old patient diagnosed with early-stage gallbladder cancer is considering surgical options. The surgical team proposes minimally invasive surgery. Which of the following statements regarding minimally invasive surgery for gallbladder cancer is incorrect?

A. Minimally invasive surgery includes laparoscopic extended cholecystectomy.
B. Short- and long-term outcomes of minimally invasive surgery are comparable to those of open surgery.
C. Minimally invasive surgery is not recommended for any stage of gallbladder cancer.
D. Laparoscopic surgery offers benefits such as reduced hospital stay and quicker recovery.
E. The role of robotic surgery in gallbladder cancer is under investigation.

Answer: C

Explanation: Minimally invasive surgery is not recommended for any stage of gallbladder cancer. This statement is incorrect as minimally invasive surgery, including laparoscopic surgery, is considered a safe and effective alternative for the treatment of gallbladder cancer, especially in early stages.

45. A 54-year-old patient presents with advanced gallbladder cancer. The medical team discusses the surgical options. Which of the following statements about the surgical management of advanced gallbladder cancer is incorrect?

    A. Radical en bloc resection offers greater long-term survival benefits over conventional cholecystectomy alone.
    B. Simple cholecystectomy is adequate for treating T1a gallbladder cancer.
    C. Radical surgery is not beneficial for patients with T2 gallbladder cancer lesions.
    D. Lymph node excision can improve survival in patients with T2 lesions.
    E. Negative surgical margins are critical in the surgical treatment of gallbladder cancer.

    Answer: C

    Explanation: Radical surgery is not beneficial for patients with T2 gallbladder cancer lesions. This statement is incorrect as patients with T2 cancer can have significantly improved 5-year survival rates with radical surgery.

46. A 60-year-old patient undergoes a laparoscopic cholecystectomy. Post-operative pathology confirms gallbladder cancer: Which of the following statements regarding laparoscopic cholecystectomy in gallbladder cancer is incorrect?

    A. Laparoscopic cholecystectomy is contraindicated if gallbladder cancer is suspected preoperatively.
    B. Patients inadvertently undergoing laparoscopic cholecystectomy for gallbladder cancer require port site resection.
    C. Laparoscopic cholecystectomy is the preferred method for all stages of gallbladder cancer.
    D. Tis and T1a gallbladder cancer can be cured with simple cholecystectomy.
    E. Radical cholecystectomy is recommended for cancers beyond T1a stage.

    Answer: C

    Explanation: Laparoscopic cholecystectomy is the preferred method for all stages of gallbladder cancer. This statement is incorrect as laparoscopic cholecystectomy should not be performed if gallbladder cancer is suspected preoperatively. It is contraindicated due to the risk of cancer spread.

47. Discussing the treatment options for a patient with stage IV gallbladder cancer, the surgical team considers aggressive surgery. Which of the following statements regarding the role of aggressive surgery in stage IV gallbladder cancer is incorrect?

    A. Aggressive surgery in stage IV gallbladder cancer has proven to be performed with safety.
    B. Hepatopancreatoduodenectomy has been investigated in clinical trials for its efficacy.
    C. Aggressive surgery is universally recommended for all patients with stage IV gallbladder cancer.

D. Attention must be paid to the high incidence of operative mortality in aggressive surgeries.
E. Extended lymph node dissection is part of the discussion in aggressive surgical approaches.

Answer: C

Explanation: Aggressive surgery is universally recommended for all patients with stage IV gallbladder cancer. This statement is incorrect because aggressive surgery for stage IV gallbladder cancer needs to be considered carefully due to high operative mortality rates, and it is not recommended for all patients.

48. A multidisciplinary team evaluates the appropriateness of laparoscopic surgery for a patient with overt gallbladder cancer. Which of the following statements about the indications for laparoscopic surgery in gallbladder cancer is incorrect?

A. Laparoscopic surgery is considered for highly selected cases of gallbladder cancer.
B. Selection criteria for laparoscopic surgery in gallbladder cancer vary among surgeons.
C. Laparoscopic surgery is indicated for patients with late-stage gallbladder cancer.
D. Favorable outcomes have been reported in selected patients undergoing laparoscopic surgery.
E. Experienced surgeons hold a positive view of laparoscopic surgery for gallbladder cancer.

Answer: C

Explanation: Laparoscopic surgery is indicated for patients with late-stage gallbladder cancer. This statement is incorrect as laparoscopic surgery for gallbladder cancer is typically performed in highly selected cases, often in early stages, and the selection criteria do not universally include late-stage cancer.

49. A 75-year-old male undergoes surgical intervention for GBC. Regarding the contents of Calot's triangle, the incorrect statement is:

A. The right hepatic artery is within Calot's triangle.
B. The cystic artery is within Calot's triangle.
C. Lymph nodes of Lund are within Calot's triangle.
D. The common bile duct is within Calot's triangle.
E. The cystic duct is within Calot's triangle.

Answer: D

Explanation: The common bile duct is not a content of Calot's triangle. The triangle typically contains the cystic artery, cystic duct, and lymph nodes of Lund.

Bibliography

1. Yu MH, Kim YJ, Park HS, Jung SI. Benign gallbladder diseases: imaging techniques and tips for differentiating with malignant gallbladder diseases. World J Gastroenterol. 2020;26(22):2967.
2. Sharma A, Sharma KL, Gupta A, Yadav A, Kumar A. Gallbladder cancer epidemiology, pathogenesis and molecular genetics: recent update. World J Gastroenterol. 2017;23(22):3978–98.
3. Hsing AW, Gao YT, Han TQ, Rashid A, Sakoda LC, Wang BS, et al. Gallstones and the risk of biliary tract cancer: a population-based study in China. Br J Cancer. 2007;97(11):1577–82.
4. Morimoto M, Matsuo T, Mori N. Management of Porcelain Gallbladder, its risk factors, and complications: a review. Diagnostics (Basel). 2021;11(6):1073.
5. Wiles R, Varadpande M, Muly S, Webb J. Growth rate and malignant potential of small gallbladder polyps—systematic review of evidence. Surgeon. 2014;12(4):221–6.
6. Wiles R, Thoeni RF, Barbu ST, Vashist YK, Rafaelsen SR, Dewhurst C, et al. Management and follow-up of gallbladder polyps. Eur Radiol. 2017;27(9):3856–66.
7. Andrén-Sandberg A. Diagnosis and management of gallbladder polyps. N Am J Med Sci. 2012;4(5):203–11.
8. Schmidt MA, Marcano-Bonilla L, Roberts LR. Gallbladder cancer: epidemiology and genetic risk associations. Chin Clin Oncol. 2019;8(4):31.
9. Rakić M, Patrlj L, Kopljar M, Kliček R, Kolovrat M, Loncar B, et al. Gallbladder cancer. Hepatobiliary Surg Nutr. 2014;3(5):221–6.
10. Valle JW, Borbath I, Khan SA, Huguet F, Gruenberger T, Arnold D. Biliary cancer: ESMO clinical practice guidelines for diagnosis, treatment and follow-up. Ann Oncol. 2016;27:v28–37.
11. Sons HU, Borchard F, Joel BS. Carcinoma of the gallbladder: autopsy findings in 287 cases and review of the literature. J Surg Oncol. 1985;28(3):199–206.
12. Goere D, Wagholikar GD, Pessaux P, Carrère N, Sibert A, Vilgrain V, et al. Utility of staging laparoscopy in subsets of biliary cancers : laparoscopy is a powerful diagnostic tool in patients with intrahepatic and gallbladder carcinoma. Surg Endosc. 2006;20(5):721–5.
13. Kanthan R, Senger JL, Ahmed S, Kanthan SC. Gallbladder cancer in the 21st century. J Oncol. 2015;2015:967472.
14. Amin MB, Greene FL, Edge SB, Compton CC, Gershenwald JE, Brookland RK, et al. The eighth edition AJCC cancer staging manual: continuing to build a bridge from a population-based to a more "personalized" approach to cancer staging. CA Cancer J Clin. 2017;67(2):93–9.
15. Pilgrim C, Usatoff V, Evans PM. A review of the surgical strategies for the management of gallbladder carcinoma based on T stage and growth type of the tumour. Eur J Surg Oncol. 2009;35(9):903–7.
16. Hickman L, Contreras C. Gallbladder cancer: diagnosis, surgical management, and adjuvant therapies. Surg Clin North Am. 2019;99(2):337–55.
17. Maker AV, Butte JM, Oxenberg J, Kuk D, Gonen M, Fong Y, et al. Is port site resection necessary in the surgical management of gallbladder cancer? Ann Surg Oncol. 2012;19(2):409–17.
18. Misra S, Chaturvedi A, Misra NC. Gallbladder cancer. Curr Treat Options Gastroenterol. 2006;9:95–106.
19. Kiran RP, Pokala N, Dudrick SJ. Incidence pattern and survival for gallbladder cancer over three decades—an analysis of 10301 patients. Ann Surg Oncol. 2007;14(2):827–32.
20. Cubertafond P, Mathonnet M, Gainant A, Launois B. Radical surgery for gallbladder cancer. Results of the French surgical association survey. Hepatogastroenterology. 1999;46(27):1567–71.
21. Pawlik TM, Gleisner AL, Vigano L, Kooby DA, Bauer TW, Frilling A, et al. Incidence of finding residual disease for incidental gallbladder carcinoma: implications for re-resection. J Gastrointest Surg. 2007;11(11):1478–86; discussion 86-7.
22. Qadan M, Kingham TP. Technical aspects of gallbladder cancer surgery. Surg Clin North Am. 2016;96(2):229–45.
23. Zaidi MY, Maithel SK. Updates on gallbladder cancer management. Curr Oncol Rep. 2018;20(2):21.
24. Agarwal AK, Kalayarasan R, Javed A, Gupta N, Nag HH. The role of staging laparoscopy in primary gall bladder cancer—an analysis of 409 patients: a prospective study to evalu-

ate the role of staging laparoscopy in the management of gallbladder cancer. Ann Surg. 2013;258(2):318–23.
25. Li Y, Song Y, Zhang Y, Liu S. Progress in gallbladder cancer with lymph node metastasis. Front Oncol. 2022;12:966835.
26. Chijiiwa K, Noshiro H, Nakano K, Okido M, Sugitani A, Yamaguchi K, et al. Role of surgery for gallbladder carcinoma with special reference to lymph node metastasis and stage using Western and Japanese classification systems. World J Surg. 2000;24(10):1271–7.
27. Mekeel KL, Hemming AW. Surgical management of gallbladder carcinoma: a review. J Gastrointest Surg. 2007;11(9):1188–93.
28. Feo CF, Ginesu GC, Fancellu A, Perra T, Ninniri C, Deiana G, et al. Current management of incidental gallbladder cancer: a review. Int J Surg. 2022;98:106234.
29. Aloia TA, Járufe N, Javle M, Maithel SK, Roa JC, Adsay V, et al. Gallbladder cancer: expert consensus statement. HPB (Oxford). 2015;17(8):681–90.
30. Jarnagin WR, Ruo L, Little SA, Klimstra D, D'Angelica M, DeMatteo RP, et al. Patterns of initial disease recurrence after resection of gallbladder carcinoma and hilar cholangiocarcinoma: implications for adjuvant therapeutic strategies. Cancer. 2003;98(8):1689–700.
31. Primrose JN, Fox RP, Palmer DH, Malik HZ, Prasad R, Mirza D, et al. Capecitabine compared with observation in resected biliary tract cancer (BILCAP): a randomised, controlled, multicentre, phase 3 study. Lancet Oncol. 2019;20(5):663–73.
32. Horgan AM, Amir E, Walter T, Knox JJ. Adjuvant therapy in the treatment of biliary tract cancer: a systematic review and meta-analysis. J Clin Oncol. 2012;30(16):1934–40.
33. Macdonald OK, Crane CH. Palliative and postoperative radiotherapy in biliary tract cancer. Surg Oncol Clin N Am. 2002;11(4):941–54.
34. Tran TB, Norton JA, Ethun CG, Pawlik TM, Buettner S, Schmidt C, et al. Gallbladder cancer presenting with jaundice: uniformly fatal or still potentially curable? J Gastrointest Surg. 2017;21(8):1245–53.
35. Hakeem AR, Papoulas M, Menon KV. The role of neoadjuvant chemotherapy or chemoradiotherapy for advanced gallbladder cancer—a systematic review. Eur J Surg Oncol. 2019;45(2):83–91.
36. Sharma A, Dwary AD, Mohanti BK, Deo SV, Pal S, Sreenivas V, et al. Best supportive care compared with chemotherapy for unresectable gall bladder cancer: a randomized controlled study. J Clin Oncol. 2010;28(30):4581–6.
37. Xiang JX, Zhang XF, Weber SM, Poultsides G, Fields RC, Hatzaras I, et al. Identification of patients who may benefit the most from adjuvant chemotherapy following resection of incidental gallbladder carcinoma. J Surg Oncol. 2021;123(4):978–85.
38. Wen Z, Si A, Yang J, Yang P, Yang X, Liu H, et al. Elevation of CA19-9 and CEA is associated with a poor prognosis in patients with resectable gallbladder carcinoma. HPB (Oxford). 2017;19(11):951–6.
39. Isambert M, Leux C, Métairie S, Paineau J. Incidentally-discovered gallbladder cancer: when, why and which reoperation? J Visc Surg. 2011;148(2):e77–84.
40. Randi G, Franceschi S, La Vecchia C. Gallbladder cancer worldwide: geographical distribution and risk factors. Int J Cancer. 2006;118(7):1591–602.
41. Aloia TA, Járufe N, Javle M, Maithel SK, Roa JC, Adsay V, Coimbra FJ, Jarnagin WR. Gallbladder cancer: expert consensus statement. HPB. 2015;17(8):681–90.
42. Lee J-S, Han H-S, Yoon Y-S, Cho J, Lee H, Lee B, Kim M, Jo Y-S. Minimally invasive surgery for gallbladder cancer at an expert center. Mini-invasive Surg. 2021;5:57.
43. Andrén-Sandberg A, Deng Y. Aspects on gallbladder cancer in 2014. Curr Opin Gastroenterol. 2014;30(3):326–31.
44. Misra S, Chaturvedi A, Misra NC. Gall bladder cancer: surgical management. Indian J Med Paediatr Oncol. 2005;26:46.
45. Lendoire J, Gil L. Controversies and future directions in the management of gallbladder cancer. Oncol Transl Med. 2023;9:163–7.
46. Yoon Y-S, Han H-S, Agarwal A, Belli G, Itano O, Gumbs A, Yoon D, Kang C, Lee SE, Wakai T, Troisi R. Survey results of the expert meeting on laparoscopic surgery for gallbladder cancer and a review of relevant literature. Dig Surg. 2018;36(1):7–12.

Chapter 10
Cholangiocarcinoma

Aqeel Shakir Mahmood, Noufel sh. Alshadood, Munthir A. Alobaidi, Saleh Abdulkareem Saleh, and Mustafa Ismail

1. A 55-year-old male with a history of ulcerative colitis presents with jaundice. Imaging reveals a mass in the biliary tract. Biopsy confirms cholangiocarcinoma. Regarding cholangiocarcinoma, identify the incorrect statement:

   A. Represents approximately 30% of all gastrointestinal cancers, with a rising incidence in recent years.
   B. Classifiable into intrahepatic (ICC) and extrahepatic cholangiocarcinoma (ECC) based on location.
   C. Perihilar cholangiocarcinoma (PCC) typically involves the hepatic duct bifurcation, situated proximal to the cystic duct insertion.
   D. PCC tumors account for about 50% of all cholangiocarcinomas.
   E. Distal cholangiocarcinomas are extrahepatic tumors located in the peripancreatic region, distal to the cystic duct insertion.

   Answer: A

   Explanation: It's a relatively rare tumor, constituting about 3% of all gastrointestinal cancers.

2. A 60-year-old female with a history of hepatitis C and liver cirrhosis presents with upper abdominal pain. Imaging suggests a liver mass, raising concerns for ICC. Which of the following is incorrect risk factor for ICC?

A. S. Mahmood
Department of General Surgery, University of Baghdad, Baghdad, Iraq

N. s. Alshadood
Baghdad Teaching Hospital, Baghdad, Iraq

M. A. Alobaidi · M. Ismail (✉)
Department of Surgery, College of Medicine, University of Baghdad, Baghdad, Iraq

S. A. Saleh
College of Medicine University of Baghdad, Baghdad, Iraq

A. S. Mahmood, A. Koulouris (eds.), *MCQs in General Surgical Oncology*, https://doi.org/10.1007/978-3-031-65738-2_10

A. Cirrhosis.
B. Chronic hepatitis C infection.
C. Liver fluke infestation.
D. Caroli disease, characterized by nonobstructive saccular or fusiform dilatation of intrahepatic bile ducts.
E. Primary biliary cirrhosis.

Answer: E

Explanation: Primary biliary cirrhosis is not well-established as a risk factor for ICC.

3. A 50-year-old patient presents with jaundice, pruritus, and weight loss. Cholangiography suggests a tumor at the hepatic duct bifurcation. In the context of the Bismuth-Corlette classification for PCC, which statement is incorrect?

A. Type 1 tumors are located below the confluence of the left and right hepatic ducts.
B. Common hepatic duct bifurcation tumors, regardless of their intrahepatic or extrahepatic origin, are referred to as Klatskin tumors or hilar cholangiocarcinoma.
C. Type 2 tumors extend up to but not beyond the confluence of the hepatic ducts.
D. Perihilar tumors, typically extrahepatic, extend from the hepatic duct bifurcation to the cystic duct insertion.
E. Type 3 tumors involve the common hepatic duct and either the right or left hepatic duct.

Answer: D

Explanation: Perihilar tumors are usually extrahepatic, located in the region extending from the hepatic duct bifurcation to near the cystic duct insertion.

4. A 55-year-old male with a history of PSC is being evaluated for cholangiocarcinoma. Which of the following is incorrectly listed as a risk factor for cholangiocarcinoma?

A. Female gender.
B. Hepatolithiasis.
C. PSC.
D. Bile duct cysts.
E. Exposure to thorotrast, a previously used radiographic contrast agent.

Answer: A

Explanation: CC has a male predominance.

5. A 45-year-old male with a long-standing history of ulcerative colitis and PSC is being evaluated for cholangiocarcinoma. Which of the following statements about the relationship between PSC and CC is incorrect?

A. The risk of developing cancer is related to the duration of PSC.
B. PSC is strongly associated with ulcerative colitis.

C. There is a strong association between PSC and cholangiocarcinoma, particularly the perihilar type.
D. The mean age of CC diagnosis in PSC patients is around 40 years.
E. Males are more susceptible to both PSC and cholangiocarcinoma.

Answer: A

Explanation: The risk of cancer in PSC patients does not correlate with the duration of the disease; cancer can occur at any time.

6. A patient diagnosed with intrahepatic cholangiocarcinoma (ICC) presents with abdominal pain and weight loss. Imaging reveals a large liver mass with regional LN involvement and evidence of distant metastasis. Identify the incorrect statement for a T3N1M1 ICC staging:

A. The tumor invades the visceral peritoneum.
B. There is evidence of regional LN metastasis.
C. The tumor exhibits vascular invasion.
D. The tumor is a solitary lesion ≤5 cm without vascular invasion.
E. There are distant metastases.

Answer: D

Explanation: A solitary tumor ≤5 cm without vascular invasion is classified as T1a, not T3N1M1.

7. During a tumor board discussion, a patient's liver tumor biopsy reveals features of both HCC and cholangiocarcinoma. Regarding combined hepatocellular cholangiocarcinoma, identify the incorrect statement:

A. It is a subtype of cholangiocarcinoma.
B. This mixed tumor contains both HCC cells and CC cells.
C. It is staged as HCC and not as ICC.
D. These tumors originate from common hepatic stem cells.
E. In advanced disease, treatment principles established for advanced CC should be applied.

Answer: C

Explanation: Such tumors would be termed as ICCs and not HCCs, since it is quite distinct from the cells from which the cancer originated. The adult hepatic stem cells, from which arise such kinds of tumors, are capable of regenerating. For ICCs, the origin of cancerous cells is from the biliary epithelial cells, while for HCCs, the origin is from the hepatocytes.

8. A patient with suspected PCC is undergoing imaging assessments. Which statement about the role of imaging in PCC is incorrect?

A. Imaging plays a significant role in tumor staging and assessing the potential for complete curative resection.
B. Ultrasound commonly shows intrahepatic bile duct dilation, with lesion detection sensitivity around 82%.
C. CT scan offers superior soft tissue contrast compared to MRI, aiding in better visualization of the tumor and biliary tree.

D. Endoscopic ultrasonography is used for fine needle aspiration (FNA) or biopsy of the tumor and lymph nodes.
E. Multidetector CT is essential for estimating the volume of the future liver remnant before surgery.

Answer: C

Explanation: MRI, not CT scan, offers superior soft tissue contrast and better visualization of CC location and biliary tree anatomy.

9. During a follow-up appointment for a patient with treated cholangiocarcinoma, the risk of recurrence is discussed. Identify the incorrect statement regarding the recurrence of cholangiocarcinoma:

A. PET has no significant role in assessing disease recurrence and prognosis.
B. The recurrence rate is 60–80% within the next 5 years.
C. Tumor recurrence typically occurs near the excision region, the hilum, and locoregional lymph nodes.
D. Follow-up imaging typically involves CT or MRI scans.
E. FDG-PET is useful for detecting recurrence, with a sensitivity of 89% and specificity of 100% when tumor markers are high despite negative imaging.
F. PET/CT plays a significant role in predicting tumor recurrence.

Answer: A

Explanation: PET/CT provides prognostic benefits for recurrence prediction and prognosis and can distinguish between post-therapy changes and recurrence.

10. A 56-year-old patient with CC is undergoing evaluation. The oncologist reviews tumor markers to monitor disease progression. Which of the following tumor markers is incorrect for the follow-up of cholangiocarcinoma?

A. NMP22.
B. CA 19-9.
C. CEA.
D. CA 125.
E. Mucins.

Answer: A

Explanation: NMP22 is primarily used for detecting transitional cell carcinoma of the bladder, not for cholangiocarcinoma.

11. During a differential diagnosis discussion for a patient with biliary strictures and obstructive jaundice, the team considers the role of serum IgG4 levels. Which statement about the relationship between serum IgG4 and CC is incorrect?

A. Elevated serum IgG4 is a characteristic feature of autoimmune pancreatitis (AIP).
B. Serum IgG4 levels are elevated in CC and used as a tumor marker.
C. IgG4-associated cholangitis (IAC) often presents with elevated serum IgG4 levels.

D. A more than twofold increase in serum IgG4 is highly specific for IgG4-related diseases.
E. Serum IgG4 is ordered to help differentiate cholangitis from cholangiocarcinoma.

Answer: B

Explanation: Elevated serum IgG4 levels are indicative of AIP and IAC but are not used as a tumor marker for cholangiocarcinoma.

12. During a review of a patient with cholangiocarcinoma, the oncology team discusses the patterns of metastasis. Which statement about metastasis in CC is incorrect?

A. The metastasis rate of ICC with T1 tumor stage is higher than that for ECC.
B. Only about one-third of patients are eligible for tumor resection due to advanced presentation.
C. The rate of LN involvement in ICC is lower than that in ECC.
D. The rate of metastasis in ICC is higher than in ECC.
E. The rate of metastasis decreases with increasing age.

Answer: A

Explanation: The metastasis rate of ICC with T1 tumor stage is lower, not higher, than that for ECC.

13. A patient with a newly diagnosed liver lesion undergoes evaluation. Imaging and biopsy confirm a diagnosis of ICC. Regarding T1 ICC staging, which of the following statements is incorrect?

A. The tumor is multiple in nature.
B. There is no vascular invasion.
C. T1a classification includes tumors that are ≤5 cm in size.
D. T1b classification is for tumors that are >5 cm in size.
E. The tumor does not invade the visceral peritoneum.

Answer: A

Explanation: T1 ICC is characterized as a solitary mass without vessel invasion.

14. In discussing the prognosis of a patient with newly diagnosed ICC, the oncology team reviews various clinical and genetic factors. Which of the following is not an independent prognostic factor for worse overall survival in ICC?

A. Multifocal liver disease.
B. Mutation in the tumor protein P53.
C. Cyclin-dependent kinase inhibitor 2A (CDKN2A) mutation.
D. Having a T2 stage ICC.
E. KRAS mutation.

Answer: D

Explanation: T2 stage ICC is not independently associated with worse overall survival compared to TP53, KRAS, CDKN2A mutations, and multifocal liver disease.

15. A patient with CC undergoes a PET/CT scan to evaluate the extent of the disease. Regarding the role of PET/CT in cholangiocarcinoma, which statement is incorrect?

    A. The scan uses fluoro-2-deoxy-D-glucose (FDG) as a tracer.
    B. PET/CT plays a role in the staging of primary cholangiocarcinoma.
    C. It helps in detecting tumor recurrence.
    D. PET/CT can differentiate between post-therapy changes (including fibrosis due to RT) and tumor recurrence.
    E. PET/CT has no role in monitoring treatment response.

Answer: E

Explanation: PET/CT can be useful for monitoring treatment response, as metabolic changes may precede anatomical changes.

16. During a case review, a patient with distal CC is discussed. Which statement about T2N1 staging for distal CC is incorrect?

    A. The tumor invades the bile duct wall distal to the cystic duct insertion.
    B. The tumor has a depth of invasion between 5 and 12 mm.
    C. There is metastasis in one to three regional lymph nodes.
    D. The tumor involves the celiac axis.
    E. There is no evidence of vascular invasion.

Answer: D

Explanation: Involvement of the celiac axis is characteristic of T4, not T2N1, distal cholangiocarcinoma.

17. A patient with suspected CC is considered for staging laparoscopy. The surgical team evaluates its effectiveness. Which of the following statements about staging laparoscopy in CC is incorrect?

    A. Staging laparoscopy has good sensitivity for detecting peritoneal metastases.
    B. Finding locally advanced disease by laparoscopy may preclude resectability by laparotomy.
    C. The sensitivity of laparoscopy for detecting ICC is approximately 85%.
    D. The sensitivity of laparoscopy for detecting hilar CC is about 25%.
    E. Staging laparoscopy can result in an infected infraumbilical port site, a Clavien-Dindo grade II postoperative complication.

Answer: D

Explanation: The sensitivity of laparoscopy for detecting hilar CC is much higher, around 95%.

18. During a multidisciplinary meeting, a patient with a suspicious biliary stricture is being discussed. Which statement about tissue diagnosis in CC is incorrect?

    A. Biopsy techniques include brush cytology and FNA.

B. CT/MRI-guided biopsy can be used for diagnosis.
C. Used in cases of strictures with clinically undefined origin.
D. Tissue diagnosis must be obtained preoperatively in every case.
E. Essential to establish a diagnosis for patients opting for nonoperative treatment.

Answer: D

Explanation: Tissue sampling before surgery is not always necessary, especially if the tumor is potentially operable and presents with findings suggestive of malignant biliary obstruction.

19. A patient with distal CC is being staged to determine the extent of disease. Which statement about the TNM staging for distal CC is incorrect?

A. N2 involves four or more regional lymph nodes.
B. T1 tumors invade the bile duct wall with a depth of 5 to 12 mm.
C. T3 tumors invade the bile duct wall with a depth greater than 12 mm.
D. T4 tumors involve the celiac axis, SMA, and common hepatic artery.
E. T2 tumors invade the bile duct wall with a depth of 5–12 mm.

Answer: B

Explanation: T1 tumors invade the bile duct wall with a depth of less than 5 mm.

20. In reviewing the case of a patient with ICC, the oncology team discusses TNM staging. Which statement about ICC TNM staging is incorrect?

A. Tis: Intraductal tumor.
B. T1: Single tumor without vascular invasion, can be ≤5 cm or >5 cm.
C. T2: Single tumor with intrahepatic vascular invasion or multiple tumors, with or without vascular invasion.
D. T3: Tumor invades one side of the branches of the portal vein or hepatic artery.
E. T4: Tumor invading local extrahepatic structures by direct involvement.

Answer: D

Explanation: Tumor invasion of unilateral branches of the portal vein or hepatic artery describes T3 staging in PCC, not ICC.

21. In a case review of a patient with ICC, the oncology team discusses the TNM staging. Which statement about T4N1M0 ICC is incorrect?

A. Regional LN involvement is present.
B. There is no evidence of distant metastasis.
C. The tumor involves direct invasion of local extrahepatic tissue.
D. The presentation includes multiple tumors, with vascular invasion.
E. The tumors invade the celiac axis, SMA, and common hepatic artery.

Answer: E

Explanation: Invasion of the celiac axis, SMA, and common hepatic artery describes T4 staging in distal cholangiocarcinoma, not ICC.

22. A 48-year-old patient presents with a recent diagnosis of PCC. Imaging suggests a localized tumor without LN involvement. Which of the following statements about T1 N0 PCC is incorrect?

    A. The tumor shows no regional LN involvement.
    B. The tumor is confined within the bile duct.
    C. The tumor may extend to the muscle layer or fibrous tissue of the biliary ducts.
    D. There is no evidence of invasion into the adjacent liver tissue.
    E. The tumor extends beyond the wall of the bile duct.

    Answer: E

    Explanation: T1 tumors are confined to the bile duct, including up to the muscle layer or fibrous tissue, but not beyond.

23. In reviewing the treatment options for a patient with newly diagnosed PCC, which of the following statements about PCC is incorrect?

    A. PCC is also known as a Klatskin tumor.
    B. It is the most commonly encountered subtype of cholangiocarcinoma.
    C. First-line chemotherapy typically involves a combination of gemcitabine and cisplatin.
    D. For localized, node-negative PCC, liver transplantation plus neoadjuvant therapy has shown superiority over resection.
    E. Gemcitabine monotherapy is the standard treatment of choice.

    Answer: E

    Explanation: The standard first-line therapy is a combination of gemcitabine and cisplatin, not gemcitabine monotherapy.

24. A patient with PCC is being considered for surgical management. In evaluating the treatment options, which of the following statements about perihilar tumor resection is incorrect?

    A. Liver transplantation plus neoadjuvant therapy is often a better alternative to resection for PCC patients.
    B. Liver transplantation with neoadjuvant therapy is particularly advantageous in localized, node-negative cases.
    C. Liver transplantation eliminates the need to preserve vascular inflow to the remaining liver.
    D. Broader resection margins are achievable with liver transplantation compared to standard resection.
    E. Liver transplantation offers an R0 resection but is associated with lower long-term survival than resection.

    Answer: E

    Explanation: Liver transplantation with neoadjuvant therapy can be a better alternative to resection, often providing improved long-term survival.

25. A 62-year-old patient is diagnosed with Bismuth type III cholangiocarcinoma. The surgical team is considering the approach for resection. Which of the following statements regarding Bismuth type III and IV CC is incorrect?

    A. IIIa: The tumor involves the confluence and extends into the right hepatic duct.
    B. IIIb: The tumor involves the confluence and extends into the left hepatic duct.
    C. IV: There is tumor involvement of bilateral intrahepatic secondary bile ducts.
    D. There is no difference in survival between patients undergoing total caudate lobectomy (TCL) and those who do not.
    E. TCL has an acceptable safety profile and high rates of curative resectability.

    Answer: D

    Explanation: TCL provides higher survival rates for Bismuth type III and IV cholangiocarcinoma, with significant curative resection potential and safety profile.

26. During a multidisciplinary team meeting, the resectability of a patient with PCC is being discussed. Which of the following is incorrect regarding factors that render CC unresectable?

    A. Distant LN metastases.
    B. T2b perihilar tumor.
    C. Peritoneal metastases.
    D. Intrahepatic metastases.
    E. Vascular encasement.

    Answer: B

    Explanation: A T2b perihilar tumor does not necessarily preclude resectability.

27. A patient with inoperable ICC is being evaluated for palliative treatment options. Which of the following is not a liver-directed therapy for inoperable cholangiocarcinoma?

    A. TACE.
    B. Hepatic arterial infusion.
    C. ERCP.
    D. Percutaneous ablation.
    E. Radioembolization.

    Answer: C

    Explanation: ERCP is not a liver-directed therapy for ICC.

28. A patient with cholangiocarcinoma, post-surgical resection with positive lymph nodes, is being considered for adjuvant therapy. Which of the following statements about adjuvant therapy in CC is incorrect?

    A. Patients receiving chemotherapy or CRT show greater benefit than those receiving radiation therapy alone.

B. The most significant benefit of adjuvant therapy is seen in patients with positive LN disease.
C. Patients with R1 resection status derive the greatest benefit from adjuvant therapies.
D. Unselected patients, regardless of node and margin status, show no significant benefit from adjuvant therapy.
E. Radiation therapy has no role in the management of patients with R1 resections.

Answer: E

Explanation: Radiation therapy can be beneficial for patients with R1 resections, with potential harm in R0 resection patients.

29. In discussing the case of a patient with perihilar bile duct cancer, the team is reviewing the TNM staging. Which statement about T3N1 staging for perihilar bile duct cancer is incorrect?

A. Involvement of one to three positive lymph nodes.
B. Lymph nodes involved may include hilar, posterior pancreaticoduodenal, common bile duct, hepatic artery, cystic duct, and portal vein lymph nodes.
C. The tumor invades the main portal vein or its branches bilaterally.
D. The tumor invades unilateral branches of the portal vein.
E. The tumor invades unilateral branches of the hepatic artery.

Answer: C

Explanation: T4, not T3N1, is characterized by invasion of the main portal vein or its branches bilaterally.

30. A patient with advanced CC is being evaluated for chemotherapy options. Which of the following is incorrect chemotherapy regimen for cholangiocarcinoma?

A. Combination of gemcitabine with S-1.
B. Mitomycin-C and 5-fluorouracil.
C. Cytarabine.
D. Gemcitabine alone.
E. Gemcitabine combined with oxaliplatin.

Answer: C

Explanation: Cytarabine is not commonly used in the chemotherapy regimen for cholangiocarcinoma.

31. In a case conference, a patient with unresectable ECC is discussed for palliative treatment options. Which statement about the treatment of unresectable ECC is incorrect?

A. Biliary drainage is achieved through stent placement.
B. PDT and RFA can prolong survival.
C. One-month mortality with PDT is significantly higher than with RFA and stent placement alone.

D. Survival is longer in patients using photothermal therapy (PTU) compared to RFA and stent placement.
E. Stent patency duration is longer in patients using PTU compared to RFA and stent placement.

Answer: C

Explanation: One-month mortality with PDT is actually lower than with RFA and stent placement alone.

32. In a tumor board meeting, the team discusses the risk factors for recurrence in a patient with recently resected ICC. Which of the following is incorrect predictor for ICC recurrence?

A. Tumor size ≥5 cm.
B. Presence of perineural invasion.
C. Evidence of vascular invasion.
D. The tumor is solitary.
E. Nodal status.

Answer: D

Explanation: The presence of multiple tumors, not a solitary tumor, is a predictor for earlier recurrence of ICC.

33. In discussing the risks of PTCp for a patient with suspected biliary obstruction, which statement about PTCp complications is incorrect?

A. Bile leakage is a potential complication.
B. Severe blood loss requiring transfusion may occur.
C. Hemobilia can be a complication of the procedure.
D. Formation of a biloma is a possible complication.
E. Pneumoperitoneum is a recognized complication.

Answer: B

Explanation: Severe blood loss requiring transfusion is not a typical complication of PTCp; hemobilia is usually temporary and does not generally require emergency intervention or blood transfusion.

34. A patient with hilar CC is being evaluated for diagnostic and palliative options. Which statement about the roles of PTCp and ERCP is incorrect?

A. PTCp is more frequently used as it better outlines tumor involvement in the proximal biliary tree than ERCP.
B. Both ERCP and PTCp are often needed to assess the feasibility of major liver resection.
C. PTCp can be used to decompress bile ducts before surgical excision as a palliative approach for jaundice.
D. ERCP can be used for stent placement as palliative therapy in unresectable hilar cholangiocarcinoma.
E. PTCp is the preferred test in the majority of cases and offers a greater overall survival benefit compared to ERCP.

Answer: E

Explanation: The choice between PTCp and ERCP depends on expertise availability and tumor anatomy, not on one providing a greater overall survival benefit.

35. During a multidisciplinary discussion about a patient with unresectable ECC, RFA is considered. Which of the following statements about RFA is incorrect?

    A. Overall survival is significantly longer in patients treated with RFA and stenting compared to stenting alone.
    B. Stent patency period is longer in patients treated with RFA and stenting than in stent-only patients.
    C. There is a significant difference in the incidence of postoperative adverse events between the RFA and stent-only groups.
    D. RFA is a safe and effective palliative treatment option for these patients.
    E. RFA can be applied either endoscopically or percutaneously.

Answer: C

Explanation: There is no significant difference in the incidence of postoperative adverse events between the RFA and stent-only groups.

36. The team evaluates a patient with unresectable CC for brachytherapy in conjunction with stenting. Which statement about this combined treatment approach is incorrect?

    A. Brachytherapy increases the duration of stent patency compared with stenting alone.
    B. Brachytherapy offers an average survival of 10 months, compared to 4–6 months without it.
    C. Brachytherapy improves localized control, enhancing complete and partial response rates, with or without external beam radiation.
    D. Overall survival is better with brachytherapy.
    E. There are no significant side effects when comparing brachytherapy with stenting alone.

Answer: E

Explanation: Radiation-associated complications, such as duodenal ulcers and later duodenal stenosis, can occur with brachytherapy.

37. A patient with unresectable hilar CC is being evaluated for biliary drainage. Which statement about the drainage of this type of cancer is incorrect?

    A. Effective drainage is often achieved when more than 50% of the liver volume, especially in Bismuth 3 strictures, is drained.
    B. Unilateral stent placement is usually sufficient.
    C. Pre-ERCP assessment of hepatic volume distribution on CT imaging can optimize endoscopic procedures.
    D. Intubation of an atrophic liver segment (30%) is not useful and may increase cholangitis cases.
    E. Drainage of 50% of liver volume is associated with longer survival.

Answer: B

Explanation: Bilateral stent placement is often needed to drain more than 50% of the liver volume in these cases.

38. The oncology team is considering chemotherapy options for a patient with advanced, unresectable cholangiocarcinoma. Which statement about chemotherapy in this setting is incorrect?

  A. Gemcitabine plus cisplatin has been proven effective.
  B. Gemcitabine plus cisplatin is superior to gemcitabine alone in patients with advanced disease.
  C. Patients receiving combined therapy may experience a significant increase in lethargy.
  D. Chemotherapy does not play a role in prolonging survival in advanced unresectable tumors.
  E. Combining S-1 with gemcitabine is a treatment option.

Answer: D

Explanation: Chemotherapy, including regimens like gemcitabine plus cisplatin, plays a role in prolonging survival in advanced unresectable cholangiocarcinoma.

39. A patient with unresectable stage IVa/IVb ICC is being evaluated for treatment options. Which statement about the management of this condition is incorrect?

  A. Capecitabine plus cisplatin (XP) chemotherapy with external radiotherapy (XP-CCRT) is well-tolerated.
  B. XP-CCRT patients have a longer overall survival than those receiving XP chemotherapy alone.
  C. Neutropenia as a side effect is more common in XP-CCRT than in the XP group alone.
  D. Neoadjuvant concurrent CRT offers more advantages than locoregional RT alone for patients with advanced and unresectable ICC, including those with distant metastases.
  E. Chemotherapy alone is the standard treatment of choice for most patients with advanced unresectable ICC.

Answer: E

Explanation: Better overall survival has been noted in XP-CCRT patients compared to XP chemotherapy alone.

40. In a multidisciplinary team meeting, the treatment plan for a patient with locally advanced, unresectable ICC is discussed. Which of the following statements is incorrect?

  A. Chemotherapy alone is superior to locoregional treatment for these types of tumors.
  B. Locoregional treatment benefits patients with locally advanced, unresectable ICC.
  C. Locoregional treatment is superior to systemic chemotherapy alone.

D. Locoregional therapy reduces the occurrence of death by decreasing liver failure cases.
E. Locoregional therapy maintains control of intrahepatic disease, thereby increasing overall survival.

Answer: A

Explanation: Locoregional treatment, not chemotherapy alone, is superior for these types of tumors.

41. A patient with an incurable biliary tract tumor is being considered for stenting. Which statement about biliary tract stenting is incorrect?

A. Stenting can be used as a palliative procedure in incurable tumors.
B. Preoperative stent placement is advised if serum bilirubin is >10 mg/dL and surgery is deferred until serum bilirubin is <3 mg/dL.
C. Complications include obstruction due to tumor ingrowth or overgrowth and cholangitis.
D. The placement of a stent is best done transcutaneously.
E. Self-expandable metallic stents (SEMS) are more effective than plastic stents for both proximal and distal obstructions.

Answer: D

Explanation: The placement of stents is typically best performed using ERCP, not transcutaneously.

42. In evaluating a patient with risk factors for gallbladder malignancy, the surgical team discusses the associated risks. Which statement about risk factors for gallbladder malignancy is incorrect?

A. Stones larger than 3 cm carry a tenfold increased risk of malignancy.
B. Symptomatic stone disease carries a lower risk of developing malignancy than asymptomatic stones.
C. Gallbladder polyps larger than 10 mm have a 25% risk of malignancy.
D. Porcelain gallbladders are malignant in 10% of cases.
E. Prophylactic cholecystectomy is advised when risk factors for gallbladder malignancy are present.

Answer: B

Explanation: Symptomatic gallstones carry a higher risk of developing malignancy compared to asymptomatic gallstones.

Bibliography

1. DeOliveira ML, Cunningham SC, Cameron JL, Kamangar F, Winter JM, Lillemoe KD, et al. Cholangiocarcinoma: thirty-one-year experience with 564 patients at a single institution. Ann Surg. 2007;245(5):755–62.

2. Palmer WC, Patel T. Are common factors involved in the pathogenesis of primary liver cancers? A meta-analysis of risk factors for intrahepatic cholangiocarcinoma. J Hepatol. 2012;57(1):69–76.
3. Bismuth H, Nakache R, Diamond T. Management strategies in resection for hilar cholangiocarcinoma. Ann Surg. 1992;215(1):31–8.
4. Clements O, Eliahoo J, Kim JU, Taylor-Robinson SD, Khan SA. Risk factors for intrahepatic and extrahepatic cholangiocarcinoma: a systematic review and meta-analysis. J Hepatol. 2020;72(1):95–103.
5. Burak K, Angulo P, Pasha TM, Egan K, Petz J, Lindor KD. Incidence and risk factors for cholangiocarcinoma in primary sclerosing cholangitis. Am J Gastroenterol. 2004;99(3):523–6.
6. Burkhart RA, Pawlik TM. Staging and prognostic models for hepatocellular carcinoma and intrahepatic cholangiocarcinoma. Cancer Control. 2017;24(3):1073274817729235.
7. Akiba J, Nakashima O, Hattori S, Tanikawa K, Takenaka M, Nakayama M, et al. Clinicopathologic analysis of combined hepatocellular-cholangiocarcinoma according to the latest WHO classification. Am J Surg Pathol. 2013;37(4):496–505.
8. Madhusudhan KS, Gamanagatti S, Gupta AK. Imaging and interventions in hilar cholangiocarcinoma: a review. World J Radiol. 2015;7(2):28–44.
9. Brandi G, Venturi M, Pantaleo MA, Ercolani G. Cholangiocarcinoma: current opinion on clinical practice diagnostic and therapeutic algorithms: a review of the literature and a long-standing experience of a referral center. Dig Liver Dis. 2016;48(3):231–41.
10. Malaguarnera G, Paladina I, Giordano M, Malaguarnera M, Bertino G, Berretta M. Serum markers of intrahepatic cholangiocarcinoma. Dis Markers. 2013;34(4):219–28.
11. Oseini AM, Chaiteerakij R, Shire AM, Ghazale A, Kaiya J, Moser CD, et al. Utility of serum immunoglobulin G4 in distinguishing immunoglobulin G4-associated cholangitis from cholangiocarcinoma. Hepatology. 2011;54(3):940–8.
12. Liao P, Cao L, Chen H, Pang SZ. Analysis of metastasis and survival between extrahepatic and intrahepatic cholangiocarcinoma: a large population-based study. Medicine (Baltimore). 2021;100(16):e25635.
13. Bagante F, Spolverato G, Weiss M, Alexandrescu S, Marques HP, Aldrighetti L, et al. Assessment of the lymph node status in patients undergoing liver resection for intrahepatic cholangiocarcinoma: the new eighth edition AJCC staging system. J Gastrointest Surg. 2018;22(1):52–9.
14. Boerner T, Drill E, Pak LM, Nguyen B, Sigel CS, Doussot A, et al. Genetic determinants of outcome in intrahepatic cholangiocarcinoma. Hepatology. 2021;74(3):1429–44.
15. Olthof SC, Othman A, Clasen S, Schraml C, Nikolaou K, Bongers M. Imaging of cholangiocarcinoma. Visc Med. 2016;32(6):402–10.
16. You Y, Shin YC, Choi DW, Heo JS, Shin SH, Kim N, et al. Proposed modification of staging for distal cholangiocarcinoma based on the lymph node ratio using Korean multicenter database. Cancers (Basel). 2020;12(3):762.
17. Bird N, Elmasry M, Jones R, Elniel M, Kelly M, Palmer D, et al. Role of staging laparoscopy in the stratification of patients with perihilar cholangiocarcinoma. Br J Surg. 2016;104(4):418–25.
18. Pelsang RE, Johlin FC. A percutaneous biopsy technique for patients with suspected biliary or pancreatic cancer without a radiographic mass. Abdom Imaging. 1997;22(3):307–10.
19. Park JY, Kim SY, Shin DH, Choi KU, Kim JY, Sol MY, et al. Validation of the T category for distal cholangiocarcinoma: measuring the depth of invasion is complex but correlates with survival. Ann Diagn Pathol. 2020;46:151489.
20. Lee AJ, Chun YS. Intrahepatic cholangiocarcinoma: the AJCC/UICC 8th edition updates. Chin Clin Oncol. 2018;7(5):52.
21. Yamamoto Y, Sugiura T, Okamura Y, Ito T, Ashida R, Ohgi K, Nakanuma Y, Uesaka K. The evaluation of the eighth edition of the AJCC/UICC staging system for intrahepatic cholangiocarcinoma: a proposal of a modified new staging system. J Gastrointest Surg. 2020;24(4):786–95.

22. Hau HM, Meyer F, Jahn N, Rademacher S, Sucher R, Seehofer D. Prognostic relevance of the eighth edition of TNM classification for resected perihilar cholangiocarcinoma. J Clin Med. 2020;9(10):3152.
23. Valle J, Wasan H, Palmer DH, Cunningham D, Anthoney A, Maraveyas A, et al. Cisplatin plus gemcitabine versus gemcitabine for biliary tract cancer. N Engl J Med. 2010;362(14):1273–81.
24. Rea DJ, Heimbach JK, Rosen CB, Haddock MG, Alberts SR, Kremers WK, et al. Liver transplantation with neoadjuvant chemoradiation is more effective than resection for hilar cholangiocarcinoma. Ann Surg. 2005;242(3):451–8; discussion 8–61, 461.
25. Cheng QB, Yi B, Wang JH, Jiang XQ, Luo XJ, Liu C, et al. Resection with total caudate lobectomy confers survival benefit in hilar cholangiocarcinoma of Bismuth type III and IV. Eur J Surg Oncol. 2012;38(12):1197–203.
26. Liu P, Song Y, Shakoor K, Peng C, Liu S. The pros and cons of the PCC staging system to guide surgical resectability and prognosis. J Cancer. 2022;13(13):3444–51.
27. Koay EJ, Odisio BC, Javle M, Vauthey JN, Crane CH. Management of unresectable intrahepatic cholangiocarcinoma: how do we decide among the various liver-directed treatments? Hepatobiliary Surg Nutr. 2017;6(2):105–16.
28. Horgan AM, Amir E, Walter T, Knox JJ. Adjuvant therapy in the treatment of biliary tract cancer: a systematic review and meta-analysis. J Clin Oncol. 2012;30(16):1934–40.
29. Ueno M, Morizane C, Ikeda M, Okusaka T, Ishii H, Furuse J. A review of changes to and clinical implications of the eighth TNM classification of hepatobiliary and pancreatic cancers. Jpn J Clin Oncol. 2019;49(12):1073–82.
30. Luvira V, Satitkarnmanee E, Pugkhem A, Kietpeerakool C, Lumbiganon P, Pattanittum P. Postoperative adjuvant chemotherapy for resectable cholangiocarcinoma. Cochrane Database Syst Rev. 2021;9(9):Cd012814.
31. Mohan BP, Chandan S, Khan SR, Kassab LL, Ponnada S, Artifon ELA, et al. Photodynamic therapy (PDT), radiofrequency ablation (RFA) with biliary stents in palliative treatment of unresectable extrahepatic cholangiocarcinoma: a systematic review and meta-analysis. J Clin Gastroenterol. 2022;56(2):e153–e60.
32. Hyder O, Hatzaras I, Sotiropoulos GC, Paul A, Alexandrescu S, Marques H, et al. Recurrence after operative management of intrahepatic cholangiocarcinoma. Surgery. 2013;153(6):811–8.
33. Chang HY, Liu B, Wang YZ, Wang WJ, Wang W, Li D, et al. Percutaneous transhepatic cholangiography versus endoscopic retrograde cholangiography for the pathological diagnosis of suspected malignant bile duct strictures. Medicine (Baltimore). 2020;99(11):e19545.
34. Zhimin G, Noor H, Jian-Bo Z, Lin W, Jha RK. Advances in diagnosis and treatment of hilar cholangiocarcinoma—a review. Med Sci Monit. 2013;19:648–56.
35. Yang J, Wang J, Zhou H, Zhou Y, Wang Y, Jin H, et al. Efficacy and safety of endoscopic radiofrequency ablation for unresectable extrahepatic cholangiocarcinoma: a randomized trial. Endoscopy. 2018;50(8):751–60.
36. Taggar AS, Mann P, Folkert MR, Aliakbari S, Myrehaug SD, Dawson LA. A systematic review of intraluminal high dose rate brachytherapy in the management of malignant biliary tract obstruction and cholangiocarcinoma. Radiother Oncol. 2021;165:60–74.
37. Vienne A, Hobeika E, Gouya H, Lapidus N, Fritsch J, Choury AD, et al. Prediction of drainage effectiveness during endoscopic stenting of malignant hilar strictures: the role of liver volume assessment. Gastrointest Endosc. 2010;72(4):728–35.
38. Valle JW, Wasan H, Johnson P, Jones E, Dixon L, Swindell R, et al. Gemcitabine alone or in combination with cisplatin in patients with advanced or metastatic cholangiocarcinomas or other biliary tract tumours: a multicentre randomised phase II study—the UK ABC-01 study. Br J Cancer. 2009;101(4):621–7.
39. Kim YI, Park JW, Kim BH, Woo SM, Kim TH, Koh YH, et al. Outcomes of concurrent chemoradiotherapy versus chemotherapy alone for advanced-stage unresectable intrahepatic cholangiocarcinoma. Radiat Oncol. 2013;8:292.

40. Yamashita S, Koay EJ, Passot G, Shroff R, Raghav KP, Conrad C, et al. Local therapy reduces the risk of liver failure and improves survival in patients with intrahepatic cholangiocarcinoma: a comprehensive analysis of 362 consecutive patients. Cancer. 2017;123(8):1354–62.
41. Machairas N, Lang H, Jayant K, Raptis DA, Sotiropoulos GC. Intrahepatic cholangiocarcinoma: limitations for resectability, current surgical concepts and future perspectives. Eur J Surg Oncol. 2020;46(5):740–6.
42. Yu MH, Kim YJ, Park HS, Jung SI. Benign gallbladder diseases: imaging techniques and tips for differentiating with malignant gallbladder diseases. World J Gastroenterol. 2020;26(22):2967.

Chapter 11
Anal Cancers

Salih Ahmed Aljiburi, Aqeel Shakir Mahmood, Saleh Abdulkareem Saleh, and Mustafa Ismail

1. A 67-year-old male presented with hematochezia; further evaluation revealed SCC. In epidemiology of anal cancer, the incorrect statement is:
   - A. Less than 1000 new cases are diagnosed annually in the United States.
   - B. Anal cancer incidence and mortality have increased dramatically in the recent decades in the United States.
   - C. Anal cancer is more common in men.
   - D. Anal cancer accounts for 1–2% of digestive tract tumors.
   - E. SCC constitutes 80–90% of all malignant anal tumors.

     Answer: C

     Explanation: Anal cancer is more common in females, potentially attributed to sexual behavior or the prevalence of human papillomavirus (HPV) infection in females. This demographic difference is a key point to remember.
2. A 77-year-old male presented with fresh bleeding and pain during defecation; further evaluation exhibits SCC in the anus. In risk factors for anal cancer, the incorrect statement is:
   - A. Autoimmune diseases are associated with an increased prevalence of anal cancer.

S. A. Aljiburi
Baghdad Teaching Hospital, Baghdad, Iraq

A. S. Mahmood
Department of General Surgery, University of Baghdad, Baghdad, Iraq

S. A. Saleh
College of Medicine University of Baghdad, Baghdad, Iraq

M. Ismail (✉)
Department of Surgery, College of Medicine, University of Baghdad, Baghdad, Iraq

A. S. Mahmood, A. Koulouris (eds.), *MCQs in General Surgical Oncology*,
https://doi.org/10.1007/978-3-031-65738-2_11

B. Anal cancer's etiology is more similar to genital malignancies than it is to gastrointestinal tract cancers.
C. Solid organ transplant is a risk factor.
D. Antiretroviral therapy (ART) eliminates the risk of developing anal cancer in HIV patients.
E. High-grade squamous intraepithelial lesions (HSIL) are associated with all CD4+ strata in patients with HIV.

Answer: D

Explanation: Initial studies did not conclusively establish that ART eliminates the risk of developing anal cancer in HIV patients. More recent research suggests a modest protective effect of ART, but the impact may be limited in a population with a high prevalence of squamous intraepithelial lesions (SIL).

3. In the context of human papillomavirus (HPV) and anal cancer, a 45-year-old male patient presents with anal cancer. His medical history includes multiple sexual partners and a recent diagnosis of HPV infection. The incorrect statement is:

A. HPV is the most common sexually transmitted disease in the United States.
B. HPV 16 presence is also associated with a poor prognosis.
C. Infection with high-risk strains of HPV is associated with more than 90% of cases of anal cancer.
D. HPV 16-associated anal SCC can be identified histologically by immunohistochemical expression of p16.
E. Quadrivalent HPV vaccine prevents HPV types 6, 11, 16, and 18.

Answer: B

Explanation: Contrary to the misconception, HPV 16 presence is associated with a good prognosis in anal cancer cases.

4. Regarding the anatomy of the anal canal, and during an examination of a patient with rectal complaints, you are assessing the anatomy of the anal canal. The incorrect statement is:

A. The length of the anatomical anal canal is 5 cm long.
B. It begins where the rectum enters the puborectalis sling.
C. It ends roughly at the palpable intersphincteric groove.
D. The dentate line is a macroscopically visible landmark that overlies the transition from glandular to squamous mucosa.
E. The anal sphincter complex is palpable as the anorectal ring on digital rectal examination.

Answer: A

Explanation: The anatomical anal canal is, on average, 2.5–3.5 cm long, while the surgical anal canal measures 5 cm. Understanding this distinction is vital for accurate assessment in clinical practice.

5. In anal intraepithelial neoplasia (AIN) of the anal canal, you are managing a 35-year-old patient with AIN and discussing treatment options. The incorrect statement is:

A. AIN I recurrence usually has an indolent course.
B. Local excision should only be considered if lesions cover less than one-third of the anal circumference.
C. In AIN II/III, wide-local excision leads to recurrence in 1/3 of cases at 1 year.
D. Anoscopy should be performed every 4–6 months in AIN II/III.
E. Watchful waiting is the standard in recurrence of AIN I.

Answer: C

Explanation: Contrary to the statement, in AIN II/III, wide-local excision can lead to recurrence in approximately 2/3 of cases at 1 year. Understanding the management and outcomes of AIN is crucial for patient care.

6. Regarding the anatomy of the anal canal, you are conducting a proctologic examination on a patient presenting with anal discomfort. The incorrect statement is:

A. The internal anal sphincter is involuntary.
B. Hemorrhoids can be a sign of portal hypertension.
C. The perianus extends 5 cm laterally from the anal verge.
D. The perianus is characterized by the presence of hair follicles and glands.
E. The anal pecten is superior to the dentate line.

Answer: E

Explanation: Above the dentate line, the epithelium is mucous membrane-like, while inferior to the dentate line, a transition zone known as the anal pecten is lined by nonkeratinized stratified squamous epithelium. Understanding the location and characteristics of the anal pecten is essential for clinical assessment.

7. In the context of anatomy of the anal canal, during an examination of a patient with anal discomfort, you are assessing the anatomy of the anal canal. The incorrect statement is:

A. The anorectal junction is located 2–3 cm in front and a little below the tip of the coccyx.
B. In males, it is surrounded by the membranous urethra anteriorly.
C. Anal columns contain the inferior rectal veins.
D. The floor of the anal sinuses contains the opening to the anal glands.
E. Under anesthesia, the pectinate line can be observed.

Answer: C

Explanation: Contrary to common understanding, anal columns contain the superior rectal veins, which is a key distinction in understanding the vascular anatomy of the anal canal.

8. In levator ani anatomy, during a surgical procedure for pelvic organ prolapse, you are considering the anatomy of the levator ani muscle. The incorrect statement is:

A. Puborectalis and the pubococcygeus are located medially and superiorly.
B. Levator ani muscle is thick anteriorly.

C. It is mostly thin and aponeurotic posteriorly.
D. Iliococcygeus is primarily innervated by the sacral S1 and S2 nerves.
E. Pubococcygeus and the puborectalis muscles are primarily innervated by the pudendal nerve.

Answer: D

Explanation: The statement about the innervation of the iliococcygeus muscle is incorrect. Iliococcygeus is primarily innervated by the sacral S3 and S4 nerves, which is an important detail in understanding pelvic floor anatomy and function.

9. In the context of SIL of the anal canal, you are reviewing the management of a 30-year-old female patient with a history of HPV infection and anal SIL. The incorrect statement is:

A. Low-grade squamous intraepithelial lesions (LSIL) represent a marker for risk of HSIL rather than a direct precursor.
B. LSIL may spontaneously regress.
C. HSIL containing HPV 16 are the least likely to regress.
D. Biopsy of small HSIL lesions contributes to its regression.
E. HPV vaccination has a role in preventing the progression of HSIL to invasive anal cancer.

Answer: E

Explanation: Contrary to popular belief, HPV vaccination does not induce regression of pre-existing HSIL, and it does not play a role in preventing the progression of HSIL to invasive anal cancer. It primarily provides protection against new HPV infections.

10. In the staging of anal cancers, you are assessing the staging and management of a 55-year-old male patient newly diagnosed with anal cancer. The incorrect statement is:

A. The probability of nodal spread is directly related to the tumor size.
B. Perianal skin cancers are staged and treated like squamous cell skin cancers.
C. There are no tumor markers that are consistently elevated in anal SCC.
D. Surgical staging is no longer performed routinely.
E. At initial presentation, most patients have a T1 or T2 lesion, and fewer than 20% are node-positive.

Answer: B

Explanation: The staging for perianal skin cancers has changed; they are now staged and treated like anal canal cancers rather than squamous cell skin cancers. Understanding this shift in staging is important for accurate diagnosis and management.

11. In the context of histopathology of the anal canal, a 55-year-old male patient presents with a suspicious anal lesion, and a biopsy is performed. The incorrect statement is:

A. The anal verge is where the squamous mucosa merges with the perianal skin.

B. The term "anal cancer," by common definition, refers to SCCs arising within the mucosa of the anus.
C. Basaloid tumors are the older terms for nonkeratinizing types of SCC.
D. Tumors originating above the dentate line spread to the superficial inguinal and external iliac (deep inguinal) nodes.
E. Adenocarcinomas arising from glandular elements within the anal canal are rare.

Answer: D

Explanation: Contrary to common belief, tumors originating above the dentate line, similar to rectal cancers, primarily drain to the mesorectal and internal iliac nodes. It is essential to distinguish this nodal spread pattern.

12. In the treatment of anal cancer, you are discussing treatment options with a 50-year-old patient diagnosed with anal canal SCC. The incorrect statement is:

A. Surgery is the initial treatment rather than upfront concurrent CRT for anal canal SCCs.
B. Concurrent use of fluorouracil plus mitomycin during RT is the preferred regime for most patients.
C. Cisplatin has less hematologic toxicity compared to mitomycin.
D. There is no role for induction chemotherapy or a continuation of chemotherapy beyond concurrent CRT.
E. Cisplatin is more active in the treatment of SCCs than is mitomycin.

Answer: A

Explanation: Contrary to the statement, initial concurrent CRT rather than upfront surgery is recommended for most patients with anal canal SCC. CRT has become the preferred method of treatment for anal canal SCCs because it can cure many patients while preserving the anal sphincter in a significant percentage of cases. Understanding the preferred treatment approach is essential for managing these patients effectively.

13. In the therapy of anal cancer, you are discussing treatment options with a 55-year-old patient diagnosed with early-stage anal cancer. The incorrect statement is:

A. Patients with active HIV/AIDS-related complications may require dose adjustment.
B. RT dose is 45 Gy for early-stage disease.
C. Isolated para-aortic LN involvement is common.
D. The total dose of RT in node-positive disease is 55–59 Gy.
E. There is no benefit in intensifying treatment for locally advanced disease.

Answer: C

Explanation: Isolated para-aortic LN involvement is rare and considered M1 (stage IV) disease in the context of anal cancer. Understanding the staging and treatment implications for such cases is crucial for accurate management.

14. In the treatment guidelines of anal cancer, you are following up with a patient who underwent treatment for anal cancer. The incorrect statement is:

A. Local excision is standard of care for patients with T1 tumors less than 1 cm in size.
B. Vigilant follow-up soon after resection is mandatory.
C. After 3 years, extended imaging surveillance is not indicated.
D. MRI is indicated at 8–12 weeks posttreatment to assess the patient's response.
E. SCCs regress slowly.

Answer: D

Explanation: Contrary to the statement, posttreatment assessment by MRI at 8–12 weeks is not recommended for evaluating the patient's response to treatment in anal cancer. Instead, physical examination, including digital rectal examination and palpation of the inguinal regions, is typically carried out during this period. Understanding the appropriate follow-up protocols is essential for patient care.

15. A 55-year-old patient presents with symptoms suggestive of anal cancer. The primary care physician is considering the initial approach to management. Which of the following statements regarding the general approach to anal cancer is incorrect?

A. Radiation therapy combined with chemotherapy is the main treatment modality for anal cancer.
B. Surgery is primarily considered for tumors that are not controlled with chemoradiotherapy.
C. Early stages of anal cancer have a poor prognosis even with treatment.
D. Differentiating anal cancer from common hemorrhoids is essential for diagnosis.
E. Diagnosis and treatment are centralized to specialized cancer clinics.

Answer: C

Explanation: Early stages of anal cancer have a poor prognosis even with treatment. This statement is incorrect as the prognosis for early stages of anal cancer is generally good with appropriate treatment.

16. A patient diagnosed with anal cancer is being discussed in a multidisciplinary team meeting where treatment options are being considered. Which of the following statements about the treatment paradigm for anal cancer is incorrect?

A. Organ preservation by chemoradiotherapy has become the standard of care.
B. Radical surgical resection is the first-line treatment for all stages of anal cancer.
C. The incidence of anal cancer is increasing, particularly in HIV-positive males.
D. Understanding of pathophysiology and treatment has evolved significantly over the last 30 years.
E. Risk factors for anal cancer have been identified and are key to management strategies.

Answer: B

Explanation: Radical surgical resection is the first-line treatment for all stages of anal cancer. This statement is incorrect as the treatment paradigm has shifted from radical surgical resection to organ preservation by chemoradiotherapy.

17. A patient with squamous cell carcinoma of the anal canal is being evaluated for treatment options. Which of the following statements about the management of squamous cell carcinoma of the anal canal is incorrect?

    A. Sphincter-saving chemoradiation has replaced abdominoperineal resection as the first-line therapy.
    B. Surgeons play a crucial role in diagnosis, posttreatment surveillance, and managing persistent or recurrent cancers.
    C. Sentinel node biopsy is irrelevant in managing squamous cell carcinoma of the anal canal.
    D. In select cases, local excision has been employed as primary treatment in conjunction with radiation and chemotherapy.
    E. The introduction of HPV vaccines presents the potential for the disease's eradication.

    Answer: C

    Explanation: Sentinel node biopsy is irrelevant in managing squamous cell carcinoma of the anal canal. This statement is incorrect as sentinel node biopsy may identify patients who will benefit from groin irradiation.

18. During a conference on anal cancer management, a debate arises about the perioperative use of opioids. Which of the following statements regarding opioids' role in cancer surgery is incorrect?

    A. Opioids are the most commonly prescribed analgesics in the perioperative period of cancer surgery.
    B. The influence of opioids on cancer recurrence or metastasis is well-established and universally understood.
    C. Recent findings on opioids' effects on cancer surgery outcomes have yielded conflicting results.
    D. Prospective randomized trials are required to investigate opioids' effects on cancer surgery outcomes further.
    E. Opioids continue to play an essential role in the perioperative period.

    Answer: B

    Explanation: The influence of opioids on cancer recurrence or metastasis is well-established and universally understood. This statement is incorrect as the question of whether opioids could influence recurrence or metastasis remains unanswered.

19. A public health initiative is being developed to address the increasing incidence of anal cancer in women. Which of the following statements regarding screening for anal cancer in women is incorrect?

    A. The incidence of anal cancer is higher in women than in men in the general population.
    B. Most anal cancers are not associated with HPV infection.
    C. Anal cancers are believed to be preceded by anal HSIL.

D. HPV-infected women and those with a history of lower genital tract neoplasia are at the highest risk.
E. Screening recommendations have been provided for women in high-risk groups.

Answer: B

Explanation: Most anal cancers are not associated with HPV infection. This statement is incorrect as most anal cancers are associated with HPV infection.

20. You are evaluating a 50-year-old patient who has recently completed treatment for anal cancer. During the follow-up visit, you discuss potential risk factors for the recurrence of the disease. In the context of risk factors for the recurrence of anal cancer, the incorrect statement is:

A. Primary tumor size >2 cm is a significant risk factor for recurrence.
B. Nodal positivity increases the risk of recurrence.
C. Poor treatment adherence can contribute to recurrence.
D. Unnecessary chemotherapy dose reductions may increase the risk of recurrence.
E. Treatment delay is a known risk factor for recurrence.

Answer: A

Explanation: Contrary to the statement, primary tumor size >5 cm, not >2 cm, is associated with a higher risk of recurrence in anal cancer patients. Understanding the specific risk factors for recurrence is vital for post-treatment management.

21. In the context of HIV in anal cancer, you are evaluating a 40-year-old patient newly diagnosed with anal cancer who also has a history of HIV infection; the incorrect statement is:

A. Newly diagnosed anal squamous cell cancer should be screened for HIV.
B. Newly diagnosed anal basal cell cancer should be screened for HIV.
C. Newly diagnosed anal adenocarcinoma should be screened for HIV.
D. Anal cancer is not a disease-defining condition for progression to acquired immunodeficiency syndrome (AIDS).
E. HIV-positive patients are treated similarly to non-HIV-positive individuals.

Answer: C

Explanation: While it is recommended to screen for HIV in patients with anal squamous cell cancer, routine testing for HIV status in patients with anal adenocarcinoma is not typically done unless the patient's history suggests that screening may be warranted. It's important to be aware of the nuances in screening protocols for different histological types of anal cancer.

Bibliography

1. Hernandez BY, McDuffie K, Zhu X, Wilkens LR, Killeen J, Kessel B, Wakabayashi MT, Bertram CC, Easa D, Ning L, Boyd J, Sunoo C, Kamemoto L, Goodman MT. Anal human papillomavirus infection in women and its relationship with cervical infection. Cancer Epidemiol Biomarkers Prev. 2005;14(11 Pt 1):2550–6. https://doi.org/10.1158/1055-9965.EPI-05-0460. PMID: 16284377; PMCID: PMC1475824
2. Kelly H, Chikandiwa A, Alemany Vilches L, Palefsky JM, de Sanjose S, Mayaud P. Association of antiretroviral therapy with anal high-risk human papillomavirus, anal intraepithelial neoplasia, and anal cancer in people living with HIV: a systematic review and meta-analysis. Lancet HIV. 2020;7(4):e262–78. https://doi.org/10.1016/S2352-3018(19)30434-5. Epub 2020 Feb 25
3. Serup-Hansen E, Linnemann D, Skovrider-Ruminski W, Høgdall E, Geertsen PF, Havsteen H. Human papillomavirus genotyping and p16 expression as prognostic factors for patients with American Joint Committee on Cancer stages I to III carcinoma of the anal canal. J Clin Oncol. 2014;32(17):1812–7. https://doi.org/10.1200/JCO.2013.52.3464. Epub 2014 May 12
4. Barleben A, Mills S. Anorectal anatomy and physiology. Surg Clin North Am. 2010;90(1):1–15., Table of Contents. https://doi.org/10.1016/j.suc.2009.09.001.
5. Scholefield JH, Harris D, Radcliffe A. Guidelines for management of anal intraepithelial neoplasia. Color Dis. 2011;13(Suppl 1):3–10.
6. Drake R, Wayne Vogl A, Mitchell AWM. Gray's anatomy for students E-Book. 2019; ISBN: 9780323611053.
7. Pandey P. Anal anatomy and normal histology. Sex Health. 2012;9(6):513–6. https://doi.org/10.1071/SH12034.
8. Ahmed A, Arbor TC, Qureshi WA. Anatomy, abdomen and pelvis: anal canal. 2023 May 22. In: StatPearls [internet]. Treasure Island, FL: StatPearls Publishing; 2023.
9. Poynten IM, Jin F, Roberts JM, Templeton DJ, Law C, Cornall AM, Molano M, Machalek DA, Carr A, Farnsworth A, Tabrizi S, Phillips S, Fairley CK, Garland SM, Hillman RJ, Grulich AE. The natural history of anal high-grade squamous intraepithelial lesions in gay and bisexual men. Clin Infect Dis. 2021;72(5):853–61. https://doi.org/10.1093/cid/ciaa166. Erratum in: Clin Infect Dis. 2022 May 30;74(10):1892
10. Welton ML, Steele SR, Goodman KA, et al. Anus. In: Amin MB, editor. AJCC cancer staging manual. 8th ed. Chicago: AJCC; 2017. p. 275.
11. Dapper H, Oechsner M, Hirche C, Münch S, Sauter C, Borm K, Peeken JC, Combs SE, Habermehl D. Dosimetric comparison of different radiation techniques (IMRT vs. 3-dimensional) of the "true" (deep) ano-inguinal lymphatic drainage of anal cancer patients. Radiat Oncol. 2018;13(1):227. https://doi.org/10.1186/s13014-018-1174-z. PMID: 30466454; PMCID: PMC6249729
12. Lam AK, Goldblum JR. Tumours of the anal canal: introduction. In: WHO Classification of Tumours Editorial Board, editor. WHO classification of tumours: digestive system tumours. 5th ed. Lyon: International Agency for Research on Cancer; 2019.
13. Das P, Bhatia S, Eng C, Ajani JA, Skibber JM, Rodriguez-Bigas MA, Chang GJ, Bhosale P, Delclos ME, Krishnan S, Janjan NA, Crane CH. Predictors and patterns of recurrence after definitive chemoradiation for anal cancer. Int J Radiat Oncol Biol Phys. 2007;68(3):794–800. https://doi.org/10.1016/j.ijrobp.2006.12.052. Epub 2007 Mar 26
14. Frazer ML, Yang G, Felder S, McDonald J, Sanchez J, Dessureault S, Imanirad I, Carballido E, Kim RD, Hoffe SE, Frakes JM. Determining optimal follow-up for patients with anal cancer following chemoradiation. Am J Clin Oncol. 2020;43(5):319–24. https://doi.org/10.1097/COC.0000000000000673.
15. Hong TS, Pretz JL, Suh WW, Herman JM, Abdel-Wahab M, Azad N, Blackstock W, Das P, Goodman KA, Jabbour SK, Jones WE III, Konski AA, Koong AC, Rodriguez-Bigas M, Small W Jr, Thomas CR Jr, Zook J. Anal cancer. In: Anal cancer [internet]. Springer; 2013. [cited 2023].
16. Salati SA, Kadi A. Anal cancer—a review. Int J Health Sci (Qassim). 2012;6(2):206–30.

17. Szmulowicz U, Wu JS. Squamous cell carcinoma of the anal canal: a review of the aetiology, presentation, staging, prognosis and methods available for treatment. Sex Health. 2012;9(6):593–609.
18. Connolly C, Buggy D. Opioids and tumour metastasis: does the choice of the anesthetic-analgesic technique influence outcome after cancer surgery? Curr Opin Anaesthesiol. 2016;29(4):468–74.
19. Moscicki AB, Darragh TM, Berry-Lawhorn JM, Roberts JM, Khan MJ, Boardman LA, Chiao E, Einstein MH, Goldstone SE, Jay N, Likes W, Stier EA, Welton ML, Wiley DJ, Palefsky JM. Screening for anal cancer in women. J Low Genit Tract Dis. 2015;19(3 Suppl 1):S27–42.
20. Gunderson LL, Moughan J, Ajani JA, Pedersen JE, Winter KA, Benson AB 3rd, Thomas CR Jr, Mayer RJ, Haddock MG, Rich TA, Willett CG. Anal carcinoma: impact of TN category of disease on survival, disease relapse, and colostomy failure in US Gastrointestinal Intergroup RTOG 98-11 phase 3 trial. Int J Radiat Oncol Biol Phys. 2013;87(4):638–45. https://doi.org/10.1016/j.ijrobp.2013.07.035. Epub 2013 Sep 10. PMID: 24035327; PMCID: PMC3938865
21. National Comprehensive Cancer Network (NCCN). NCCN clinical practice guidelines in oncology. Available at: https://www.nccn.org/professionals/physician_gls (Accessed 18 May 2022).

Part II
Surgical Endocrine Oncology

Chapter 12
Breast Cancers

Salih Ahmed Aljiburi, Saleh Abdulkareem Saleh, Sajjad G. Al-Badri, and Aqeel Shakir Mahmood

1. A 50-year-old woman presents with a palpable breast lump. On evaluation, she is diagnosed with breast cancer. Which statement about breast cancer is incorrect?

   A. The most common cancer in women worldwide.
   B. Accounts for 15% of all cancer deaths in females.
   C. Accounts for about 25% of all new cancer diagnoses.
   D. The incidence is higher in developing countries than in developed countries.
   E. The global incidence of breast cancer is increasing.

   Answer: D

   Explanation: The incidence of breast cancer is higher in developed countries than in developing countries, with an age-standardized incidence rate of about 74 per 100,000 in developed areas and 31 per 100,000 in less developed areas of the world.

2. A 45-year-old woman with a family history of breast cancer seeks counseling for risk assessment. Which of the following general risk factors for breast cancer is incorrect?

   A. Increasing age.
   B. Previous high-dose radiation to the chest area.
   C. Alcohol consumption.
   D. Young age at menarche.
   E. Bilateral oophorectomy.

S. A. Aljiburi
Baghdad Teaching Hospital, Baghdad, Iraq

S. A. Saleh · S. G. Al-Badri
College of Medicine University of Baghdad, Baghdad, Iraq

A. S. Mahmood (✉)
Department of General Surgery, University of Baghdad, Baghdad, Iraq

A. S. Mahmood, A. Koulouris (eds.), *MCQs in General Surgical Oncology*,
https://doi.org/10.1007/978-3-031-65738-2_12

Answer: E

Explanation: Bilateral oophorectomy reduces the risk of breast cancer, and the earlier in life the oophorectomy is performed, the greater the risk reduction.

3. A 38-year-old woman with a family history of breast cancer undergoes genetic testing. Which of the following highly penetrant breast cancer gene mutations is incorrect?

   A. BRCA1.
   B. CHEK2.
   C. TP53.
   D. CDH1.
   E. STK11.

   Answer: B

   Explanation: CHEK2 is a protein kinase involved in cell cycle regulation at the G2 phase. It is considered a moderate to low breast cancer susceptibility gene, associated with a twofold increase in the risk of breast cancer.

4. A 42-year-old woman presents with a palpable breast lump that is later diagnosed as a phyllodes tumor. Which statement about phyllodes tumors is incorrect?

   A. The median age of incidence is 40–45 years.
   B. Most patients present with a smooth, firm, mobile, and palpable breast lump.
   C. It is regarded as a benign lesion.
   D. Wide local excision with ≥1 cm free tumor margin is recommended.
   E. Mostly, it spreads hematogenously.

   Answer: C

   Explanation: Phyllodes tumors are histologically graded into benign, borderline, and malignant based on characteristic features. Only borderline and malignant tumors are known to metastasize.

5. A 58-year-old woman presents with eczema-like changes on her nipple and areola. A biopsy confirms Paget's disease of the breast. Which statement about Paget's disease is incorrect?

   A. It occurs due to the migration of malignant ductal cells toward the skin through lactiferous ducts.
   B. Risk factors include old age, radiation exposure, and BRCA1/2 mutations.
   C. Histology shows malignant intraepithelial adenocarcinoma cells of variable sizes.
   D. All cases need to undergo mastectomy to decrease recurrence.
   E. Peak incidence is between 50 and 60 years old.

   Answer: D

   Explanation: Simple mastectomy has been the standard care for Paget's disease of the breast. However, recent studies show that breast conservation therapy with radiation therapy is oncologically safe and can be performed for many cases.

6. A 46-year-old woman presents with a breast mass. On ultrasound examination, irregular findings are noted. Which ultrasound finding is incorrect regarding breast cancer ultrasound findings?

   A. Homogeneous texture.
   B. Irregular and poorly defined mass.
   C. Speculated margin.
   D. Posterior acoustic shadowing.
   E. Microcalcifications.

   Answer: A

   Explanation: Malignant breast masses that suggest breast cancer appear heterogeneous in texture and are often hypoechoic lesions.

7. A 48-year-old woman is found to have LCIS during a breast biopsy. Which statement about LCIS is incorrect?

   A. Majority of women with LCIS who develop cancer develop ductal carcinoma.
   B. The time to develop invasive cancer is about 5 years.
   C. The lifelong risk of developing an invasive cancer is about 1% per year.
   D. If found on core needle biopsy, excision should be done.
   E. If found on isolation or excisional biopsy, no further surgical intervention is required.

   Answer: B

   Explanation: The time to develop invasive cancer in LCIS is about 10–15 years.

8. A 55-year-old woman is diagnosed with invasive breast cancer. Which statement about breast cancer incidence and characteristics is incorrect?

   A. Invasive lobular carcinoma (ILC) is the most common and accounts for 80% of all cases.
   B. ILC has a linear arrangement and grows in ducts and lobules circumferentially.
   C. ILC has a lower rate of HER-2 overexpression and a higher rate of hormone receptor positivity.
   D. Medullary, mucinous, tubular, and adenoid carcinoma are associated with a good prognosis.
   E. Micropapillary carcinoma and angiosarcoma are aggressive subtypes.

   Answer: A

   Explanation: Invasive ductal carcinoma (IDC) is the most common and represents 80% of all cases, while ILC is the second most common and accounts for about 8–15% only.

9. A 58-year-old postmenopausal woman presents with mammographic abnormalities and is diagnosed with ductal carcinoma in situ (DCIS). Which statement about DCIS is incorrect?

   A. Represents 20% of all newly diagnosed breast cancers.
   B. Occurs in young women with inherited BRCA mutations.

C. The average age of diagnosis is between 30 and 35 years.
D. Risk factors include increased breast density, obesity, nulliparity, and late age at first birth.
E. The progression into invasive breast cancer is not obligatory and cannot be predicted.

Answer: C

Explanation: The average age of diagnosis for DCIS is between 54 and 56 years, with the majority of cases found in postmenopausal women.

10. A 48-year-old woman presents with a breast mass. Biopsy reveals medullary breast cancer. Which statement about medullary breast cancer is incorrect?

A. It is a rare subtype of invasive ductal carcinoma (IDC).
B. It is associated with the BRCA1 mutation.
C. The mean age of presentation is 60–70 years.
D. It is usually triple negative.
E. Tumors are well-circumscribed and moderately firm.

Answer: C

Explanation: The median age of presentation for medullary breast cancer is younger than that of IDC, ranging from 45 to 54 years.

11. A 45-year-old woman presents with microcalcifications on mammography, leading to a diagnosis of DCIS. Which statement about DCIS is incorrect?

A. Mostly presents as a palpable mass or bloody nipple discharge.
B. Diagnosis should be confirmed by stereotactic core biopsy.
C. Breast-conserving surgery is safe for DCIS and should be followed by radiation therapy.
D. An excisional margin width of 1–2 mm is sufficient for women undergoing radiation therapy.
E. The incidence of LN involvement is 1–2%.

Answer: A

Explanation: About 90% of DCIS lesions are identified radiographically by the presence of microcalcifications, not as a palpable mass or bloody nipple discharge.

12. A 52-year-old woman inquires about breast cancer screening. Which statement about breast cancer screening is incorrect?

A. Screening reduces mortality from breast cancer by up to 30% in the screened population.
B. It detects smaller, low-grade tumors and less frequently LN involvement.
C. It may lead to unnecessary biopsy for benign lesions.
D. The EU recommends screening the 30–50 age group at an interval of 2 years.
E. Mammography is less beneficial for women under 50 years.

Answer: D

Explanation: The EU recommends screening the 50–69 age group with a 2-year interval.

13. A 50-year-old woman undergoing a breast biopsy for another lesion is incidentally found to have lobular carcinoma in situ (LCIS). Which statement about LCIS is incorrect?

    A. Is a premalignant lesion.
    B. The risk of cancer is conferred to both the ipsilateral and contralateral breasts.
    C. Found incidentally on biopsy performed for another lesion.
    D. The mean age of diagnosis is between 44 and 46 years.
    E. E-cadherin staining is used to differentiate between DCIS and LCIS.

    Answer: A

    Explanation: LCIS is not considered a premalignant lesion; it is a noninvasive abnormal proliferation of cells in the terminal duct and lobule of the breast and is not indicative of cancer itself.

14. A 52-year-old woman with early breast cancer seeks treatment options. Which indication for breast-conserving surgery is incorrect?

    A. Early breast cancer without skin or fascia involvement.
    B. Tumor size not exceeding 30–40% of the original breast volume.
    C. Unifocal lesions or multifocal lesions situated in the same quadrant.
    D. Tumors that can be removed with microscopically clear surgical resection margins regardless of cosmetic outcome.
    E. Tumors downsized by neoadjuvant chemotherapy or systemic endocrine treatment.

    Answer: D

    Explanation: Acceptable cosmetic outcome, including the shape, contour, and size of the remaining breast, is an important consideration even for tumors that can be removed with microscopically clear surgical margins.

15. A 55-year-old woman is being evaluated for breast cancer treatment options. Which statement about absolute contraindications for breast-conserving surgery is incorrect?

    A. Presence of any contraindication to adjuvant radiation therapy.
    B. Extensive skin or chest wall involvement affecting more than 40% of the original breast volume.
    C. Breast-conserving surgery leading to significant breast deformity and a poor aesthetic outcome.
    D. Presence of extensive malignant microcalcifications or inflammatory carcinoma.
    E. Multifocal or multicentric cancers are always an absolute contraindication.

    Answer: E

    Explanation: Multifocal (two or more foci in the same quadrant) or multicentric (different quadrant) cancers are considered relative contraindications, and with the introduction of oncoplastic surgery techniques, these cases have become more manageable. However, there are still a risk of incomplete resection and a higher likelihood of re-excision and recurrence.

16. A 38-year-old woman with breast cancer is being evaluated for potential risk factors for locoregional recurrence. Which risk factor has incorrect association with an increased risk of locoregional recurrence?

    A. Old-age patient.
    B. Advanced nodal disease.
    C. Multifocal primary tumor pattern.
    D. Presence of lymphovascular invasion.
    E. Residual disease after preoperative systemic therapy.

    Answer: A

    Explanation: Young age patients, those less than 40 years old, are at an increased risk for locoregional recurrence.

17. A 44-year-old woman with breast cancer is discussing treatment options with her oncologist. Which indication for mastectomy is incorrect?

    A. Multicentric disease (different quadrant or more than 4 cm apart).
    B. Extensive DCIS >4 cm.
    C. Recurrence after breast-conserving surgery and chemotherapy.
    D. Patient preference.
    E. Tumor size not exceeding 30–40% of the original breast volume.

    Answer: E

    Explanation: Early breast cancer that is less than 30–40% of the original breast volume is an indication for breast-conserving surgery, not mastectomy.

18. A 56-year-old man presents with a breast mass, and further evaluation reveals male breast cancer. Which statement about male breast cancer is incorrect?

    A. Risk factors involve Klinefelter syndrome, prostate cancer, and BRCA1/2 mutations.
    B. Mostly presents as a painless palpable mass retro- or periareolar and ill-defined.
    C. Evaluation should be performed with core needle biopsy.
    D. Median age of onset is 50 years.
    E. Invasive ductal carcinoma is the most common type.

    Answer: D

    Explanation: The median age of onset for male breast cancer is 67 years, which is 5–10 years older than female breast cancer.

19. A 30-year-old pregnant woman is diagnosed with breast cancer. Which statement about pregnancy-associated breast cancer is incorrect?

    A. Diagnosis is made during pregnancy or within the first postpartum year.
    B. Trastuzumab and endocrine therapies are safe during pregnancy.
    C. Gadolinium is contraindicated during pregnancy, so MRI is not recommended.
    D. Surgery is the initial treatment and can be done anytime during pregnancy.
    E. Thromboprophylaxis with heparin is required due to a high risk of thromboembolic events.

    Answer: B

Explanation: Trastuzumab and endocrine therapies are contraindicated during pregnancy due to the high risk of pregnancy, fetal, and newborn complications.

20. A pregnant woman is diagnosed with breast cancer, and her treatment options are being discussed. Which statement about pregnancy-associated breast cancer management is incorrect?

    A. Ultrasound is the first-choice imaging modality for breast during pregnancy.
    B. Chemotherapy can be given from the second and third trimesters from 14 weeks on.
    C. Anthracyclines and taxanes are contraindicated.
    D. The last chemotherapy course should be given latest at week 35 of gestation.
    E. Axillary staging is performed with axillary LN dissection.

    Answer: C

    Explanation: Anthracyclines and taxanes are safe during pregnancy and can be considered in the treatment plan for pregnancy-associated breast cancer.

21. A 48-year-old woman is considering nipple-sparing mastectomy for her breast cancer treatment. Which statement about nipple-sparing mastectomy is incorrect?

    A. Biopsy of subareolar tissue is recommended in all nipple-sparing mastectomies.
    B. The most frequently used incisions are inframammary, radial, and periareolar.
    C. Selection criteria involve tumor size less than 6 cm and a distance from the nipple of 2 cm.
    D. Under-nipple areolar complex sharp dissection is recommended.
    E. Nipple loss is increased in large ptotic breasts.

    Answer: C

    Explanation: The recommended selection criteria for nipple-sparing mastectomy involve a tumor size less than 4.5 cm in diameter, a 4 cm distance from the nipple, and without nipple-areolar complex involvement.

22. A 40-year-old woman with breast cancer is considering nipple-sparing mastectomy (NSM). Which statement about contraindications for NSM is incorrect?

    A. Tumors less than 2 cm from the nipple-areolar complex.
    B. Multicentric disease or positive subareolar histology.
    C. Presence of extensive DCIS.
    D. Inflammatory breast cancer.
    E. BRCA gene mutation.

    Answer: E

    Explanation: NSM is safe in patients with genetic mutations, including BRCA gene mutations.

23. A 56-year-old woman with breast cancer is discussing reconstruction options. Which statement about implant-based reconstruction is incorrect?

A. It is the most widely used reconstruction procedure.
B. Patients with small to medium breasts, slim physique, and minimal breast ptosis are the best candidates.
C. Risk factors for complications include smoking, obesity, and age more than 65 years.
D. Early complications include hematoma, infection, and skin flap necrosis.
E. Chemotherapy administration or previous radiation therapy does not increase the incidence of complications.

Answer: E

Explanation: Chemotherapy administered during expansion or previous radiation therapy does not significantly affect or increase the incidence of complications in implant-based reconstruction.

24. A 48-year-old woman is considering autologous tissue-based breast reconstruction. Which statement about autologous tissue-based reconstruction is incorrect?

A. It can be used in combination with an implant to increase breast volume or on its own as an extended procedure.
B. It can be combined with lipomodeling to avoid the use of an implant.
C. The latissimus dorsi (LD) flap can be used as a pedicled rotational flap.
D. LD flap has a high risk of complications when adjuvant radiation therapy is needed.
E. Contraindications include congenital absence of muscle or neurovascular damage to the thoracodorsal pedicle.

Answer: D

Explanation: The LD flap is a reliable and surgically safe technique even when adjuvant radiation therapy is needed.

25. A 45-year-old woman with breast cancer is considering reconstruction options after mastectomy. Which of the following is incorrect about indications for autologous tissue-based reconstruction?

A. Risk-reducing mastectomy.
B. Small size, ptotic contralateral breast.
C. Poor aesthetic outcome with implant-based reconstruction.
D. Patients who prefer to avoid implant-based reconstruction.
E. Unilateral breast reconstruction.

Answer: B

Explanation: Large size, not a small size, ptotic contralateral breast, is an indication for autologous tissue-based reconstruction.

26. A 52-year-old woman with breast cancer is discussing immediate breast reconstruction with her surgeon. In which of the following situations in immediate breast reconstruction recommendations is incorrect?

A. T3–T4 tumor stage.
B. Inflammatory breast cancer.
C. Axillary LN metastasis.
D. After adjuvant radiation therapy.

E. If it delays the therapeutic surgery.

Answer: D

Explanation: Immediate breast reconstruction is generally not recommended before or after adjuvant radiation therapy.

27. A 48-year-old woman has undergone autologous flap reconstruction following mastectomy. Which complication has incorrect association with autologous flap reconstruction?

A. Flap necrosis.
B. Seroma.
C. Chronic breast pain.
D. Abdominal weakness or hernia.
E. Infection.

Answer: C

Explanation: Chronic back pain is a complication of autologous flap reconstruction, while chronic breast pain is a complication of implant-based reconstruction.

28. A 50-year-old woman with invasive breast cancer is discussing her treatment options with her surgeon. Which statement about SLNB indications, contraindications, and recommendations is incorrect?

A. Indicated in patients with invasive breast cancer and clinically negative axilla.
B. Contraindicated in patients with DCIS who undergo planned mastectomy.
C. Not recommended in patients with inflammatory breast cancer.
D. Using radiolabeled colloids is safe during pregnancy.
E. Recommended for multifocal and/or multicentric breast cancer.

Answer: B

Explanation: SLNB is indicated in patients with extensive DCIS undergoing planned mastectomy to avoid further surgery in case there is invasive tumor in the mastectomy specimen. However, it is not recommended routinely in DCIS patients with breast conservation surgery.

29. A 45-year-old woman with positive SLNB results is considering further treatment options. Which criterion is incorrect regarding axillary LN node dissection in such patients?

A. Tumor size ≤5 cm.
B. ≤2 positive sentinel LNs.
C. Lumpectomy with whole breast irradiation.
D. Receiving systemic therapy.
E. Patients who have mastectomy.

Answer: E

Explanation: Patients who undergo mastectomy or those who will not receive radiation that covers the axilla require axillary LN dissection for positive SLNB.

30. A 55-year-old woman is planning her breast cancer treatment and potential reconstruction. Which statement about radiation therapy after mastectomy is incorrect?

   A. It may impair the results of implant-based reconstructive surgery.
   B. It increases the capsular formation by 2.5-fold if applied to implant-based reconstruction.
   C. Early reconstruction is advised if radiation therapy is expected.
   D. It may lead to explantation, infection, and poor aesthetic outcome.
   E. Radiation therapy should not be considered an absolute contraindication for reconstruction.

   Answer: C

   Explanation: Late reconstruction is recommended when radiation therapy is predicted, and autologous flap-based reconstruction is preferred.

31. A 47-year-old woman with breast cancer is being evaluated for her treatment plan. Which statement about indications for referring breast cancer to radiation oncology is incorrect?

   A. In situ or invasive carcinoma treated with breast-conserving therapy.
   B. Positive margins after mastectomy.
   C. Tumors with more than 5 cm, irrespective of the surgical treatment offered.
   D. Locally advanced and inflammatory breast cancer.
   E. LN-positive breast cancer.

   Answer: A

   Explanation: LN-positive breast cancer should be referred to radiation oncology due to the potential for metastasis.

32. A 55-year-old woman with breast cancer is discussing her chemotherapy options with her oncologist. Which statement about chemotherapy for breast cancer is incorrect?

   A. Indicated for negative high-risk estrogen receptor and negative HER-2 diseases.
   B. Consists of six to eight courses of treatment given over 5 to 6 months.
   C. Taxanes and anthracyclines are the most efficient regimen.
   D. It is the only possible systemic treatment for triple-negative breast cancer.
   E. Neoadjuvant therapy is often used for cancer that has spread to the lymph nodes.

   Answer: A

   Explanation: Chemotherapy is indicated for positive estrogen receptor, positive HER-2, grade 3 carcinomas, high Ki-67 levels, triple-negative type, and cancer involving more than three lymph nodes.

33. A 49-year-old woman is diagnosed with locally advanced breast cancer (LABC) and is discussing her treatment options. Which statement about LABC is incorrect?

   A. Involves inflammatory breast cancer and cancer growing into the thoracic wall.

B. If metastasis is excluded, it is potentially curable, starting with neoadjuvant systemic therapy.
C. Baseline ultrasound, MRI, whole-body CT, and bone scan are needed before therapy.
D. Mastectomy with axillary LN dissection is the gold standard.
E. Skin-sparing mastectomy and immediate breast reconstruction are contraindicated.

Answer: E

Explanation: Skin-sparing mastectomy and immediate breast reconstruction are considered oncologically safe procedures except for inflammatory diseases.

34. A 40-year-old woman with LABC is discussing her treatment options after receiving neoadjuvant chemotherapy. Which statement about potential candidates for breast conservation after neoadjuvant chemotherapy in LABC is incorrect?

A. Multifocal disease.
B. No inflammatory skin involvement.
C. Radiographic abnormalities resectable with lumpectomy.
D. No contraindication for adjuvant chemotherapy.
E. Accept higher risk of local recurrence in conversion from mastectomy to breast conservation.

Answer: A

Explanation: Patients with unifocal, not multifocal disease, are potential candidates for breast conservation after neoadjuvant chemotherapy.

35. A 47-year-old woman is diagnosed with inflammatory breast cancer. Which statement about inflammatory breast cancer is incorrect?

A. It is the most aggressive entity of breast cancer.
B. Classified as T4d and characterized by diffuse induration and erythema of the skin.
C. Median survival is less than 10 years.
D. Primary systemic chemotherapy is the first-choice treatment followed by mastectomy.
E. Mastectomy is usually performed 2–3 weeks after completion of chemotherapy.

Answer: C

Explanation: The median survival for inflammatory breast cancer is less than 4 years even with multimodality treatment options.

36. A 55-year-old woman has been diagnosed with metastatic breast cancer, and her treatment options are being discussed. Which statement about metastatic breast cancer is incorrect?

A. Metastasis eventually affects 25% of women with breast cancer and results in their death.

B. The treatment goal is to prolong survival, alleviate symptoms, and maintain life quality.
C. Surgery may be considered for solitary brain metastasis.
D. Stereotactic RT is suitable for up to ten metastases.
E. The median survival with metastatic breast cancer is about 3 years.

Answer: D

Explanation: Stereotactic RT is considered for one to five macroscopic radiographically detected metastases, not up to ten metastases.

37. Regarding risk factors for local recurrence after conventional mastectomy for stage I and II disease, a 46-year-old woman who underwent conventional mastectomy for stage I breast cancer is being assessed for potential risk factors for local recurrence. Which risk factor has incorrect association with an increased risk of local recurrence?

A. Young age.
B. Extensive (more than four) nodal involvement.
C. High grade.
D. Extracapsular extension.
E. Positive estrogen receptor status.

Answer: E

Explanation: Negative estrogen receptor status is associated with a significant risk for local recurrence.

38. A 55-year-old woman diagnosed with breast cancer is considering mastectomy options. Which statement about skin-sparing mastectomy is incorrect?

A. It reduces postmastectomy deformity.
B. It reduces the need for contralateral symmetrization surgery.
C. It should leave only an extremely small amount of breast tissue behind with clear superficial resection margins.
D. Dissection at the superficial fascial level is avoided.
E. An ultrathin flap has more complications like lymphedema and prolonged hospital stay.

Answer: D

Explanation: Superficial fascial dissection is advisable during skin-sparing mastectomy, with the flap thickness typically ranging from 7 to 8 mm, which may vary according to the adiposity of the patient.

39. A 42-year-old woman is discussing her mastectomy options with her surgeon. Which risk factor has incorrect association with an increased risk of complications after skin-sparing mastectomy?

A. Young age.
B. Previous radiation therapy to the breast.
C. Large and ptotic breast.
D. Immediate reconstruction with a fixed-volume implant.
E. Smoking.

Answer: A

Explanation: Elderly age patients have a higher risk of complications after skin-sparing mastectomy, possibly due to thinner skin compared to younger patients.

40. A 50-year-old woman who underwent breast cancer treatment presents with arm swelling and discomfort. You suspect breast cancer-related lymphedema. Which statement about breast cancer lymphedema is incorrect?

    A. The most notorious long-term morbidity after breast cancer treatment.
    B. Twenty percent of patients who undergo SLNB develop lymphedema.
    C. Radiation therapy to the axilla and supraclavicular field increases the risk of development.
    D. Conservative treatment involves lymphatic draining and supportive gloves.
    E. Surgical options include liposuction and excision of the edematous area.

    Answer: B

    Explanation: Lymphedema is less frequently reported in women who underwent sentinel lymph node biopsy (SLNB), which occurs in about 3% of cases, while 20% of patients who had axillary LN dissection develop this complication.

41. A 45-year-old woman is scheduled for breast surgery to remove a suspicious lesion. Wire needle localization is planned. Which statement about wire needle localization is incorrect?

    A. Placed using mammography or ultrasound guidance.
    B. Placement should be on the 2 days before breast surgery.
    C. Multiple wires occasionally required to bracket tumors greater than or equal to 2 cm.
    D. Wire migration can lead to pneumothorax or hemothorax, or breast implant puncture.
    E. Retained wire fragments can occur if the wire is accidentally cut during the procedure.

    Answer: B

    Explanation: Placement of the wire should be on the same day as breast surgery, not 2 days before.

42. A patient is scheduled for breast surgery, and non-wire localization devices are being considered for tumor localization. Which statement about non-wire localization devices is incorrect?

    A. Low risk of dislodgment or migrating to another location.
    B. Increased flexibility in timing.
    C. Reduced length of stay on the day of surgery.
    D. Localization access is independent of the surgical approach.
    E. Can be placed 5 days maximally before the procedure.

    Answer: E

    Explanation: Non-wire localization devices can be placed between 5 and 30 days before the procedure, depending on the type of device, providing flexibility in scheduling and coordination between team personnel.

43. A 55-year-old woman with a breast mass is scheduled for lumpectomy. Surgical considerations are essential. Which statement regarding lumpectomy surgical considerations is incorrect?

   A. The incision may be located within the Langer lines over the mass or radially.
   B. Following the incision, subcutaneous flaps are created surrounding the tumor.
   C. Intraoperative specimen imaging is then performed to verify the presence of the biopsy clip and any preoperatively placed markers.
   D. "Shave margins" or an additional 1 mm excision of tissue shown to reduce margin positivity and re-excision rates, possibly.
   E. Placing radiopaque clips is not needed as the tumor is removed.

   Answer: E

   Explanation: Placing radiopaque clips in the tumor cavity is important to guide future radiation treatment as well as follow-up imaging.

44. A 60-year-old woman is scheduled for a mastectomy due to breast cancer. Understanding the procedure is crucial. Which statement about mastectomy is incorrect?

   A. Elliptical incision and raising uniform flaps.
   B. The flaps differ in thickness but range between 5 mm and 1.0 cm.
   C. Ideally, all breast tissue gets excised, including blood supply, to ensure completeness.
   D. The flaps extend to the clavicle superiorly, the lateral edge of the sternum medially, the inframammary fold inferiorly, and the anterior edge of the LD laterally.
   E. Simple mastectomy involves removing all breast tissue without necessitating a complete axillary node dissection.

   Answer: B

   Explanation: During mastectomy, all breast tissue should be excised, but the flaps should preserve the blood supply overlying the skin.

Bibliography

1. Torre LA, Bray F, Siegel RL, Ferlay J, Lortet-Tieulent J, Jemal A. Global cancer statistics, 2012. CA Cancer J Clin. 2015;65(2):87–108.
2. Vermeulen RF, Beurden MV, Korse CM, Kenter GG. Impact of risk-reducing salpingo-oophorectomy in premenopausal women. Climacteric. 2017;20(3):212–21.
3. Shiovitz S, Korde LA. Genetics of breast cancer: a topic in evolution. Ann Oncol. 2015;26(7):1291–9.
4. Khosravi-Shahi P. Management of non-metastatic phyllodes tumors of the breast: review of the literature. Surg Oncol. 2011;20:143–8.

5. Caliskan M, Gatti G, Sosnovskikh I, Rotmensz N, Botteri E, Musmeci S, Rosali dos Santos G, Viale G, Luini A. Paget's disease of the breast: the experience of the European Institute of Oncology and review of the literature. Breast Cancer Res Treat. 2008;112:513–21.
6. Gokhale S. Ultrasound characterization of breast masses. Indian J Radiol Imaging. 2009;19(03):242–7.
7. Chuba PJ, Hamre MR, Yap J, et al. Bilateral risk for subsequent breast cancer after lobular carcinoma in situ: analysis of surveillance, epidemiology, and end results data. J Clin Oncol. 2005;23:5534.
8. Arpino G, Bardou VJ, Clark GM, Elledge RM. Infiltrating lobular carcinoma of the breast: tumor characteristics and clinical outcome. Breast Cancer Res. 2004;6(3):R149–56.
9. Ernster VL, Barclay J, Kerlikowske K, Wilkie H, Ballard-Barbash R. Mortality among women with ductal carcinoma in situ of the breast in the population-based surveillance, epidemiology and end results program. Arch Intern Med. 2000;160(7):953.
10. Foschini MP, Eusebi V. Rare (new) entities of the breast and medullary carcinoma. Pathology. 2009;41(1):48–56.
11. Dershaw DD, Abramson A, Cha I, et al. Ductal carcinoma in situ: mammographic findings and clinical implications. Radiology. 1989;170:411.
12. Perry NM. Multi-disciplinary aspects of quality assurance in the diagnosis of breast disease. 2006. (This is a revised version of the original EUSOMA position paper published in 2001 [European Journal of Cancer 2001;37:159–172].) Available from http://www.eusoma.org/Engx/Guidelines/Other/OtherQA_D.aspx?cont=QA_D
13. Goldschmidt RA, Victor TA. Lobular carcinoma in situ of the breast. In: Seminars in surgical oncology. New York: John Wiley & Sons, Inc.; 1996. (Vol. 12, No. 5, pp. 314-320).
14. Masetti R, Di Leone A, Franceschini G, et al. Oncoplastic techniques in the conservative surgical treatment of breast cancer: an overview. Breast J. 2006;12(Suppl.2):S174–80.
15. Patani N, Carpenter R. Oncological and aesthetic considerations of conservational surgery for multifocal/multicentric breast cancer. Breast J. 2010;16(3):222–32.
16. Fredriksson I, Liljegren G, Palm-Sjövall M, Arnesson LG, Emdin SO, Fornander T, Lindgren A, Nordgren H, Idvall I, Holmqvist M, Holmberg L. Risk factors for local recurrence after breast-conserving surgery. J Br Surg. 2003;90(9):1093–102.
17. Zurrida S, Bassi F, Arnone P, Martella S, Del Castillo A, Ribeiro Martini R, Semenkiw ME, Caldarella P. The changing face of mastectomy (from mutilation to aid to breast reconstruction). Int J Surg Oncol. 2011;5:2011.
18. Nahleh ZA, Srikantiah R, Safa M, Jazieh AR, Muhleman A, Komrokji R. Male breast cancer in the veterans affairs population: a comparative analysis. Cancer. 2007;109(8):1471–7.
19. Xia LY, Hu QL, Zhou Q. Use of trastuzumab in treating breast cancer during pregnancy: a systematic review and meta-analysis. BMC Womens Health. 2021;21:1–2.
20. Framarino-dei-Malatesta M, Sammartino P, Napoli A. Does anthracycline-based chemotherapy in pregnant women with cancer offer safe cardiac and neurodevelopmental outcomes for the developing fetus? BMC Cancer. 2017;17:1–9.
21. Voltura AM, Tsangaris TN, Rossion GD, et al. Nipplesparing mastectomy: critical assessment of 51 procedures and implications for selection criteria. Ann Surg Oncol. 2008;15:3396–401.
22. Lee SC, Mendez-Broomberg K, Eacobacci K, Vincoff NS, Gupta E, McElligott SE. Nipple-sparing mastectomy: what the radiologist should know. Radiographics. 2022;42(2):321–39.
23. Spear SL, Meshabi AN. Implant based reconstruction. Clin Plast Surg. 2007;34(1):63–73.
24. Li L, Yang Y, Li W, Zhao X, He J, Mei S, Guo X, Zhang X, Ran J. Latissimus dorsi myocutaneous flap repair is effective after neoadjuvant chemotherapy for locally advanced breast cancer. World J Surg Oncol. 2022;20(1):134.
25. Bertozzi N, Pesce M, Santi PL, Raposio E. Oncoplastic breast surgery: comprehensive review. Eur Rev Med Pharmacol Sci. 2017;21(11):2572–85.
26. Shea-Budgell M, Quan ML, Mehling B, et al. Breast reconstruction following prophylactic or therapeutic mastectomy for breast cancer: recommendations from an evidence-based provincial guideline. Plast Surg. 2014;22(2):103–11.

27. Wijayanayagam A, Kumar AS, Rd F, et al. Optimizing the total skin-sparing mastectomy. Arch Surg. 2008;143:38–45.
28. Triantafillidou SE. The evolution of the current indications for sentinel lymph node biopsy in breast cancer. Hell J Surg. 2018;90(4):186–94.
29. Giuliano AE, Hunt KK, Ballman KV, et al. Axillary dissection vs no axillary dissection in women with invasive breast cancer and sentinel node metastasis: a randomized clinical trial. JAMA. 2011;305(6):569–75.
30. Kelley BP, Ahmed R, Kidwell KM, Kozlow JH, Chung KC, Momoh AO. A systematic review of morbidity associated with autologous breast reconstruction before and after exposure to radiotherapy: are current practices ideal? Ann Surg Oncol. 2014;21(5):1732–8.
31. Wu S, He Z, Li F, Wang J, Guo J, Lin Q, Guan X. The clinical value of adjuvant radiotherapy in patients with early stage breast cancer with 1 to 3 positive lymph nodes after mastectomy. Chin J Cancer. 2010;29(7):668–76.
32. Schmidt M. Chemotherapy in early breast cancer: when, how and which one? Breast Care. 2014;9(3):154–60.
33. Lim W, Ko BS, Kim HJ, Lee JW, Eom JS, Son BH, Lee TJ, Ahn SH. Oncological safety of skin sparing mastectomy followed by immediate reconstruction for locally advanced breast cancer. J Surg Oncol. 2010;102(1):39–42.
34. Carrara GF, Scapulatempo-Neto C, Abrahão-Machado LF, Brentani MM, Nunes JS, Folgueira MA, Vieira RA. Breast-conserving surgery in locally advanced breast cancer submitted to neoadjuvant chemotherapy. Safety and effectiveness based on ipsilateral breast tumor recurrence and long-term follow-up. Clinics. 2017;72:134–42.
35. Van Uden DJ, Van Laarhoven HW, Westenberg AH, de Wilt JH, Blanken-Peeters CF. Inflammatory breast cancer: an overview. Crit Rev Oncol Hematol. 2015;93(2):116–26.
36. Jardel P, Kammerer E, Villeneuve H, Thariat J. Stereotactic radiation therapy for breast cancer in the elderly. Transl Cancer Res. 2020;9(Suppl 1):S86.
37. Tokin C, Weiss A, Wang-Rodriguez J, et al. Oncologic safety of skin-sparing and nipplesparing mastectomy: a discussion and review of the literature. Int J Surg Oncol. 2012. article ID: 921821:1–8.
38. Krohn IT, Cooper DR, Bassett JG. Radical mastectomy: thick vs thin skin flaps. Arch Surg. 1982;117(6):760–3.
39. Paprottka FJ, Schlett CL, Luketina R, Paprottka K, Klimas D, Radtke C, Hebebrand D. Risk factors for complications after skin-sparing and nipple-sparing mastectomy. Breast Care. 2019;5(5):289–97.
40. Fu MR. Breast cancer-related lymphedema: symptoms, diagnosis, risk reduction, and management. World J Clin Oncol. 2014;5(3):241.
41. Kapoor MM, Patel MM, Scoggins ME. The wire and beyond: recent advances in breast imaging preoperative needle localization. Radiographics. 2019;39(7):1886–906.
42. Aydogan T, Sezgin E, Ilvan S, Yilmaz OC, Aslan N, Golshan M, Aydogan F. Comparison of radio-guided occult lesion localization (ROLL) and magnetic occult lesion localization (MOLL) for non-palpable lesions: a phantom model study. Clin Breast Cancer. 2020;20(1):e9–13.
43. Rahman GA. Breast conserving therapy: a surgical technique where little can mean more. J Surg Tech Case Rep. 2011;3(1):1–4.
44. Freeman MD, Gopman JM, Salzberg CA. The evolution of mastectomy surgical technique: from mutilation to medicine. Gland Surg. 2018;7(3):308.

Chapter 13
Pancreatic Cancer

Raafat Raoof Alturfi, Sabah Noori Abdulraheem, Noufel sh. Alshadood, Haider A. H. Ahmed, and Aqeel Shakir Mahmood

1. A 60-year-old patient presents with suspected pancreatic cancer. Understanding the epidemiology is crucial. Which statement about pancreatic cancer epidemiology is incorrect?
   A. Worldwide, pancreatic cancer is the seventh leading cause of cancer deaths in both men and women.
   B. Incidence is rare below 45 years of age.
   C. Sixty percent of tumors are potentially resectable at diagnosis.
   D. It affects males slightly more commonly than females (1.3:1).
   E. Incidence rates vary by sex and race.
   Answer: C
   Explanation: Only 15–20% of newly diagnosed cases are potentially resectable.

2. A patient is diagnosed with a periamullary tumor, which refers to a tumor located near the ampulla of Vater. Understanding the origin of the tumor is essential for determining the appropriate treatment plan. Which of the following statements about the origin of periamullary tumors is incorrect?

R. R. Alturfi
Department of Digestive Surgery, Gastroenterology and Hepatology Teaching Hospital, Baghdad, Iraq

S. N. Abdulraheem · N. s. Alshadood
Baghdad Teaching Hospital, Baghdad, Iraq

H. A. H. Ahmed
Medical City Complex, Baghdad, Iraq

A. S. Mahmood (✉)
Department of General Surgery, University of Baghdad, Baghdad, Iraq

A. S. Mahmood, A. Koulouris (eds.), *MCQs in General Surgical Oncology*,
https://doi.org/10.1007/978-3-031-65738-2_13

A. The pancreas can be the origin of periamullary tumors.
B. The ampulla of Vater complex can be the origin of periamullary tumors.
C. The distal common bile duct (CBD) can be the origin of periamullary tumors.
D. The duodenum can be the origin of periamullary tumors.
E. The gallbladder is commonly associated with periamullary tumors.

Answer: E

Explanation: Gallbladder tumors are not related to periamullary tumors. Periamullary tumors originate from structures near the ampulla of Vater, such as the pancreas, ampulla of Vater, distal common bile duct, or duodenum.

3. A 70-year-old patient is diagnosed with a primary ampullary tumor. Understanding its biological behavior is important. Which statement about primary ampullary tumors' biological behavior is incorrect?

A. Primary ampullary tumors are rare.
B. They have a better prognosis than periampullary malignancies of pancreatic or extrahepatic biliary origin.
C. Histology resembles that of adenomas and adenocarcinomas of intestinal origin rather than pancreaticobiliary origin.
D. The average age at diagnosis of sporadic ampullary carcinomas is 60 to 70 years old.
E. No genetic component is observed in these tumors.

Answer: E

Explanation: K-ras mutations are an early event in ampullary carcinogenesis, with an incidence (37 percent) that is similar to that in colon cancer (up to 50%).

4. A 55-year-old patient with a history of smoking and alcoholism presents with suspected pancreatic cancer. Understanding risk factors is crucial. Which of the following is not a risk factor for pancreatic cancer?

A. Smoking.
B. Insulin resistance.
C. Aspirin use.
D. Heavy alcoholism.
E. Chronic pancreatitis.

Answer: C

Explanation: Studies of other large cohorts have not found any link between aspirin use and higher pancreatic cancer risk, even among individuals using aspirin ≥30 times monthly for over 20 years.

5. A patient presents with symptoms suggestive of pancreatic exocrine tumors, and understanding the symptomatology is crucial. Which statement about the symptomatology of pancreatic exocrine tumors is incorrect?

A. Jaundice is a relatively early sign in tumors arising from the pancreatic head.
B. Jaundice is present in about 90% of cases.
C. Abdominal pain is very frequent, with a gnawing visceral quality even with small tumors less than 2 cm.
D. Weight loss is a very well-recognized symptom.
E. The initial presentation of pancreatic cancer varies according to tumor location.

Answer: B

Explanation: Jaundice is present in only about half of the cases (56%).

6. A 55-year-old patient presents with clinical manifestations suggestive of ampullary cancer. Accurate knowledge of these manifestations is critical. Which statement about the clinical manifestations of ampullary cancers is incorrect?

A. The most common presenting symptom of ampullary carcinoma is weight loss.
B. Jaundice is less likely to be a clinical manifestation of ampullary cancer than periampullary tumors.
C. Ampullary cancers may present with steatorrhea, diarrhea, and mild weight loss.
D. Large lesions may produce gastric outlet obstruction associated with severe nausea and vomiting.
E. Nonspecific symptoms such as abdominal pain and fever are somewhat frequent.

Answer: A

Explanation: The most common presenting symptom of ampullary carcinoma is obstructive jaundice.

7. A 60-year-old patient presents with a pancreatic tumor. Histopathological evaluation is crucial for diagnosis. Which statement about pancreatic ductal adenocarcinoma pathology is incorrect?

A. Poorly circumscribed gray-white hard gritty lesions.
B. Arises most commonly in the pancreatic body.
C. Although named ductal, mostly not originating in the main duct or branched duct but in the small ducts of acinar tissues.
D. Most pancreatic ductal adenocarcinomas are moderately to poorly differentiated.
E. Extension typically involves adjacent structures and shows a striking tendency toward perineural invasion.

Answer: B

Explanation: Pancreatic ductal adenocarcinoma usually arises in the head of the pancreas, with a head to body/tail ratio of 3:1.

8. A patient presents with a pancreatic tumor, and identifying the key features is essential. Which statement about pancreatic tumors and their key features is incorrect?

A. Serous cystadenoma—older female, pancreatic body.
B. Intraductal tubulopapillary neoplasm—old age, solid tumors.
C. Mucinous cystic neoplasm—cystic, body/tail of pancreas.
D. Solid pseudopapillary neoplasms—young age females less than 20 years.
E. IMPN—young age female, solid.

Answer: B

Explanation: Intraductal papillary mucinous neoplasms (IPMN) are cystic neoplasms that are clearly derived from the pancreatic ducts. They typically occur in older adults (mean age approximately 65 years).

9. A patient is diagnosed with a pancreatic neuroendocrine tumor (NET), and understanding its characteristics is crucial. Which statement about pancreatic NETs is incorrect?

A. Could be functional and nonfunctional.
B. Functional pancreatic NETs are usually well-differentiated.
C. Usually have a worse prognosis than pancreatic exocrine tumors.
D. Have an increasing incidence because of advances in imaging and endoscopy.
E. Pancreatic NETs represent less than 3% of primary pancreatic neoplasms.

Answer: C

Explanation: Pancreatic NETs generally have a better prognosis than pancreatic exocrine tumors.

10. A 65-year-old patient is diagnosed with an ampullary neoplasm. Understanding the histology and biological behavior of these tumors is crucial. Which statement about ampullary and periampullary neoplasms is incorrect?

A. Ampullary carcinomas are thought to arise from ampullary adenomas, a premalignant precursor lesion displaying the adenoma-carcinoma sequence.
B. Ampullary tumors usually have a worse prognosis than periampullary tumors and pancreaticobiliary tumors.
C. The histology of primary ampullary neoplasms more often resembles that of adenomas and adenocarcinomas of intestinal origin rather than pancreaticobiliary origin.
D. The average age at diagnosis of sporadic ampullary carcinomas is 60 to 70 years old.
E. Ampullary carcinomas arise in the setting of an inherited polyposis syndrome, usually present at an earlier age.

Answer: B

Explanation: Ampullary tumors usually have a better prognosis than periampullary tumors and pancreaticobiliary tumors.

11. A patient has been diagnosed with exocrine pancreatic cancer, and genetic assessment is essential. Which statement about the molecular pathogenesis of exocrine pancreatic cancer is incorrect?

    A. All patients diagnosed with pancreatic cancer should undergo assessment of their risk of a familial predisposition to cancer with a detailed personal and family cancer history.
    B. BRCA1, as well as BRCA2 mutations, have the potential for an increased risk of pancreatic cancer.
    C. Up to 20% of patients with pancreatic cancer have germline mutations in known cancer predisposition syndromes.
    D. Both FAP and HNPCC have an increased risk of developing pancreatic cancer.
    E. Testing and gene profiling of tumor tissue (i.e., with next-generation sequencing) should be undertaken as quickly as possible after diagnosis.

    Answer: B

    Explanation: BRCA2 mutations, but not BRCA1 mutations, have the potential for an increased risk of pancreatic cancer.

12. A patient is diagnosed with serous cystadenoma in the pancreas. Understanding its characteristics is crucial. Which statement about serous cystadenoma is incorrect?

    A. It is the most common benign pancreatic tumor.
    B. It arises from the pancreatic exocrine portion.
    C. It can be reliably cured with surgical removal alone.
    D. Based on imaging alone, the benign nature can be confirmed with certainty.
    E. It has a premalignant potential.

    Answer: E

    Explanation: Serous adenomas are benign lesions in the pancreas and do not have a malignant potential.

13. A patient is diagnosed with a pancreatic tumor, and understanding its pathology is essential. Which statement about pancreatic tumors' pathology is incorrect?

    A. Exocrine pancreatic tumors are the majority.
    B. Ductal adenocarcinoma comprises 85% of all pancreatic exocrine tumors.
    C. Neuroendocrine tumors (NETs) account for less than 5% of pancreatic tumors.
    D. Colloid carcinoma is a subtype of endocrine pancreatic tumors.
    E. Adenosquamous carcinoma has the poorest prognosis among pancreatic ductal adenocarcinoma subtypes.

    Answer: D

    Explanation: Colloid carcinoma is a subtype of exocrine pancreatic tumors.

14. A 60-year-old patient is being evaluated for suspected pancreatic cancer. Proper staging workup is essential to determine resectability. Which statement regarding the staging workup of pancreatic cancer is incorrect?

    A. CT abdomen and pelvis with IV contrast and triphasic study is the gold standard modality for proper preoperative locoregional staging and assessment of resectability.
    B. Routine staging chest CT for patients suspected of having pancreatic cancer who have no symptoms to suggest pulmonary metastases is not recommended.
    C. Routine use of PET/CT for staging of pancreatic cancer is advisable.
    D. EUS-guided fine needle aspiration biopsy (FNAB) is the best modality for obtaining a tissue diagnosis.
    E. Up to one-third of patients thought to be resectable by state-of-the-art imaging will be found to be unresectable based upon laparoscopic findings.

    Answer: C

    Explanation: Routine use of PET/CT for staging of pancreatic cancer is not recommended.

15. A 70-year-old patient presents with symptoms suggestive of pancreatic cancer. Understanding the differential diagnosis is essential for accurate diagnosis. Which statement about the differential diagnosis of pancreatic cancer is incorrect?

    A. There is a large list of differentials for pancreatic cancer because the symptoms are nonspecific.
    B. A solid pancreatic lesion is uncommonly found as an incidental finding on CT scans done for another reason.
    C. The positive predictive value (PPV) of jaundice, abdominal pain, and abdominal mass for the diagnosis of pancreatic cancer is low, with the possible exception of jaundice in an older patient.
    D. The most common primary sites for pancreatic metastases are renal cell carcinoma and melanoma.
    E. Differentiating a primary exocrine pancreatic carcinoma from other less common periampullary malignancies is straightforward.

    Answer: E

    Explanation: Differentiating a primary exocrine pancreatic carcinoma from other less common periampullary malignancies can be challenging.

16. A 58-year-old patient presents with symptoms suggestive of pancreatic cancer. Diagnostic imaging is crucial for further evaluation. Which statement about pancreatic cancer imaging modalities is incorrect?

    A. For patients with jaundice, the initial imaging study is often transabdominal ultrasound (US).

B. If a pancreatic mass is seen on transabdominal US, an abdominal CT scan is typically next obtained to confirm the presence of the mass and to assess disease extent.
C. If a pancreatic cancer is suspected, a “pancreatic protocol” (i.e., multiphase contrast-enhanced, helical) CT of the abdomen and pelvis is warranted.
D. Oral contrast is mandatory for proper preoperative assessment of respectability.
E. MRI has similar sensitivity and specificity to CT scan regarding the identification of the mass and metastatic spread.

Answer: D

Explanation: CT abdomen and pelvis with IV contrast and triphasic study is the protocol of choice for locoregional staging of pancreatic cancers. There is no need for oral contrast in preoperative settings.

17. A 63-year-old patient is being evaluated for suspected pancreatic cancer. A precise diagnostic approach is crucial for accurate diagnosis and management. Which statement regarding the diagnostic approach for pancreatic cancer is incorrect?

A. CA 19-9 level sensitivity is not affected by tumor size.
B. A typical finding on imaging is satisfactory before proceeding to surgery if resectability is eligible.
C. Pancreatic biopsy is usually done by FNA/cytology if histological confirmation is needed in atypical cases of irresectable tumors.
D. Endoscopic US can be used for locoregional staging as an alternative to CT scan.
E. ERCP is indicated if biliary decompression is needed.

Answer: A

Explanation: CA 19-9 level sensitivity is limited for small lesions.

18. A 56-year-old patient with a pancreatic mass requires histological confirmation. Choosing the appropriate biopsy method is essential. Which statement about pancreatic mass FNA/tru-cut biopsy is incorrect?

A. Percutaneous FNA biopsy of the pancreas may disseminate tumor cells intraperitoneally or along the needle path.
B. FNA/tru-cut biopsy of pancreatic masses is dependent on tumor size and operator expertise, with sensitivity reaching more than 85%.
C. FNA/biopsy is indicated in cases when histological confirmation is needed but resectability is not amenable.
D. EUS-guided FNA is the preferred modality for obtaining a tissue diagnosis.
E. If FNA specimens are inadequate or nondiagnostic, EUS-guided fine needle (core) biopsy may be considered.

Answer: A

Explanation: The risk that percutaneous FNA biopsy of the pancreas may disseminate tumor cells intraperitoneally or along the needle path is only theoretical and quite low or absent.

19. A 60-year-old patient is undergoing evaluation for pancreatic cancer. The medical team is assessing the extent of the disease to determine whether it is advanced and incurable. Which of the following statements regarding signs of advanced and incurable pancreatic cancer is incorrect?

    A. Liver metastases are a sign of advanced pancreatic cancer.
    B. Ascites is indicative of advanced disease.
    C. Presence of an abdominal mass suggests advanced pancreatic cancer.
    D. Supraclavicular lymph nodes involvement indicates advanced disease.
    E. Jaundice is a sign of advanced and incurable pancreatic cancer.

    Answer: E

    Explanation: Jaundice is a relatively early sign of pancreatic tumors, often caused by the obstruction of the bile duct by the tumor. It does not necessarily indicate advanced or incurable disease, unlike the other signs listed.

20. A 64-year-old patient with pancreatic cancer is evaluated for resectability. Which of the following features is incorrect indicative of irresectable disease?

    A. Encasement of SMA by more than 180°.
    B. Inseparability from adjacent organs (e.g., spleen).
    C. Short segment of vascular venous involvement.
    D. Metastases to lymph nodes beyond the peripancreatic region.
    E. SMA thrombosis.

    Answer: C

    Explanation: If venous occlusion is present, a suitable segment of portal vein (above) and SMV (below the site of venous involvement) must be present to allow for venous reconstruction. However, in most centers, surgery will be preceded by some form of neoadjuvant treatment for patients with venous occlusion.

21. A 59-year-old patient presents with obstructive jaundice, and ampullary carcinoma is suspected. Select the incorrect statement regarding the diagnostic workup for ampullary carcinoma.

    A. A transabdominal ultrasound is a reasonable first test in patients presenting with obstructive jaundice.
    B. ERCP is the preferred modality for diagnosis.
    C. It may be difficult to completely exclude carcinoma on endoscopic findings alone.
    D. Contrast-enhanced CT scan is the most accurate modality available to assess the T stage of ampullary tumors.

E. MRCP is indicated if the patient cannot tolerate invasive procedures or there is obstruction that limits cannulation of pancreaticobiliary channels.

Answer: D

Explanation: EUS is the most accurate modality available to assess the T stage of ampullary tumors, although it is not done routinely.

22. A 58-year-old patient is diagnosed with pancreatic adenocarcinoma, and the management plan is being discussed. Choose the incorrect statement regarding the management of pancreatic cancer.

A. Surgical resection is the only potentially curative treatment for pancreatic adenocarcinoma.
B. Forty percent of patients are candidates for pancreatectomy.
C. Patients with borderline resectable or locally advanced unresectable pancreatic cancer, but no metastatic disease, are potential candidates for downstaging with neoadjuvant therapy.
D. Neoadjuvant therapy is increasingly considered an acceptable option for patients with potentially resectable pancreatic cancer.
E. Encasement (more than one-half of the vessel circumference) is an absolute contraindication for surgery.

Answer: B

Explanation: Unfortunately, because of the late presentation, only 15 to 20 percent of patients are candidates for pancreatectomy. Although uncommon, some patients with initially unresectable or borderline resectable disease may be downstaged to resectable disease with neoadjuvant treatment.

23. A 65-year-old patient is scheduled for a Whipple procedure due to pancreatic cancer. Which statement regarding the conventional Whipple procedure is incorrect?

A. Removal of the entire pancreas.
B. Removal of the gallbladder and common bile duct.
C. Partial gastrectomy.
D. Duodenectomy.
E. Removal of the first 15 cm of the jejunum.

Answer: A

Explanation: Conventional Whipple procedure includes the removal of the head of the pancreas and not the entire pancreas.

24. A 62-year-old patient with pancreatic cancer is discussing treatment options. Identify the incorrect statement about pancreaticoduodenectomy (Whipple procedure).

A. It is the only curative treatment for pancreatic cancer cases.
B. Extended lymphadenectomy, when performed, is superior to conventional lymphadenectomy.

C. Pylorus-preserving pancreaticoduodenectomy has the same results as pylorectomy.
D. Vascular resection and reconstruction at the time of pancreaticoduodenectomy is controversial.
E. Minimally invasive (laparoscopic, robotic-assisted) pancreaticoduodenectomy is technically feasible.

Answer: B

Explanation: The evidence to support a benefit from extended lymphadenectomy is conflicting, with some trials suggesting benefit limited to the setting of positive nodes, others suggesting no survival benefit in any subgroup, and two suggesting worse quality of life following extended lymphadenectomy.

25. A 58-year-old man with a history of type 2 diabetes and chronic pancreatitis presents with jaundice, weight loss, and abdominal pain radiating to the back. Imaging studies suggest a mass at the head of the pancreas, and further evaluation including biopsy confirms adenocarcinoma. The patient undergoes a pancreaticoduodenectomy (Whipple procedure). Postoperatively, the surgical team discusses the prognosis and future management with the patient and his family. Which of the following statements regarding the outcomes of Whipple procedure is incorrect?

A. The prognosis of cases remains poor even with negative surgical margins.
B. Newer multiagent adjuvant chemotherapy regimens significantly increase both median and 5-year survival after surgical resection.
C. Perioperative mortality of pancreaticoduodenectomy in most modern series is less than 3%.
D. There is a significant association between hospital volume and postoperative mortality.
E. There is improvement over time regarding outcomes of this procedure.

Answer: C

Explanation: In most modern series, the perioperative mortality of pancreaticoduodenectomy (Whipple procedure) is less than 3%, not 25%. This procedure has seen improvements in outcomes over time, and there is indeed a significant association between hospital volume and postoperative mortality in pancreaticoduodenectomy cases. However, it's important to note that even with negative surgical margins, the prognosis for patients undergoing this procedure can still be poor due to the aggressive nature of pancreatic cancer. The use of newer multiagent adjuvant chemotherapy regimens has also shown promise in increasing survival rates after surgical resection.

26. A 64-year-old patient presents with a tumor located in the body of the pancreas. Which statement regarding pancreatic body/tail tumors is incorrect?

A. The majority have locally advanced or metastatic disease at the time of presentation.

B. Usually, they do not cause obstruction of the intrapancreatic portion of the common bile duct.
C. They have a worse prognosis compared to those with cancers involving the head of the pancreas.
D. Surgical resection consists of total pancreatectomy, usually combined with splenectomy.
E. Most commonly include ductal adenocarcinoma.

Answer: D

Explanation: Surgical resection of cancers located in the body or tail of the pancreas consists of a distal subtotal pancreatectomy, usually combined with splenectomy.

27. A 60-year-old patient is scheduled for pancreatic cancer resection surgery. Which statement regarding perioperative care is incorrect?

A. Biliary decompression/drainage is advised if bilirubin >250 μmol/L.
B. Oral bowel preparation is recommended.
C. Nasogastric tube does not improve outcomes and is not recommended routinely.
D. Early removal of the drain after 72 h in patients with a low risk of developing pancreatic fistula.
E. Removal of the urinary catheter is advised on the first postoperative day, along with early mobilization.

Answer: B

Explanation: Oral bowel preparations are not needed for pancreatic cancer resection procedures.

28. A 68-year-old man with a recent diagnosis of pancreatic cancer is being evaluated for treatment options. The tumor is located in the head of the pancreas and appears to be borderline resectable on imaging. The patient has a good performance status with manageable comorbidities. In the context of treatment decision-making for pancreatic cancer, which of the following statements is incorrect?

A. The decision to pursue surgery for pancreatic cancer should be based on a comprehensive assessment, including but not limited to the stage of the disease.
B. The patient's performance status and comorbidities are critical factors in determining eligibility for surgical intervention.
C. Neoadjuvant chemotherapy is the preferred approach for managing borderline resectable pancreatic tumors to potentially increase the chances of a successful resection.
D. For patients with locally advanced unresectable pancreatic cancer, palliative chemotherapy can be offered to manage symptoms and potentially improve survival.
E. Engaging in multidisciplinary tumor board discussions is crucial for formulating a comprehensive and individualized treatment plan for pancreatic cancer patients.

Answer: A

Explanation: The decision to pursue surgery for pancreatic cancer should not be based solely on the stage of the disease. It is essential to consider a variety of factors, including the patient's performance status, comorbidities, and the tumor's resectability. Neoadjuvant chemotherapy is often recommended for borderline resectable tumors to potentially increase the chances of successful surgery. For locally advanced unresectable disease, palliative chemotherapy is an option to improve quality of life and survival. Multidisciplinary tumor board discussions are essential in planning the treatment approach for pancreatic cancer patients.

29. A 52-year-old woman with a strong family history of pancreatic cancer is being evaluated for her risk of developing the disease. Her mother and maternal uncle were diagnosed with pancreatic cancer in their 60s. She is considering genetic counseling and testing. In the context of pancreatic cancer and genetic risk factors, which of the following statements is incorrect?

    A. Individuals with a family history of pancreatic cancer have no increased risk of developing the disease compared to the general population.
    B. Mutations in BRCA1 and BRCA2 genes are associated with an elevated risk of pancreatic cancer.
    C. Hereditary pancreatitis, a genetic condition, significantly increases the risk of developing pancreatic cancer over time.
    D. Patients with Lynch syndrome (hereditary nonpolyposis colorectal cancer, HNPCC) are at an increased risk of pancreatic cancer.
    E. Genetic counseling and testing are recommended for individuals with a strong family history of pancreatic cancer to assess their risk and guide screening strategies.

    Answer: A

    Explanation: Individuals with a family history of pancreatic cancer do have an increased risk of developing the disease. Genetic factors such as mutations in BRCA1, BRCA2, and genes associated with hereditary pancreatitis and Lynch syndrome can significantly elevate the risk of pancreatic cancer. Therefore, genetic counseling and testing are important for individuals with a strong family history of the disease to identify potential genetic risks and inform appropriate screening and preventive measures.

30. A 64-year-old man undergoes a pancreaticoduodenectomy (Whipple procedure) for pancreatic adenocarcinoma. Postoperatively, he is closely monitored for potential complications associated with the surgery. In the context of pancreatic cancer treatment-related complications, which of the following statements is incorrect?

    A. Whipple procedure is associated with a low risk of postoperative pancreatic fistula.

B. Delayed gastric emptying is a frequent complication following pancreatic surgery and can impact patient recovery and nutrition.
C. Pancreatic exocrine insufficiency is a common consequence of pancreatic resection, often necessitating enzyme replacement therapy to aid digestion.
D. Anastomotic leakage at the surgical site is a serious complication of pancreatic surgery that can lead to significant morbidity.
E. Biliary stricture can occur as a complication after pancreaticoduodenectomy, necessitating endoscopic or surgical intervention for management.

Answer: A

Explanation: Pancreaticoduodenectomy (Whipple procedure) is a complex surgical procedure associated with a significant risk of postoperative complications. One of the most common complications is the development of a postoperative pancreatic fistula, which occurs when there is a leak of pancreatic fluid from the surgical site. This is a well-recognized risk and is not considered a low-risk complication. Delayed gastric emptying, pancreatic exocrine insufficiency, anastomotic leakage, and biliary stricture are other potential complications that can occur following pancreatic surgery and require careful management to optimize patient outcomes.

31. A 70-year-old woman with metastatic pancreatic cancer is experiencing significant pain and a decrease in quality of life. The oncology team is discussing the integration of palliative care into her treatment plan. In the context of palliative care in pancreatic cancer, which of the following statements is incorrect?

A. Palliative care should be initiated only in the terminal stages of pancreatic cancer when other treatments are no longer effective.
B. Palliative care encompasses a holistic approach, including symptom management, psychological support, and end-of-life care.
C. Integrating palliative care alongside active cancer treatment from the time of diagnosis can improve the patient's quality of life and overall well-being.
D. Effective symptom control and pain management are central components of palliative care, aiming to alleviate the patient's suffering.
E. The palliative care team is multidisciplinary, consisting of healthcare professionals such as palliative care physicians, nurses, social workers, and chaplains.

Answer: A

Explanation: Palliative care is not limited to the terminal stages of pancreatic cancer but can be integrated alongside active cancer treatment from the time of diagnosis. It aims to improve the quality of life for patients by addressing physical symptoms, emotional and spiritual needs, and providing support for both patients and their families. The multidisciplinary palliative care team works collaboratively to provide comprehensive care throughout the course of the illness.

32. A 72-year-old man with locally advanced pancreatic cancer is experiencing obstructive jaundice and gastric outlet obstruction. The surgical oncology team is considering palliative surgical options to alleviate his symptoms. In the context of palliative surgery in pancreatic cancer, which of the following statements is incorrect?

   A. Palliative surgery is often performed with the primary goal of achieving curative intent in patients with locally advanced pancreatic cancer.
   B. Various techniques can be utilized for palliative bypass surgery to alleviate obstructive jaundice, including biliary bypass or endoscopic stent placement.
   C. The primary aim of palliative surgery in pancreatic cancer is to relieve symptoms and enhance the patient's quality of life.
   D. Surgical gastrojejunostomy is a palliative option for relieving gastric outlet obstruction in patients with pancreatic cancer.
   E. In cases of unresectable pancreatic cancer, palliative surgical procedures such as cholecystostomy or hepaticojejunostomy may be considered to manage symptoms.

   Answer: A

   Explanation: Palliative surgery in pancreatic cancer is not typically performed with curative intent, especially in patients with locally advanced disease. Instead, the primary goal of palliative surgery is to alleviate symptoms such as obstructive jaundice or gastric outlet obstruction and improve the patient's quality of life. Techniques like biliary bypass or stent placement, gastrojejunostomy, cholecystostomy, and hepaticojejunostomy are aimed at symptom relief rather than curing the disease.

33. A 66-year-old woman with borderline resectable pancreatic cancer has completed neoadjuvant chemotherapy. The multidisciplinary team is discussing the potential role of CRT in her treatment plan. In the context of CRT in pancreatic cancer, which of the following statements is incorrect?

   A. CRT is routinely used as the initial treatment modality for all stages of pancreatic cancer.
   B. CRT may be considered for patients with borderline resectable disease after completion of neoadjuvant therapy to enhance the chances of successful resection.
   C. For locally advanced unresectable pancreatic cancer, CRT can be utilized to control disease progression and alleviate symptoms.
   D. Intensity-modulated radiation therapy is a technique that allows for more precise delivery of radiation to the tumor, minimizing exposure to surrounding healthy tissue.
   E. In certain cases, CRT may be combined with systemic chemotherapy to improve treatment efficacy and patient outcomes.

Answer: A

Explanation: CRT is not commonly used as the initial treatment for all patients with pancreatic cancer. It is typically considered for specific stages and situations, such as locally advanced unresectable disease or after neoadjuvant therapy.

34. A 59-year-old man with metastatic pancreatic cancer is being evaluated for potential treatment options. The oncology team is discussing the role of immunotherapy in his treatment plan, considering his advanced stage of disease. In the context of pancreatic cancer immunotherapy, which of the following statements is incorrect?

    A. Immunotherapy has demonstrated significant efficacy in treating all stages of pancreatic cancer, revolutionizing the treatment landscape.
    B. Clinical trials have investigated the use of checkpoint inhibitors targeting PD-1/PD-L1 in pancreatic cancer.
    C. Combination therapies involving immunotherapy and chemotherapy are being explored to enhance treatment efficacy.
    D. For certain patients with advanced pancreatic cancer, immunotherapy may be considered as a potential treatment option.
    E. Ongoing research in pancreatic cancer immunotherapy aims to identify new strategies and improve patient outcomes.

    Answer: A

    Explanation: While immunotherapy holds promise in the treatment of pancreatic cancer, it has not shown significant efficacy in treating all stages of the disease. Its role is still being explored in clinical trials and research.

35. A 65-year-old woman with unresectable pancreatic cancer is experiencing severe pain, jaundice, and ascites. The oncology team is discussing various palliative therapy options to manage her symptoms and improve her quality of life. In the context of palliative therapy for pancreatic cancer cases, which of the following statements is incorrect?

    A. Celiac plexus block is often preferred over radiation therapy for pain relief, as it generally provides faster relief from pain.
    B. Palliation of jaundice in patients with unresectable pancreatic cancer is typically achieved through endoscopic stenting rather than palliative radiation therapy.
    C. Management of ascites may involve intermittent paracentesis or the placement of a long-term drainage catheter to relieve discomfort.
    D. All patients with locally advanced or metastatic pancreatic cancer should be referred for a consultation with a nutritionist and/or dietician to address nutritional needs and support.
    E. Pancreatic cancer cases are not associated with an increased risk of developing VTE.

Answer: E

Explanation: Patients with pancreatic cancer have an increased risk of developing VTE due to factors like tumor-related hypercoagulability. Education about VTE symptoms and prophylactic measures are important in managing these cases.

Bibliography

1. Siegel RL, Miller KD, Wagle NS, Jemal A. Cancer statistics, 2023. CA Cancer J Clin. 2023;73(1):17–48.
2. Wellner UF, Bolm L, Vladimirov M, Keck T. Präoperative Diagnostik bei periampullären Adenokarzinomen [Preoperative diagnostics in periampullary adenocarcinomas]. Chirurg. 2021;92(9):771–5. German. https://doi.org/10.1007/s00104-021-01452-3.
3. Ahn DH, Bekaii-Saab T. Ampullary cancer: an overview. Am Soc Clin Oncol Educ Book. 2014:112–5. https://doi.org/10.14694/EdBook_AM.2014.34.112.
4. Jacobs EJ, Connell CJ, Rodriguez C, Patel AV, Calle EE, Thun MJ. Aspirin use and pancreatic cancer mortality in a large United States cohort. J Natl Cancer Inst. 2004;96(7):524–8. https://doi.org/10.1093/jnci/djh084.
5. Holly EA, Chaliha I, Bracci PM, Gautam M. Signs and symptoms of pancreatic cancer: a population-based case-control study in the San Francisco Bay area. Clin Gastroenterol Hepatol. 2004;2(6):510–7. https://doi.org/10.1016/s1542-3565(04)00171-5.
6. Zheng-Pywell R, Reddy S. Ampullary cancer. Surg Clin North Am. 2019;99(2):357–67. https://doi.org/10.1016/j.suc.2018.12.001. Epub 2019 Feb 10
7. Haeberle L, Esposito I. Pathology of pancreatic cancer. Transl Gastroenterol Hepatol. 2019;4:50. https://doi.org/10.21037/tgh.2019.06.02.
8. Jabłońska B, Szmigiel P, Mrowiec S. Pancreatic intraductal papillary mucinous neoplasms: current diagnosis and management. World J Gastrointest Oncol. 2021;13(12):1880–95. https://doi.org/10.4251/wjgo.v13.i12.1880.
9. Ma ZY, Gong YF, Zhuang HK, Zhou ZX, Huang SZ, Zou YP, Huang BW, Sun ZH, Zhang CZ, Tang YQ, Hou BH. Pancreatic neuroendocrine tumors: a review of serum biomarkers, staging, and management. World J Gastroenterol. 2020;26(19):2305–22. https://doi.org/10.3748/wjg.v26.i19.2305.
10. Rizzo A, Dadduzio V, Lombardi L, Ricci AD, Gadaleta-Caldarola G. Ampullary carcinoma: an overview of a rare entity and discussion of current and future therapeutic challenges. Curr Oncol. 2021;28(5):3393–402. https://doi.org/10.3390/curroncol28050293. PMID: 34590592; PMCID: PMC8482111
11. Hruban RH, Canto MI, Griffin C, Kern SE, Klein AP, Laheru D, Yeo CJ. Treatment of familial pancreatic cancer and its precursors. Curr Treat Options Gastroenterol. 2005;8(5):365–75. https://doi.org/10.1007/s11938-005-0039-3.
12. Adsay NV, Pierson C, Sarkar F, Abrams J, Weaver D, Conlon KC, Brennan MF, Klimstra DS. Colloid (mucinous noncystic) carcinoma of the pancreas. Am J Surg Pathol. 2001;25(1):26–42. https://doi.org/10.1097/00000478-200101000-00003.
13. Maisonneuve P, Lowenfels AB. Risk factors for pancreatic cancer: a summary review of meta-analytical studies. Int J Epidemiol. 2015;44(1):186–98. https://doi.org/10.1093/ije/dyu240.
14. Ghaneh P, Hanson R, Titman A, Lancaster G, Plumpton C, Lloyd-Williams H, Yeo ST, Edwards RT, Johnson C, Abu Hilal M, Higginson AP, Armstrong T, Smith A, Scarsbrook A, McKay C, Carter R, Sutcliffe RP, Bramhall S, Kocher HM, Cunningham D, Pereira SP, Davidson B, Chang D, Khan S, Zealley I, Sarker D, Al Sarireh B, Charnley R, Lobo D, Nicolson M, Halloran C, Raraty M, Sutton R, Vinjamuri S, Evans J, Campbell F, Deeks J, Sanghera B, Wong WL, Neoptolemos JP. PET-PANC: multicentre prospective diagnostic accuracy and

health economic analysis study of the impact of combined modality 18fluorine-2-fluoro-2-deoxy-d-glucose positron emission tomography with computed tomography scanning in the diagnosis and management of pancreatic cancer. Health Technol Assess. 2018;22(7):1–114. https://doi.org/10.3310/hta22070. PMID: 29402376; PMCID: PMC5817411
15. Fargo MV, Grogan SP, Saguil A. Evaluation of jaundice in adults. Am Fam Physician. 2017;95(3):164–8.
16. Lee ES, Lee JM. Imaging diagnosis of pancreatic cancer: a state-of-the-art review. World J Gastroenterol. 2014;20(24):7864–77. https://doi.org/10.3748/wjg.v20.i24.7864. PMID: 24976723; PMCID: PMC4069314
17. Kiliç M, Göçmen E, Tez M, Ertan T, Keskek M, Koç M. Value of preoperative serum CA 19-9 levels in predicting resectability for pancreatic cancer. Can J Surg. 2006;49(4):241–4. PMID: 16948881; PMCID: PMC3207573
18. Johnson DE, Pendurthi TK, Balshem AM, Ross E, Litwin S, Eisenberg BL, Hoffman JP. Implications of fine-needle aspiration in patients with resectable pancreatic cancer. Am Surg. 1997;63(8):675–9. discussion 679-80
19. Bakkevold KE, Arnesjø B, Kambestad B. Carcinoma of the pancreas and papilla of Vater: presenting symptoms, signs, and diagnosis related to stage and tumour site. A prospective multicentre trial in 472 patients. Norwegian pancreatic cancer trial. Scand J Gastroenterol. 1992;27(4):317–25. https://doi.org/10.3109/00365529209000081.
20. Li H, Zeng MS, Zhou KR, Jin DY, Lou WH. Pancreatic adenocarcinoma: the different CT criteria for peripancreatic major arterial and venous invasion. J Comput Assist Tomogr. 2005;29(2):170–5. https://doi.org/10.1097/01.rct.0000155060.73107.83.
21. Mertz HR, Sechopoulos P, Delbeke D, Leach SD. EUS, PET, and CT scanning for evaluation of pancreatic adenocarcinoma. Gastrointest Endosc. 2000;52(3):367–71. https://doi.org/10.1067/mge.2000.107727.
22. Allen PJ, Kuk D, Castillo CF, Basturk O, Wolfgang CL, Cameron JL, Lillemoe KD, Ferrone CR, Morales-Oyarvide V, He J, Weiss MJ, Hruban RH, Gönen M, Klimstra DS, Mino-Kenudson M. Multi-institutional validation study of the American joint commission on cancer (8th edition) changes for T and N staging in patients with pancreatic adenocarcinoma. Ann Surg. 2017;265(1):185–91. https://doi.org/10.1097/SLA.0000000000001763. PMID: 27163957; PMCID: PMC5611666
23. Masiak-Segit W, Rawicz-Pruszyński K, Skórzewska M, Polkowski WP. Surgical treatment of pancreatic cancer. Pol Przegl Chir. 2018;90(2):45–53. https://doi.org/10.5604/01.3001.0011.7493.
24. Nimura Y, Nagino M, Takao S, Takada T, Miyazaki K, Kawarada Y, Miyagawa S, Yamaguchi A, Ishiyama S, Takeda Y, Sakoda K, Kinoshita T, Yasui K, Shimada H, Katoh H. Standard versus extended lymphadenectomy in radical pancreatoduodenectomy for ductal adenocarcinoma of the head of the pancreas: long-term results of a Japanese multicenter randomized controlled trial. J Hepatobiliary Pancreat Sci. 2012;19(3):230–41. https://doi.org/10.1007/s00534-011-0466-6.
25. Kneuertz PJ, Pitt HA, Bilimoria KY, Smiley JP, Cohen ME, Ko CY, Pawlik TM. Risk of morbidity and mortality following hepato-pancreato-biliary surgery. J Gastrointest Surg. 2012;16(9):1727–35. https://doi.org/10.1007/s11605-012-1938-y. Epub 2012 Jul 4
26. Egawa S, Okada T, Motoi F, Rikiyama T, Katayose Y, Unno M. Distal pancreatectomy (with video). J Hepatobiliary Pancreat Sci. 2012;19(2):135–40. https://doi.org/10.1007/s00534-011-0471-9.
27. Bozzetti F, Mariani L. Perioperative nutritional support of patients undergoing pancreatic surgery in the age of ERAS. Nutrition. 2014;30(11–12):1267–71. https://doi.org/10.1016/j.nut.2014.03.002. Epub 2014 Mar 14
28. Kinsella TJ, Seo Y, Willis J, Stellato TA, Siegel CT, Harpp D, Willson JK, Gibbons J, Sanabria JR, Hardacre JM, Schulak JP. The impact of resection margin status and postoperative CA19-9 levels on survival and patterns of recurrence after postoperative high-dose radiotherapy with 5-FU-based concurrent chemotherapy for resectable pancreatic cancer. Am J Clin Oncol. 2008;31(5):446–53. https://doi.org/10.1097/COC.0b013e318168f6c4.

29. Janssen QP, van Dam JL, Doppenberg D, Prakash LR, van Eijck CHJ, Jarnagin WR, O'Reilly EM, Paniccia A, Besselink MG, MHG K, Tzeng CD, Wei AC, Zureikat AH, Groot Koerkamp B, Trans-Atlantic Pancreatic Surgery (TAPS) Consortium. FOLFIRINOX as initial treatment for localized pancreatic adenocarcinoma: a retrospective analysis by the trans-Atlantic pancreatic surgery consortium. J Natl Cancer Inst. 2022;114(5):695–703. https://doi.org/10.1093/jnci/djac018. PMID: 35157075; PMCID: PMC9086789
30. Versteijne E, Suker M, Groothuis K, Akkermans-Vogelaar JM, Besselink MG, Bonsing BA, Buijsen J, Busch OR, Creemers GM, van Dam RM, Eskens FALM, Festen S, de Groot JWB, Groot Koerkamp B, de Hingh IH, Homs MYV, van Hooft JE, Kerver ED, SAC L, Neelis KJ, Nuyttens J, Paardekooper GMRM, Patijn GA, van der Sangen MJC, de Vos-Geelen J, Wilmink JW, Zwinderman AH, Punt CJ, van Eijck CH, van Tienhoven G, Dutch Pancreatic Cancer Group. Preoperative chemoradiotherapy versus immediate surgery for resectable and borderline resectable pancreatic cancer: results of the Dutch randomized phase III PREOPANC trial. J Clin Oncol. 2020;38(16):1763–73. https://doi.org/10.1200/JCO.19.02274. Epub 2020 Feb 27. PMID: 32105518; PMCID: PMC8265386
31. Tzeng CW, Fleming JB, Lee JE, Wang X, Pisters PW, Vauthey JN, Varadhachary G, Wolff RA, Katz MH. Yield of clinical and radiographic surveillance in patients with resected pancreatic adenocarcinoma following multimodal therapy. HPB (Oxford). 2012;14(6):365–72. https://doi.org/10.1111/j.1477-2574.2012.00445.x. Epub 2012 Feb 28. PMID: 22568412; PMCID: PMC3384860
32. Chu LC, Goggins MG, Fishman EK. Diagnosis and detection of pancreatic cancer. Cancer J. 2017;23(6):333–42. https://doi.org/10.1097/PPO.0000000000000290.
33. Seufferlein T, Bachet JB, Van Cutsem E, Rougier P, ESMO Guidelines Working Group. Pancreatic adenocarcinoma: ESMO-ESDO clinical practice guidelines for diagnosis, treatment and follow-up. Ann Oncol. 2012;23(Suppl 7):vii33-40. https://doi.org/10.1093/annonc/mds224.
34. Kim R, Chabot J, Saif MW. Adjuvant treatment for ampullary cancer. Highlights from the "2011 ASCO annual meeting". Chicago, IL, USA; June 3-7, 2011. JOP. 2011;12(4):362–3.
35. House MG, Choti MA. Palliative therapy for pancreatic/biliary cancer. Surg Clin North Am. 2005;85(2):359–71. https://doi.org/10.1016/j.suc.2005.01.022.

Chapter 14
Thyroid Cancers

Talib A. Majeed, Sajjad G. Al-Badri, Saleh Abdulkareem Saleh, and Aqeel Shakir Mahmood

1. A 45-year-old woman with a family history of thyroid cancer is being evaluated for potential risk factors. She has a history of obesity, has never smoked, and has no known exposure to radiation or harmful chemicals. In the context of thyroid cancer risk factors, which of the following statements is incorrect?
   A. Obesity is considered a risk factor for the development of thyroid cancer, with studies showing a positive association between body mass index and thyroid cancer risk.
   B. Smoking has been associated with a decreased risk of thyroid cancer, although the mechanism behind this association is not fully understood.
   C. A strong correlation between reproductive issues, such as menstrual irregularities or infertility, and the development of thyroid cancer has been consistently demonstrated in studies.
   D. Exposure to radiation, particularly during childhood, significantly increases the risk of malignancies arising from thyroid follicular cells.
   E. Exposure to the herbicide Agent Orange, used during the Vietnam War, has been linked to an increased risk of thyroid cancer among veterans.

   Answer: C

   Explanation: A strong correlation between reproductive issues and the development of thyroid cancer has been demonstrated in few studies.
2. A 55-year-old woman is being evaluated for a thyroid nodule discovered during a routine physical examination. She has no family history of thyroid cancer, and

T. A. Majeed
GIT and Liver Hospital, Medical City Baghdad, Baghdad, Iraq

S. G. Al-Badri · S. A. Saleh
College of Medicine, University of Baghdad, Baghdad, Iraq

A. S. Mahmood (✉)
Department of General Surgery, University of Baghdad, Baghdad, Iraq

A. S. Mahmood, A. Koulouris (eds.), *MCQs in General Surgical Oncology*,
https://doi.org/10.1007/978-3-031-65738-2_14

her medical history is unremarkable. The patient is concerned about her risk of thyroid cancer and seeks information from her healthcare provider. In the context of thyroid cancer risk factors and epidemiology, which of the following statements is incorrect?

A. Thyroid cancers accounted for approximately 2.3% of all new cancer diagnoses in recent years.
B. The incidence of thyroid cancer has increased more than threefold since the late twentieth century, with some attributing this rise to improved detection methods.
C. The incidence of thyroid cancer is approximately three times higher in women than in men, reflecting a gender disparity in risk.
D. Overdiagnosis of small, indolent papillary thyroid carcinomas (PTC) may contribute to the observed increase in thyroid cancer incidence.
E. The incidence of thyroid cancer peaks in individuals during their third and fourth decades of life, with a median age at diagnosis of around 50 years.

Answer: E

Explanation: While thyroid cancer incidence has indeed increased significantly since the late twentieth century, and there is a notable gender disparity in risk, the peak incidence of thyroid cancer occurs in the fifth and sixth decades of life, not the third and fourth. Overdiagnosis of small papillary thyroid carcinomas is a concern in the field, as it may contribute to the rising incidence without necessarily improving patient outcomes. The statement about the peak incidence of thyroid cancer occurring in the third and fourth decades of life is incorrect.

3. A 45-year-old woman presents to your clinic with a palpable thyroid nodule. After conducting an ultrasound, a 0.8 cm hypoechoic nodule is found in the right lobe of her thyroid gland. FNAB results are consistent with PTMC. Considering the management of PTMC, which of the following statements is incorrect?

A. They are considered to be T1 lesions.
B. PTMCs are 2 cm or more in diameter.
C. Up to 50% of all DTC diagnoses are PTMCs.
D. The disease-specific mortality rate for these carcinomas is under 1%.
E. PTMCs are reasonably managed through active surveillance (active monitoring), with follow-up every 6–12 months.

Answer: B

Explanation: PTMCs are 1 cm or less in diameter.

4. A 47-year-old woman presents with a rapidly growing, painless, solitary thyroid nodule. She also reports new-onset hoarseness. Physical examination reveals no other significant findings. The patient is concerned about the possibility of thyroid cancer. In the context of the presentation of thyroid carcinoma, which of the following statements is incorrect?

A. Rapid growth of a thyroid nodule is a concerning sign and can be indicative of malignancy.
B. Sudden onset of pain in a thyroid nodule is more strongly associated with inflammatory or benign conditions rather than malignancy.
C. New-onset hoarseness can be a significant sign of thyroid carcinoma, suggesting possible involvement of the recurrent laryngeal nerve.
D. Heat intolerance and palpitations are more commonly associated with hyperfunctioning benign thyroid nodules rather than malignant nodules.
E. Thyroid carcinoma most commonly presents as a painless, palpable, solitary thyroid nodule, often detected incidentally.

Answer: D

Explanation: Thyroid carcinoma typically presents as a painless, solitary thyroid nodule, and rapid growth or new-onset hoarseness can be concerning signs of malignancy. Sudden onset of pain is more commonly associated with benign conditions. While heat intolerance and palpitations are symptoms of hyperthyroidism, they are more likely to be associated with benign hyperfunctioning thyroid nodules rather than malignant nodules. Therefore, the statement that these symptoms suggest a malignant nodule is incorrect.

5. A 40-year-old woman undergoes a total thyroidectomy for papillary thyroid carcinoma. She is started on levothyroxine therapy for thyroid hormone replacement. Six months postoperatively, she returns for follow-up. Her serum thyroglobulin levels are undetectable, and she has no evidence of recurrent disease on imaging. Considering the postoperative management of thyroid carcinoma, which of the following statements is incorrect?

A. Patients are given thyroid replacement therapy with T4 (Synthroid) or triiodothyronine (T3, Cytomel).
B. Recombinant human TSH is not used for follow-up thyroid scanning.
C. Patients are maintained on thyroid suppression, usually monotherapy with levothyroxine (T4).
D. Patients are regularly monitored every 6–12 months with serial imaging and serum TG measurements.
E. Rising TSH level after thyroid ablation suggests recurrence.

Answer: E

Explanation: Rising TSH level after thyroid ablation suggests recurrence.

6. A 28-year-old female presents with a painless, slowly enlarging mass in her neck. She is euthyroid and has no significant past medical history. Ultrasound of the neck reveals a suspicious thyroid nodule, and FNAB is consistent with PTC. Which of the following statements regarding the clinical features of PTC is incorrect?

A. Most patients are euthyroid.
B. Present with a slow-growing painless mass in the neck.
C. Dysphagia, dyspnea, and dysphonia are developed in early disease.
D. LN metastases are common, especially in children and young adults.

E. Distant metastases are uncommon at initial presentation.

Answer: C

Explanation: Dysphagia, dyspnea, and dysphonia are not common in the early stages of PTC; these symptoms are typically associated with locally advanced or invasive disease. The patient's presentation with a painless neck mass and euthyroid status is characteristic of early-stage PTC.

7. A 34-year-old woman presents with a thyroid nodule detected during a routine physical examination. She has no symptoms of dysphagia, dyspnea, or dysphonia. Fine needle aspiration cytology (FNAC) confirms PTC. Which of the following statements regarding the clinical features and management of PTC is incorrect?

A. The most common site of distant metastasis is the brain.
B. Diagnosis is established by FNAC of the thyroid mass or lymph node.
C. During thyroidectomy, enlarged central neck nodes should be removed.
D. After complete neck ultrasound to evaluate the contralateral lobe should be done.
E. PTC has an excellent prognosis with a > 95% 10-year survival rate.

Answer: A

Explanation: The most common site of distant metastasis is the lung.

8. A 55-year-old man presents with a neck mass that has been gradually increasing in size over the past year. He reports no symptoms of dysphagia or dyspnea. On examination, a firm, non-tender nodule is palpated in the right lobe of the thyroid. FNAB results are consistent with FTC. Considering the management and characteristics of FTC, which of the following statements is incorrect?

A. Its prognosis can be influenced by factors like older age, male sex, and multifocal or bilateral disease.
B. The American Thyroid Association considers tumors with minor capsular or vascular invasion to be at low risk for recurrence.
C. Metastasis to the lungs and bones is significantly increased (approximately 20%).
D. Total thyroidectomy is recommended if the tumor diameter is over 6 cm.
E. Radioiodine scanning and ablation have become commonplace after thyroidectomy, for diagnosing and treating residual thyroid tissue.

Answer: D

Explanation: Total thyroidectomy is recommended if the tumor diameter is over 4 cm.

9. A 55-year-old woman is diagnosed with follicular thyroid carcinoma (FTC) after a thyroidectomy. The tumor shows capsular and vascular invasion on histopathological examination. She lives in a region with adequate dietary iodine intake. Genetic testing is being considered to guide further management. In the context of FTC, which of the following statements is incorrect?

A. Follicular carcinoma is the second most common type of thyroid malignancy, following papillary carcinoma.

B. The incidence of FTC is higher in regions with adequate dietary intake of iodine, whereas papillary carcinoma is more common in iodine-deficient areas.
C. Mutations in genes such as RAS and PAX8/PPARγ are associated with follicular carcinoma, whereas RET/PTC mutations are more commonly linked to papillary carcinoma.
D. Neoplastic cells in follicular carcinoma are resistant to thyroid-stimulating hormone (TSH), which impacts their iodine uptake and thyroglobulin production.
E. The distinction between follicular carcinoma and benign follicular adenomas is based on the presence of capsular and/or vascular invasion in the former.

Answer: D

Explanation: FTC is the second most common type of thyroid cancer and is more prevalent in areas with sufficient dietary iodine. It is associated with genetic mutations, particularly in the RAS gene and the PAX8/PPARγ fusion gene. Neoplastic cells in follicular carcinoma are sensitive to TSH, which allows them to take up iodine and produce thyroglobulin, a feature used in both diagnosis and treatment. The presence of capsular and/or vascular invasion distinguishes follicular carcinoma from benign follicular adenomas. Therefore, the statement that neoplastic cells are TSH-resistant is incorrect.

10. A 38-year-old woman presents with a palpable thyroid nodule. FNAB confirms the diagnosis of PTC. She has no history of radiation exposure but is concerned about the implications of her diagnosis. In the context of PTC, which of the following statements is incorrect?

A. PTC is the most common type of thyroid malignancy, accounting for approximately 80% of all thyroid cancers.
B. PTC originates from parafollicular cells, also known as C cells, which are responsible for calcitonin production.
C. The incidence of PTC is approximately three times higher in women than in men, reflecting a gender disparity in risk.
D. A history of radiation exposure, particularly during childhood, is a well-established risk factor for the development of PTC.
E. Psammoma bodies, which are concentrically calcified structures, are found in about 50% of PTC cases and are considered a characteristic histologic feature.

Answer: B

Explanation: PTC is indeed the most common type of thyroid cancer and has a higher incidence in women. It is associated with a history of radiation exposure. Psammoma bodies are a characteristic feature found in many cases of PTC. However, PTC arises from follicular cells, not parafollicular cells. Parafollicular cells are responsible for producing calcitonin and are associated with medullary thyroid carcinoma (MTC), not PTC. Therefore, the statement that PTC originates from parafollicular cells is incorrect.

11. A 53-year-old woman presents with a solitary thyroid nodule. FNAB is inconclusive, and she undergoes a lobectomy. Histopathology reveals FTC. She is concerned about the nature of her diagnosis and its implications. In the context of FTC, which of the following statements is incorrect?

    A. FTC is the second most common type of thyroid malignancy, following papillary carcinoma.
    B. The incidence of follicular carcinoma is higher in men, occurring three times more frequently than in women.
    C. The neoplastic cells in follicular carcinoma are sensitive to TSH, which can influence their growth and function.
    D. Mutations in the RAS gene are commonly linked to the development of FTC.
    E. Unlike papillary thyroid carcinoma, FTC does not exhibit characteristic nuclear features such as Orphan Annie eye nuclei or psammoma bodies.

    Answer: B

    Explanation: FTC is indeed the second most common type of thyroid cancer. It is characterized by its TSH sensitivity and is often associated with RAS gene mutations. Unlike papillary thyroid carcinoma, it lacks specific nuclear features. However, the incidence of follicular carcinoma is higher in women, not men, with a female-to-male ratio of approximately 3:1. Therefore, the statement that follicular carcinoma occurs three times more frequently in men than in women is incorrect.

12. A 40-year-old woman is being evaluated for a thyroid nodule discovered during a routine physical examination. She has a history of radiation therapy to the neck region for Hodgkin's lymphoma at the age of 25. The patient is concerned about her risk of thyroid cancer due to her past radiation exposure. In the context of radiation exposure and thyroid cancer risk, which of the following statements is incorrect?

    A. Radiation exposure, particularly during childhood, significantly increases the risk for PTC.
    B. The risk of thyroid cancer rises in individuals exposed to a mean dose of over 0.05–0.1 Gy (50–100 mGy) of radiation.
    C. The risk of developing thyroid cancer decreases with increasing age at the time of radiation exposure.
    D. The risk of thyroid cancer is highest approximately 1–2 years after radiation exposure.
    E. Low-dose radiation exposure from diagnostic imaging studies has not been conclusively linked to an increased risk of thyroid cancer.

    Answer: D

    Explanation: Radiation exposure is a well-established risk factor for thyroid cancer, particularly papillary thyroid carcinoma (PTC). The risk is dose-dependent and is higher in individuals exposed to radiation doses over 0.05–0.1 Gy. The risk decreases with increasing age at exposure. However, the risk of thyroid cancer is not highest 1–2 years after radiation exposure; instead, it typically peaks several years to decades later. Low-dose radiation exposure from diagnostic imaging studies has not been conclusively linked to an increased risk of thyroid cancer, although ongoing research is evaluating this potential association.

13. A 50-year-old man presents with a palpable thyroid nodule discovered during a routine physical examination. He has no history of radiation exposure and no symptoms of hyperthyroidism. Neck ultrasonography is performed, and the nodule appears solid and hypoechoic. In the context of evaluating thyroid nodules, which of the following statements is incorrect?

    A. Neck ultrasonography is the primary imaging modality for evaluating thyroid nodules and guiding further management.
    B. Routine use of CT scan and MRI is not indicated in the initial workup of a solitary thyroid nodule, as ultrasonography provides sufficient detail for assessment.
    C. An autonomously functioning (i.e., hyperfunctioning) or "hot" nodule on a radionuclide thyroid scan is generally less likely to be malignant.
    D. The presence of carcinoma cannot be definitively excluded based solely on the results of a radioiodine scan.
    E. Not all thyroid nodules detected on ultrasonography require further evaluation with FNAB, as the decision is based on specific ultrasound features and clinical criteria.

    Answer: B

    Explanation: Neck ultrasonography is the cornerstone of thyroid nodule evaluation, providing detailed information on nodule characteristics and guiding the decision for FNAB based on established criteria. While CT scan and MRI can provide additional information in certain cases, they are not routinely used in the initial workup of a solitary thyroid nodule. An autonomously functioning "hot" nodule is generally less likely to be malignant, but carcinoma cannot be ruled out based on radioiodine scans alone. The decision to perform FNAB is based on a combination of ultrasound features and clinical risk factors.

14. A 40-year-old woman is diagnosed with a thyroid nodule following a routine physical examination. FNAB reveals PTC. She has no history of radiation exposure and no family history of thyroid cancer. In the context of DTC, which of the following statements is incorrect?

    A. Papillary thyroid carcinoma (PTC) is a slow-growing tumor that arises from follicular cells and is the most common type of thyroid cancer.
    B. Women are diagnosed with PTC approximately three times more frequently than men, reflecting a gender disparity in incidence.
    C. Follicular carcinoma, not PTC, is the most common type of thyroid malignancy, accounting for the majority of thyroid cancer cases.
    D. PTC is associated with a history of radiation exposure, particularly during childhood, which increases the risk of developing this type of cancer.

E. The presence of psammoma bodies, which are calcified structures, is a characteristic histologic feature of PTC.

Answer: C

Explanation: PTC is the most common type of thyroid cancer, accounting for approximately 80% of all thyroid malignancies. It is more prevalent in women and is associated with a history of radiation exposure. Follicular carcinoma is less common than PTC. The presence of psammoma bodies is a distinctive histologic feature of PTC. Therefore, the statement that follicular carcinoma is the most common thyroid malignancy is incorrect.

15. A 60-year-old woman presents with a palpable thyroid nodule. Ultrasound reveals a solitary, hypoechoic nodule in the left lobe of the thyroid. FNAB shows numerous Hürthle cells. Considering the characteristics and diagnosis of Hürthle cell carcinoma, which of the following statements is incorrect?

A. Differentiated from Hürthle cell adenoma by the presence of capsular invasion.
B. On gross evaluation, Hürthle cell carcinomas appear brown and solid.
C. Can be diagnosed with FNAB.
D. About 75–100% of the tumor is composed of oxyphilic, oncocytic, Askanazy, or large cells.
E. Can be found in benign thyroid conditions.

Answer: C

Explanation: Because Hürthle cell carcinoma is defined by capsular or vascular invasion, FNAB specimens alone cannot classify a tumor as malignant or benign.

16. A 45-year-old woman with a family history of thyroid cancer presents with a palpable thyroid nodule. She has a history of diarrhea and flushing episodes. FNAB of the nodule reveals MTC. Which of the following statements is incorrect regarding MTC?

A. Associated with multiple endocrine neoplasia (MEN) type 1 (MET1).
B. Tumors arise from the parafollicular C cells of the thyroid gland.
C. About 75–80% of MTCs develop sporadically, and 20–25% occur familially.
D. Familial cases are commonly multifocal throughout the thyroid gland.
E. Genetic testing is now the mainstay in the diagnosis of the familial medullary thyroid carcinoma (FMTC) syndromes.

Answer: A

Explanation: The FMTC syndromes consist of MEN 2A and MEN 2B.

17. A 30-year-old man presents with a painless thyroid mass and a family history of thyroid cancer. Genetic testing reveals a mutation associated with MEN type 2A. Which of the following statements regarding the diagnosis and symptoms of MTC is incorrect?

A. MTC in MEN 2A almost always develops by the age of 10 years.
B. Sporadic cases typically manifest with painless solitary thyroid nodules.
C. Genetic testing for MEN and FMTC syndromes is useful.

D. All patients with MEN 2B have a germline mutation resulting in a threonine-for-methionine substitution in codon 918 of exon 16.
E. Symptoms of pain, dysphagia, and hoarseness can develop with local invasion.

Answer: A

Explanation: MTC usually develops by the age of 10 years in MEN 2B, and MTC in MEN 2A can appear in the first or second decade of life, almost always developing by the third or fourth decade. MTC in FMTC usually develops during adulthood.

18. A 60-year-old man presents with a newly diagnosed PTC. His medical history is notable for head and neck radiation therapy during childhood. Imaging studies reveal suspicious lymphadenopathy, and molecular testing shows the presence of the BRAF V600E mutation. In the context of high-risk features of PTC, which of the following statements is incorrect?

A. A personal history of head and neck radiation is considered a high-risk feature for the development and progression of PTC.
B. The presence of the BRAF V600E mutation, especially when coexisting with a TERT promoter mutation, is associated with a more aggressive course of PTC.
C. Age below 18 years or above 55 years at diagnosis is considered a high-risk factor for PTC prognosis.
D. A tumor size of 3 cm in diameter is considered a high-risk feature for PTC.
E. The presence of suspicious lymphadenopathy is indicative of a higher risk of disease spread and a worse prognosis in PTC.

Answer: D

Explanation: Tumor size >4 cm in diameter is considered a high-risk feature of papillary thyroid cancer.

19. A 45-year-old woman is diagnosed with PTC after presenting with a palpable neck mass. FNAB confirms the diagnosis, and ultrasound imaging shows involvement of the central compartment lymph nodes. The patient is concerned about the prognosis and potential spread of the disease. In the context of PTC, which of the following statements is incorrect?

A. PTC has a propensity to spread to the cervical lymph nodes, with the central compartment being the most frequent site of lymph node involvement.
B. Metastasis to a Delphian (prelaryngeal) lymph node is considered a poor prognostic sign and may indicate more aggressive disease.
C. Approximately 5–10% of patients with PTC develop distant metastases, with the lungs and bones being common sites.
D. About 15–20% of patients with PTC develop distant metastases, indicating a higher rate of spread than typically observed.
E. Papillary thyroid microcarcinoma is defined as PTC that is 1 cm or less in diameter and often has an indolent clinical course.

Answer: D

Explanation: PTC is known for its tendency to spread to cervical lymph nodes, particularly in the central compartment. Metastasis to the Delphian lymph node is a poor prognostic indicator. While distant metastases do occur in PTC, they are less common, with an estimated occurrence in approximately 5–10% of patients, not 15–20% as stated in option D. Papillary thyroid microcarcinoma is a subset of PTC that is 1 cm or less in diameter and is generally associated with a favorable prognosis.

20. A 35-year-old woman presents with a palpable thyroid nodule. Ultrasound reveals a hypoechoic lesion with microcalcifications. FNAB is suggestive of PTC. Which of the following statements about PTC is incorrect?

    A. Most common thyroid malignancy in iodine-sufficient areas.
    B. Most common thyroid cancer in children.
    C. More often in women, 30–40 years.
    D. Grossly: hard and whitish and remain flat on sectioning with a blade.
    E. Usually, unifocal.

    Answer: E

    Explanation: Multifocality is common (up to 85% of cases) on microscopic examination.

21. A 42-year-old man presents with an asymptomatic neck mass discovered during a routine physical examination. Ultrasound-guided FNAB reveals characteristic nuclear features suggestive of PTC. Which of the following statements about PTC is incorrect?

    A. Usually encapsulated.
    B. PTC contains branching papillae of cuboidal epithelial cells.
    C. Associated with Orphan Annie eye nuclei.
    D. Diagnosis of PTC is based on these nuclear characteristics even in the absence of papillary structures.
    E. Microscopic, calcified deposits representing clumps of sloughed cells.

    Answer: A

    Explanation: PTC is rarely encapsulated and is more commonly characterized by an infiltrative growth pattern.

22. A 55-year-old woman presents with a rapidly enlarging thyroid mass and symptoms of compressive dysphagia. She has a history of well-differentiated thyroid cancer treated with total thyroidectomy and radioactive iodine therapy 10 years ago. Which of the following statements is incorrect regarding the types of well-differentiated thyroid cancer?

    A. PTC is a type of well-differentiated thyroid cancer.
    B. Follicular carcinoma of the thyroid is a type of well-differentiated thyroid cancer.
    C. Follicular variant of papillary carcinoma is a type of well-differentiated thyroid cancer.
    D. Hürthle cell carcinoma is a type of well-differentiated thyroid cancer.
    E. Anaplastic carcinoma is a type of well-differentiated thyroid cancer.

    Answer: E

Explanation: Anaplastic carcinoma is a poorly differentiated carcinoma of the thyroid.

23. A 45-year-old woman has undergone total thyroidectomy for well-differentiated thyroid cancer. She is now being evaluated for postoperative management options. Which of the following statements regarding postoperative management of well-differentiated thyroid cancer is incorrect?

    A. Postoperative RAI therapy reduces recurrence.
    B. Postoperative RAI therapy provides a small improvement in survival.
    C. Metastatic DTC can be detected and treated by 131I in about 75% of patients.
    D. RAI effectively treats >70% of lung micrometastasis.
    E. The success rate is about 40% for lung macro metastasis.

    Answer: E

    Explanation: The success rates drop to <10% with pulmonary macro metastasis.

24. A 50-year-old woman with well-differentiated thyroid cancer is being evaluated for postoperative management. Her tumor was 3 cm in size with evidence of vascular invasion, and she has no distant metastases. Which of the following statements regarding the indications for radioactive iodine (RAI) ablation in well-differentiated thyroid cancer is incorrect?

    A. All patients with stage III or IV disease.
    B. All patients with stage II disease <45 years.
    C. Most patients 45 years or older with stage II disease.
    D. Is contraindicated in stage I.
    E. Aggressive histology and nodal metastasis.

    Answer: D

    Explanation: RAI ablation is indicated for patients with stage I disease who have aggressive histology, nodal metastases, multifocal disease, and extrathyroid or vascular invasion.

25. A 40-year-old woman has undergone total thyroidectomy for well-differentiated thyroid cancer. She is now being prepared for postoperative RAI ablation. Which of the following statements regarding the preparation for RAI ablation is incorrect?

    A. T4 therapy should be discontinued for 3 weeks before scanning with I131.
    B. T3 needs to be discontinued for 2 weeks because it has a shorter half-life.
    C. A low-iodine diet also is recommended during this 2-week period.
    D. Administering a screening dose of 1 to 3 mCi of 123I and measuring uptake 24 h later is the usual protocol.
    E. A "hot" spot in the neck after initial screening usually represents residual normal tissue in the thyroid bed.

    Answer: A

    Explanation: Therapy should be discontinued for 6 weeks before scanning with I131.

26. A 55-year-old man with a history of total thyroidectomy for differentiated thyroid cancer is undergoing routine follow-up. His current TG level is 3 ng/mL while on thyroxine therapy. Which of the following statements regarding the follow-up of patients with differentiated thyroid cancer is incorrect?

    A. TG level > 6 ng/mL is highly suggestive of metastasis.
    B. A TG should be <2 ng/mL when the patient is taking T4 after total thyroidectomy.
    C. TG should be <5 ng/mL when the patient is hypothyroid after total thyroidectomy.
    D. TG and anti-Tg antibody levels should be measured initially at 6-month intervals.
    E. TG measurements in FNAC aspirates are useful in the detection of nodal metastatic disease.

    Answer: A

    Explanation: A TG level > 2 ng/mL is highly suggestive of metastatic disease or persistent normal thyroid tissue.

27. During a neck dissection for PTC, a 45-year-old woman is found to have thyroid tissue in a lateral cervical lymph node. Which of the following statements regarding lateral aberrant thyroid is incorrect?

    A. Any thyroid tissue found laterally separate from the thyroid gland metastasis in a cervical lymph.
    B. Aberrant thyroid tissue never occurs in a lateral position.
    C. Aberrant thyroid tissues are found along the course of the thyroglossal tract.
    D. Lateral aberrant thyroid is typically discovered incidentally on imaging.
    E. FTC is most commonly associated with lateral aberrant thyroid.

    Answer: E

    Explanation: In reality, PTC is most commonly associated with lateral aberrant thyroid, as it has a higher propensity for lymphatic spread, including to lateral cervical lymph nodes. The patient's finding of thyroid tissue in a lateral cervical lymph node during surgery for PTC is consistent with this association.

28. A 38-year-old woman with a history of well-differentiated thyroid cancer is being evaluated for RAI therapy with 131I. She is currently trying to conceive. Which of the following statements regarding 131I therapy is incorrect?

    A. I131 is an effective agent for delivering high radiation doses to the thyroid tissue.
    B. It emits mainly beta radiation (90%), which penetrates only 0.5 mm of the tissue.
    C. I131 emits beta particles and X-rays.
    D. Beta rays are utilized for their destructive effects on thyroid cells.
    E. Can be used during pregnancy.

    Answer: E

    Explanation: RAI (I131) is contraindicated in pregnancy.

29. A 60-year-old man presents with a rapidly enlarging thyroid mass, dysphagia, and hoarseness. Biopsy confirms anaplastic thyroid carcinoma. Which of the following statements regarding the spread of thyroid cancers is incorrect?

    A. PTC spreads lymphatically.
    B. Follicular carcinoma spreads hematogenously.
    C. Medullary carcinoma spreads both lymphatically and hematogenously.
    D. Anaplastic carcinoma spreads hematogenously.
    E. Medullary carcinoma's most common site of metastasis is the liver.

    Answer: D

    Explanation: Anaplastic carcinoma has direct invasion spread.

30. A 47-year-old woman with a history of thyroidectomy for PTC presents with new-onset bone pain. Imaging reveals multiple lung and bone lesions. Which of the following statements regarding thyroid cancer metastasis is incorrect?

    A. PTC's most common site of metastasis is the lungs.
    B. Follicular carcinoma's most common site of metastasis is the bones.
    C. Anaplastic carcinoma's most common site of metastasis is the lungs.
    D. Follicular carcinoma has osteolytic metastasis.
    E. Medullary carcinoma has osteoblastic metastasis.

    Answer: E

    Explanation: Medullary carcinoma has osteolytic metastasis.

31. A 55-year-old woman presents with a solitary thyroid nodule. She has a history of living in an iodine-deficient area. FNAB suggests FTC. Which of the following statements regarding FTC is incorrect?

    A. Accounts for 10% of thyroid cancer.
    B. Occurs more commonly in iodine-deficient areas.
    C. More common in women with a mean age of 50 years.
    D. Genes implicated in FTC: p53, PTEN, Ras, PAX8/PPAR1.
    E. Usually multiple without a capsule.

    Answer: E

    Explanation: FTC is usually a solitary lesion surrounded by a capsule.

32. A 60-year-old man presents with a thyroid nodule that has recently increased in size. He has a long-standing history of goiter. FNAB suggests FTC. Which of the following statements regarding FTC is incorrect?

    A. Histologically, follicles are present, but the lumen may be devoid of colloid.
    B. Malignancy is defined by the presence of capsular and vascular invasion.
    C. Maybe associated with a history of rapid size increase and long-standing goiter.
    D. Cervical lymphadenopathy is very common at initial presentation.
    E. Preoperative clinical diagnosis of cancer is difficult unless distant metastases are present.

    Answer: D

    Explanation: Cervical lymphadenopathy is uncommon at initial presentation (about 5%).

33. A 45-year-old woman is diagnosed with FTC after a lobectomy for a suspicious thyroid nodule. Further management is being discussed. Which of the following statements regarding the treatment of FTC is incorrect?

    A. Follicular lesion is treated with hemithyroidectomy.
    B. Thyroid cancer is treated with total thyroidectomy.
    C. Prophylactic nodal dissection is advised.
    D. Cumulative mortality: 15% at 10 years and 30% at 20 years.
    E. The most important prognostic factors: age and distant metastasis.

    Answer: C

    Explanation: Prophylactic nodal dissection is unwarranted because nodal involvement is infrequent.

34. A 55-year-old man presents with a neck mass and diarrhea. FNAB of the thyroid mass is suggestive of MTC. Which of the following statements regarding MTC is incorrect?

    A. Neuroendocrine carcinoma arising from parafollicular "C" cells of the thyroid.
    B. "C" cells are concentrated superolaterally in the thyroid.
    C. Most MTCs (75–80%) arise sporadically.
    D. High levels of serum calcitonin and CEA.
    E. LN metastasis occurs late.

    Answer: E

    Explanation: Cervical lymph nodes are often involved at the time of presentation (LN involvement, thyroid, and blood-borne metastases occur early).

35. A 50-year-old woman presents with a thyroid mass and symptoms of diarrhea. FNAC suggests MTC. Which of the following statements regarding MTC is incorrect?

    A. Diagnosed by FNAC.
    B. Radioiodine scan is used in the diagnosis.
    C. Tumor marker: Calcitonin is raised in almost all cases of MTC.
    D. Calcitonin excess in MTC is not associated with hypocalcemia.
    E. Diarrhea at the time of presentation.

    Answer: B

    Explanation: Radioiodine scan (I131 scan) is of no use as MTC is TSH independent.

36. A 45-year-old woman is being positioned for a thyroidectomy. Which of the following statements regarding patient positioning during thyroidectomy is incorrect?

    A. The patient should be in the supine semi-Fowler position with neck extension.
    B. A roll can be placed transversally under the scapula to increase anterior neck exposure.
    C. Neck extension can lead to postoperative pain.

D. Normal extension can lead to vertigo, headache, and postoperative nausea.
E. Patients with cervical spine disease should be assessed by orthopedics or neurosurgeon preoperatively.

Answer: D

Explanation: Extensive hyperextension during thyroidectomy can lead to vertigo, headache, and postoperative nausea.

37. During a thyroidectomy for a 55-year-old man with a large multinodular goiter, the surgical team is making decisions about the incision and exposure. Which of the following statements regarding incision and exposure of the thyroid during thyroidectomy is incorrect?

A. A Kocher incision is made on the anterior aspect of the midneck.
B. The incision should be in an existing skin crease.
C. In patients with obesity, large gland, or kyphoscoliosis, a longer incision may be needed.
D. Subplatysmal flaps are dissected and placed laterally to enlarge the field.
E. Enlarged prelaryngeal lymph nodes should be excised due to metastatic possibility.

Answer: D

Explanation: After platysma dissection, the subplatysmal flaps should be elevated above the level of the thyroid cartilage superiorly, laterally over the sternocleidomastoid muscle, and inferiorly to the level of the superior border of the manubrium sterni.

38. A 40-year-old woman with a history of exposure to head and neck radiation during childhood presents with a thyroid nodule. FNAB suggests DTC. Which of the following criteria is incorrect regarding high-risk DTC?

A. Tumor size between 1 and 4 cm.
B. Tumor with gross extrathyroid extension.
C. Clinical evidence of apparent LN or distant metastasis.
D. Thyroid cancer in a patient with prior head and neck radiation.
E. Family history of differentiated thyroid cancer in a first-degree relative.

Answer: A

Explanation: The tumor size should be $\geq$4 cm to be considered high-risk differentiated thyroid cancer; tumors between 1 and 4 cm are considered low-risk differentiated thyroid cancer.

39. During a total thyroidectomy for a 50-year-old man with papillary thyroid carcinoma, the surgical team is cautious about preserving the parathyroid glands. Which of the following statements regarding parathyroid preservation during thyroidectomy is incorrect?

A. Superior parathyroid glands (PTGs) are located anteriorly, while the inferior PTGs are located posteriorly in relation to the recurrent laryngeal nerve.
B. To avoid PTG injury, thyroid dissection should be as close to the capsule as possible.
C. The inferior thyroid artery must be ligated closely to the thyroid capsule.

D. PTGs should not be removed during thyroidectomy unless there is gross metastatic invasion or ischemic injury occurring during dissection.

Answer: A

Explanation: The superior PTGs are located posterior to the recurrent laryngeal nerve, while the inferior PTGs are located anterior to the recurrent laryngeal nerve.

40. A 45-year-old patient with locally advanced thyroid cancer is being evaluated for surgical treatment options. Which of the following statements regarding the surgical management of locally advanced thyroid cancer is incorrect?

A. Intraoperative neuromonitoring is beneficial for assessing the functional status of the recurrent laryngeal nerve.
B. A staging system based on the degree of invasion aids in managing laryngo-tracheal invasion.
C. Surgical management aims to maximize local control while minimizing the morbidity of radical resection.
D. Total thyroidectomy is not recommended for locally advanced thyroid cancer due to high recurrence rates.
E. Various factors such as tumor biology and previous treatment responses affect the extent of surgical resection.

Answer: D

Explanation: Total thyroidectomy is not recommended for locally advanced thyroid cancer due to high recurrence rates. This statement is incorrect as total thyroidectomy can be part of the treatment for locally advanced thyroid cancer to achieve local control.

41. A 55-year-old patient diagnosed with differentiated thyroid cancer is discussing surgical options with the surgical team. Which of the following statements about advances in the surgical treatment of differentiated thyroid cancer is incorrect?

A. Minimally invasive video-assisted thyroidectomy has comparable perioperative morbidity to conventional open thyroidectomy.
B. Robotic thyroidectomy offers significant cosmetic advantages over traditional surgery.
C. Therapeutic central lymph node dissection is performed only when metastatic lymph nodes are not identified.
D. The role of elective prophylactic central lymph node dissection in the absence of overt nodal metastasis remains a subject of debate.
E. Video assistance and robotics have revolutionized thyroid surgery.

Answer: C

Explanation: Therapeutic central lymph node dissection is performed only when metastatic lymph nodes are not identified. This statement is incorrect as therapeutic central lymph node dissection should be performed when metastatic lymph nodes are identified.

42. During a conference on thyroid cancer, a discussion arises about the management strategies for papillary thyroid microcarcinoma. Which of the following

statements about controversies in thyroid surgery for differentiated thyroid cancer is incorrect?

A. Active surveillance is a management option for papillary thyroid microcarcinoma.
B. The extent of thyroid surgery for low-risk differentiated thyroid cancer is a subject of ongoing debate.
C. Molecular testing plays no role in guiding decision-making about the necessity and extent of initial surgery.
D. Innovative thyroidectomy techniques include robotic and transoral approaches.
E. Patient preferences are crucial in decision-making regarding the extent of surgery and long-term surveillance.

Answer: C

Explanation: Molecular testing plays no role in guiding decision-making about the necessity and extent of initial surgery. This statement is incorrect as molecular testing can guide decision-making regarding the necessity and extent of surgery.

43. A patient with differentiated thyroid cancer is being counseled about surgical options. Which of the following statements regarding total thyroidectomy for differentiated thyroid cancer is incorrect?

A. Total thyroidectomy followed by radioiodine ablation and thyroid hormone suppression is appropriate for most patients.
B. Total thyroidectomy is associated with higher recurrence rates compared to partial thyroidectomy.
C. The approach reduces the risk of cancer recurrence and facilitates postoperative monitoring.
D. Surgeon volume is associated with patient outcomes following total thyroidectomy.
E. Retrospective analyses support total thyroidectomy for reducing recurrence risk and addressing multifocal intrathyroidal cancer.

Answer: B

Explanation: Total thyroidectomy is associated with higher recurrence rates compared to partial thyroidectomy. This statement is incorrect as total thyroidectomy, when indicated, can reduce the risk of cancer recurrence compared to less extensive surgery.

44. A patient with a bilateral nodular goiter is considering surgical treatment options. Which of the following statements about total thyroidectomy in the treatment of thyroid disease is incorrect?

A. Total thyroidectomy is indicated for bilateral nodular goiter, Graves' disease, and chronic thyroiditis.
B. The rapid frozen diagnosis being equivocal for carcinoma is a contraindication for total thyroidectomy.

C. Cosmetic outcomes are a significant concern for patients undergoing thyroid surgery.
D. Minimally invasive procedures for thyroid disease aim to improve cosmetic outcomes.
E. Total thyroidectomy has been performed for both malignant and benign thyroid diseases.

Answer: B

Explanation: The rapid frozen diagnosis being equivocal for carcinoma is a contraindication for total thyroidectomy. This statement is incorrect as an equivocal diagnosis for carcinoma may be an indication for total thyroidectomy to ensure complete removal and facilitate further treatment.

Bibliography

1. Kitahara CM, Linet MS, Beane Freeman LE, Check DP, Church TR, Park Y, Purdue MP, Schairer C, Berrington de González A. Cigarette smoking, alcohol intake, and thyroid cancer risk: a pooled analysis of five prospective studies in the United States. Cancer Causes Control. 2012;23:1615–24.
2. Pizzato M, Li M, Vignat J, Laversanne M, Singh D, La Vecchia C, Vaccarella S. The epidemiological landscape of thyroid cancer worldwide: GLOBOCAN estimates for incidence and mortality rates in 2020. Lancet Diabetes Endocrinol. 2022;10(4):264–72.
3. Pearce EN, Braverman LE. Papillary thyroid microcarcinoma outcomes and implications for treatment. J Clin Endocrinol Metabol. 2004;89(8):3710–2.
4. Welker MJ, Orlov D. Thyroid nodules. Am Fam Physician. 2003;67(3):559–67.
5. Matthews TJ, Chua E, Gargya A, Clark J, Gao K, Elliott M. Elevated serum thyroglobulin levels at the time of ablative radioactive iodine therapy indicate a worse prognosis in thyroid cancer: an Australian retrospective cohort study. J Laryngol Otol. 2016;130(Suppl 4):S50–S3. https://doi.org/10.1017/S0022215116008331.
6. Staniforth JU, Erdirimanne S, Eslick GD. Thyroid carcinoma in graves' disease: a meta-analysis. Int J Surg. 2016;27:118–25.
7. Al-Brahim N, Asa SL. Papillary thyroid carcinoma: an overview. Arch Pathol Lab Med. 2006;130(7):1057–62.
8. Park H, Heo J, Ki CS, Shin JH, Oh YL, Son YI, Kim JS, Kim SW, Chung JH, Kim TY, Kim TH, Kim JH. Selection criteria for completion thyroidectomy in follicular thyroid carcinoma using primary tumor size and TERT promoter mutational status. Ann Surg Oncol. 2023;30(5):2916–25. https://doi.org/10.1245/s10434-022-13089-5. PMID: 36637642; PMCID: PMC9838536
9. McHenry CR, Phitayakorn R. Follicular adenoma and carcinoma of the thyroid gland. Oncologist. 2011;16(5):585–93.
10. Limaiem F, Rehman A, Anastasopoulou C, Mazzoni T. Papillary thyroid carcinoma. 2023 Jan 1. In: StatPearls [internet]. Treasure Island, FL: StatPearls Publishing; 2023.
11. Rahbari R, Zhang L, Kebebew E. Thyroid cancer gender disparity. Future Oncol. 2010;6(11):1771–9. https://doi.org/10.2217/fon.10.127. PMID: 21142662; PMCID: PMC3077966
12. Iglesias ML, Schmidt A, Ghuzlan AA, Lacroix L, Vathaire F, Chevillard S, Schlumberger M. Radiation exposure and thyroid cancer: a review. Arch Endocrinol Metab. 2017;61(2):180–7.

13. Bomeli SR, LeBeau SO, Ferris RL. Evaluation of a thyroid nodule. Otolaryngol Clin N Am. 2010;43(2):229–38. https://doi.org/10.1016/j.otc.2010.01.002. PMID: 20510711; PMCID: PMC2879398, vii
14. Gonzalez-Gonzalez R, Bologna-Molina R, Carreon-Burciaga RG, Gómezpalacio-Gastelum M, Molina-Frechero N, Salazar-Rodríguez S. Papillary thyroid carcinoma: differential diagnosis and prognostic values of its different variants: review of the literature. ISRN Oncol. 2011;2011:915925. https://doi.org/10.5402/2011/915925. PMID: 22432054; PMCID: PMC3302055
15. Yutan E, Clark OH. Hürthle cell carcinoma. Curr Treat Options in Oncol. 2001;2:331–5.
16. Wells SA Jr, Pacini F, Robinson BG, Santoro M. Multiple endocrine neoplasia type 2 and familial medullary thyroid carcinoma: an update. J Clin Endocrinol Metab. 2013;98(8):3149–64.
17. Quayle FJ, Moley JF. Medullary thyroid carcinoma: including MEN 2A and MEN 2B syndromes. J Surg Oncol. 2005;89(3):122–9.
18. Haugen BR, Alexander EK, Bible KC, Doherty GM, Mandel SJ, Nikiforov YE, Pacini F, Randolph GW, Sawka AM, Schlumberger M, Schuff KG, Sherman SI, Sosa JA, Steward DL, Tuttle RM, Wartofsky L. 2015 American Thyroid Association management guidelines for adult patients with thyroid nodules and differentiated thyroid cancer: the American Thyroid Association guidelines task force on thyroid nodules and differentiated thyroid cancer. Thyroid. 2016;26(1):1–133. https://doi.org/10.1089/thy.2015.0020. PMID: 26462967; PMCID: PMC4739132
19. Schmid KW. Lymphknoten- und Organmetastasen des Schilddrüsenkarzinoms. Metastasen in der Schilddrüse [Lymph node and distant metastases of thyroid gland cancer. Metastases in the thyroid glands]. Pathologe. 2015;36(Suppl 2):171–5. Germanica. https://doi.org/10.1007/s00292-015-0071-6.
20. Del Rio P, Loderer T, Giuffrida M, Cozzani F, Rossini M, Bonfili D, Bonati E. Multifocality in patients treated for papillary thyroid carcinoma: a preliminary analysis of related risk factors. Acta Biomed. 2021;92(5):e2021017.
21. Coca-Pelaz A, Shah JP, Hernandez-Prera JC, Ghossein RA, Rodrigo JP, Hartl DM, Olsen KD, Shaha AR, Zafereo M, Suarez C, Nixon IJ, Randolph GW, Mäkitie AA, Kowalski LP, Vander Poorten V, Sanabria A, Guntinas-Lichius O, Simo R, Zbären P, Angelos P, Khafif A, Rinaldo A, Ferlito A. Papillary thyroid cancer-aggressive variants and impact on management: a narrative review. Adv Ther. 2020;37(7):3112–28. https://doi.org/10.1007/s12325-020-01391-1. Epub 2020 Jun 1. PMID: 32488657; PMCID: PMC7467416
22. Patel KN, Shaha AR. Poorly differentiated and anaplastic thyroid cancer. Cancer Control. 2006;13(2):119–28.
23. Tuttle RM, Leboeuf R. Postoperative Management of well-differentiated thyroid cancer. Endocrine surgery: principles and practice. 2009:137–48.
24. Sawka AM, Thephamongkhol K, Brouwers M, Thabane L, Browman G, Gerstein HC. A systematic review and metaanalysis of the effectiveness of radioactive iodine remnant ablation for well-differentiated thyroid cancer. J Clin Endocrinol Metabol. 2004;89(8):3668–76.
25. Berlin JA, Gross JM, O'Donoghue JE. Radioiodine therapy for thyroid cancer: a review of the literature. J Nucl Med. 2012;53(7):1163–72.
26. American Thyroid Association. Management of thyroid cancer: 2015 guidelines of the American Thyroid Association. Thyroid. 2015;25(11):1675–730.
27. Noussios G, Anagnostis P, Goulis DG, Lappas D, Natsis K. Ectopic thyroid tissue: anatomical, clinical, and surgical implications of a rare entity. Eur J Endocrinol. 2011;165(3):375–82.
28. Tran P, Desimone S, Barrett M, Bachrach B. I-131 treatment of graves' disease in an unsuspected first trimester pregnancy; the potential for adverse effects on the fetus and a review of the current guidelines for pregnancy screening. Int J Pediatr Endocrinol. 2010;2010:858359.
29. Ahmed S, Ghazarian MP, Cabanillas ME, Zafereo ME, Williams MD, Vu T, Schomer DF, Debnam JM. Imaging of anaplastic thyroid carcinoma. AJNR Am J Neuroradiol. 2018;39(3):547–51.

30. Macedo F, Ladeira K, Pinho F, Saraiva N, Bonito N, Pinto L, Goncalves F. Bone metastases: an overview. Oncol Rev. 2017;11(1):321. https://doi.org/10.4081/oncol.2017.321. PMID: 28584570; PMCID: PMC5444408
31. Baloch ZW, LiVolsi VA. Our approach to follicular-patterned lesions of the thyroid. J Clin Pathol. 2007;60(3):244–50.
32. Sobrinho-Simoes M, Eloy C, Magalhaes J, Lobo C, Amaro T. Follicular thyroid carcinoma. Mod Pathol. 2011;24:S10–S8.
33. Grani G, Lamartina L, Durante C, Filetti S, Cooper DS. Follicular thyroid cancer and Hürthle cell carcinoma: challenges in diagnosis, treatment, and clinical management. Lancet Diabetes Endocrinol. 2018;6(6):500–14.
34. Tuttle RM, Ball DW, Byrd D, Daniels GH, Dilawari RA, Doherty GM, Duh QY, Ehya H, Farrar WB, Haddad RI, Kandeel F. Medullary carcinoma. J Natl Compr Cancer Netw. 2010;8(5):512–30.
35. Pacini F, Castagna MG, Cipri C, Schlumberger M. Medullary thyroid carcinoma. Clin Oncol (R Coll Radiol). 2010;22(6):475–85.
36. Rosato L, Avenia N, Bernante P, De Palma M, Gulino G, Nasi PG, Pelizzo MR, Pezzullo L. Complications of thyroid surgery: analysis of a multicentric study on 14,934 patients operated on in Italy over 5 years. World J Surg. 2004;28:271–6.
37. Gil Z, Patel SG. Surgery for thyroid cancer. Surg Oncol Clin N Am. 2008;17(1):93–120.
38. Barczyński M, Konturek A, Hubalewska-Dydejczyk A, Gołkowski F, Cichoń S, Nowak W. Five-year follow-up of a randomized clinical trial of total thyroidectomy versus Dunhill operation versus bilateral subtotal thyroidectomy for multinodular nontoxic goiter. World J Surg. 2010;34:1203–13.
39. Uslu A, Okut G, Tercan IC, Erkul Z, Aykas A, Karatas M, Simsek C, Tatar E. Anatomical distribution and number of parathyroid glands, and parathyroid function, after total parathyroidectomy and bilateral cervical thymectomy. Medicine. 2019;98:23.
40. An S, Kim K. Surgical management of locally advanced thyroid cancer. Curr Opin Otolaryngol Head Neck Surg. 2010;18(2):119–23.
41. Venkat R, Guerrero MA. Recent advances in the surgical treatment of differentiated thyroid cancer: a comprehensive review. Sci World J. 2013;2013:425136.
42. Wang TS, Sosa JA. Thyroid surgery for differentiated thyroid cancer—recent advances and future directions. Nat Rev Endocrinol. 2018;14(11):670–83.
43. Sosa JA, Udelsman R. Total thyroidectomy for differentiated thyroid cancer. J Surg Oncol. 2006;94:701–7.
44. Chonkich GD, Petti GH, Goral W. Total thyroidectomy in the treatment of thyroid disease. Laryngoscope. 1987;97(8 Pt 1):1044–6.

Chapter 15
Parathyroid Carcinoma

Raafat Raoof Alturfi, Waseem M. Al Hamidy, Munthir A. Alobaidi, and Mustafa Ismail

1. A 58-year-old patient presents with persistent hypercalcemia and is undergoing evaluation for parathyroid disease. In parathyroid carcinoma (PC), which of the following is incorrect?

   A. Rare tumor that can occur sporadically or as a part of a syndrome.
   B. A greater number of parathyroid tumors are hormonally active for parathyroid hormone (PTH).
   C. The symptoms of hypercalcemia in parathyroid benign tumors are often more marked than in cases of PC patients.
   D. Incidence is equal between males and females.
   E. Many initially present with parathyrotoxicosis.

   Answer: C

   Explanation: The symptoms of hypercalcemia are often more marked in cases of PC patients than in parathyroid benign tumors, making it a crucial diagnostic distinction.

2. A 45-year-old patient is being evaluated for familial syndromes that might increase the risk of developing PC. Regarding the syndromes that increase the risk of PC, the incorrect statement is:

   A. MEN1 is associated with an increased risk of parathyroid cancer.
   B. MEN2A is associated with an increased risk of parathyroid cancer.

R. R. Alturfi
Department of Digestive Surgery, Gastroenterology and Hepatology Teaching Hospital, Baghdad, Iraq

W. M. Al Hamidy
Gastroenterology and Hepatology Teaching Hospital, Medical City, Baghdad, Iraq

M. A. Alobaidi · M. Ismail (✉)
Department of Surgery, College of Medicine, University of Baghdad, Baghdad, Iraq

A. S. Mahmood, A. Koulouris (eds.), *MCQs in General Surgical Oncology*,
https://doi.org/10.1007/978-3-031-65738-2_15

C. Familial hyperparathyroidism is associated with an increased risk of parathyroid cancer.
D. Hyperparathyroidism-jaw tumor syndrome is associated with an increased risk of parathyroid cancer.
E. MEN2B is associated with an increased risk of parathyroid cancer.
   Answer: E
   Explanation: MEN2B is not associated with an increased risk of parathyroid cancer, unlike the other syndromes listed.

3. A 50-year-old patient is undergoing genetic testing for HRPT2 mutations due to a family history of hyperparathyroidism. Regarding HRPT2 mutation and PC, which of the following is incorrect?

   A. Mutations are common with familial isolated hyperparathyroidism.
   B. Calcium and PTH levels are the main biochemical screening tests for hyperparathyroidism.
   C. High level of calcium is much typical of early PC associated with germline HRPT2 mutations.
   D. Additional surveillance measures, particularly neck ultrasonography, may improve sensitivity and lead to early detection of tumors.
   E. Parafibromin is an important tumor suppressor of parathyroid gland tissue and mutations in the HRPT2 gene are associated with high-grade PC.
      Answer: C
      Explanation: High levels of calcium are not typical of early PC associated with germline HRPT2 mutations, as these tumors can be normocalcemic or mildly hypercalcemic.

4. A 45-year-old patient is diagnosed with PC, and genetic testing is being considered. Regarding genetic and PC, which of the following is incorrect?

   A. HRPT2 mutations have a role in sporadic PC.
   B. Molecular pathogenesis of PC is affected by mutation of the HRPT2 (CDC73) which is a tumor suppressor gene.
   C. HRPT2 mutations have a role in the hyperparathyroidism-jaw tumor syndrome.
   D. Checking HRPT has no role in sporadic cases of parathyroid cancer.
   E. HRPT2 has a role in some isolated familial hyperparathyroidism cases.
      Answer: D
      Explanation: In sporadic cases of PC, checking for HRPT2 mutations is not typically performed; however, sporadic PC can sometimes have HRPT2 germline mutations, raising the possibility of hyperparathyroidism-jaw tumor syndrome.

5. A 30-year-old patient has a strong family history of hyperparathyroidism and jaw tumors. They are concerned about the possibility of developing PC. Which of the following is incorrect regarding hyperparathyroidism-jaw tumor (HPT-JT) syndromes?

A. Autosomal recessive disease related to familial hyperparathyroidism.
B. Strong association between HRPT2 mutations and HPT-JT.
C. PC occurs with higher frequency in HPT-JT than in sporadic PHPT.
D. Patients that have sporadic PC may have the HPT-JT syndrome.
E. HPT-JT-associated diseases include cystic parathyroid adenomatosis, ossifying fibroma.

Answer: D

Explanation: Patients with sporadic PC are not typically associated with HPT-JT syndrome. HPT-JT is an autosomal dominant type of familial hyperparathyroidism.

6. A 50-year-old patient is undergoing genetic counseling due to a family history of parathyroid disorders. The geneticist is evaluating the potential genetic factors that could be associated with an increased risk of PC. Regarding the genes associated with PC, the incorrect statement is:

A. CCND1/PRAD1 is associated with PC.
B. APC is associated with PC.
C. HRPT2 is associated with PC.
D. MEN1 is associated with PC.
E. RET is associated with PC.

Answer: B

Explanation: APC is not associated with PC; it is primarily associated with CRC. The other genes listed have roles in the development of parathyroid cancer.

7. A 52-year-old male patient presents with memory deficits and paresthesia. Laboratory findings reveal elevated calcium levels. Regarding possible clinical presentations of PC, the incorrect statement is:

A. A 55-year-old female patient with lab calcium of 14.5 mg/dL.
B. A 47-year-old asymptomatic patient with a calcium level of 13.4 mg/dL.
C. A 45-year-old female patient with a known cause of chronic kidney disease on dialysis.
D. A 50-year-old male patient with a cervical mass and fatigue.
E. A 52-year-old male patient with memory deficit and paresthesia.

Answer: C

Explanation: Most PC patients present with signs and symptoms of hyperparathyroidism. A patient with a known cause of kidney disease and hyperparathyroidism is usually due to secondary hyperparathyroidism related to renal failure, making this presentation less likely to be PC.

8. A 52-year-old patient with hyperparathyroidism is experiencing various symptoms. Regarding symptoms of hyperparathyroidism, which of the following is incorrect?

A. Clinical symptoms are mainly related to tumor spread rather than high secretion of PTH.
B. Hypercalcemia.

C. Renal failure.
D. Cardiac arrhythmia.
E. Neurocognitive dysfunction.

Answer: A

Explanation: Clinical symptoms of hyperparathyroidism are mainly related to the high secretion of PTH, which leads to various systemic effects.

9. A 48-year-old patient undergoes a parathyroidectomy, and an immunohistochemical panel is used to analyze the tissue. Regarding the role of immunohistochemical panel in PC, which is incorrect?

A. Useful in the identification of parathyroid tissue.
B. Differentiates between parathyroid cancer and other tumors like thyroid cancer.
C. Has no role in small biopsies or ectopic locations suspected to be of parathyroid origin.
D. Differentiates between parathyroid adenoma and carcinoma.
E. Identification of supernumerary parathyroid glands.

Answer: C

Explanation: Immunohistochemical panels are useful in various aspects of parathyroid pathology, including the identification of parathyroid tissue and differentiation between different parathyroid conditions, but they may have limited utility in small biopsies or ectopic locations suspected to be of parathyroid origin.

10. A 60-year-old female patient is diagnosed with primary hyperparathyroidism (PHPT), and her treatment options are being discussed. Which of the following is incorrect regarding PHPT?

A. Benign solitary adenoma is accountable for 80%–90% of all cases of PHPT.
B. Ultrasonography and sestamibi scan are considered typical imaging for parathyroid lesions.
C. Common, occur in females more than males with an age range of 50–70 years.
D. Minimally invasive intervention isn't useful if the patient having a preoperative scan is suspicious for a single solitary lesion.
E. Minimally invasive intervention is useful in the majority of cases of PHPT.

Answer: D

Explanation: Minimally invasive intervention is mostly useful when there is a preoperative scan suspicious for a single solitary lesion, or when the lesion is a benign solitary adenoma, which is the most common cause of PHPT.

11. A 45-year-old patient with a cervical mass undergoes surgical evaluation, and pathology results are awaited. In PC and atypical parathyroid adenoma, which of the following is incorrect?

A. Hypercalcemia crisis has a higher incidence in atypical adenoma than PC.
B. PC size is larger than atypical parathyroid adenoma.

C. Mean serum calcium is much higher in PC than in atypical adenoma.
D. PTH level is much higher in PC than in adenoma.
E. PC usually doesn't have a distinct capsule and adheres to nearby structures, while loss of parafibromin expression is the same as in atypical adenoma.

Answer: A

Explanation: Hypercalcemia crisis is more commonly associated with PC than atypical adenoma.

12. A 45-year-old patient is being evaluated for PHPT and is discussing diagnostic options with their endocrinologist. In parathyroid gland pathologies, which of the following is incorrect?

A. PC is least likely to be a cause of PHPT than parathyroid adenoma.
B. Diagnosis of parathyroid cancer can be made using radiological imaging.
C. Knowledge of the unusual anatomic locations for enlarged parathyroid glands is crucial to operative success during both initial and reoperative parathyroid surgery.
D. Eighty-four percent of individuals have four parathyroid glands.
E. Localization studies should not be used to establish the diagnosis of PHPT.

Answer: B

Explanation: The diagnosis of parathyroid cancer is made by pathology, typically during surgical excision. Radiological imaging alone cannot definitively diagnose parathyroid cancer.

13. A surgeon is explaining parathyroid gland anatomy to a medical student. Regarding parathyroid glands' surgical anatomy, which is incorrect?

A. The superior glands originate from the third branchial pouch. The inferior glands originate from the fourth branchial pouch.
B. Ectopic parathyroid glands occur along with tissues that have similar embryological origin.
C. Ectopic parathyroid gland may be any one of the four glands or a supernumerary gland (more than four).
D. Supernumerary glands may be responsible for persistent hyperparathyroidism after parathyroidectomy.
E. The most common location for supernumerary parathyroid glands is within the thymus or near the thyrothymic ligament.

Answer: A

Explanation: The superior parathyroid glands originate from the fourth branchial pouch, while the inferior glands originate from the third branchial pouch.

14. A medical student is learning about the vascular supply of parathyroid glands. Which of the following is incorrect?

A. The parathyroid glands are supplied by branches from the external carotid artery.
B. The superior parathyroid glands are supplied by the inferior thyroid artery.
C. The inferior parathyroid glands are supplied by the inferior thyroid artery.

D. Each parathyroid gland has its own end arterial supply.
E. Parathyroid veins drain into the thyroid vein plexus and hence to superior, middle, and inferior thyroid veins.

Answer: A

Explanation: The parathyroid glands are supplied by branches from the thyrocervical trunk of the subclavian artery, including the inferior thyroid artery that supplies both the superior and inferior parathyroid glands. They are not supplied by branches from the external carotid artery.

15. A 50-year-old patient with suspected PC is undergoing preoperative diagnostic evaluations. In preoperative diagnostic studies of PC, which of the following is incorrect?

A. The most sensitive imaging for pathologic parathyroid gland is sestamibi scintigram.
B. The most sensitive technique for the detection of possible signs of malignancy was CT scan.
C. The most widely used imaging for PC is ultrasonography.
D. Ultrasound is more sensitive than a sestamibi scan for the detection of PC.
E. Usage of nuclear magnetic resonance and PET scan was unusual.

Answer: D

Explanation: Ultrasound is not more sensitive than a sestamibi scan for the detection of PC. CT scan is the most sensitive technique for detecting possible signs of malignancy, followed by ultrasound and sestamibi scan.

16. A 55-year-old patient is being evaluated for PHPT and is discussing treatment options with their endocrinologist. Regarding the approach for PHPT, which of the following is incorrect?

A. Persistent or recurrent PHPT is an indication for re-exploration.
B. Symptomatic cervical disc disease is an absolute contraindication for parathyroidectomy.
C. Asymptomatic PHPTH is an indication for surgery in certain circumstances.
D. Parathyroid cancer is considered an indication for surgical exploration.
E. Patients with familial hypocalciuric hypercalcemia should not undergo parathyroidectomy.

Answer: B

Explanation: Symptomatic cervical disc disease is a relative contraindication for parathyroidectomy, meaning it should be carefully considered and evaluated on an individual basis.

17. A pathologist is examining tissue samples from a suspicious parathyroid lesion. Regarding the diagnosis of PC, the incorrect statement is:

A. The absence of fibrous bands arranged in a trabecular design is required for diagnosis.
B. Infiltration of surrounding structures is a key diagnostic feature.
C. Vascular invasion is necessary for diagnosing PC.

D. Metastasis is a criterion used to diagnose PC.
E. Capsular invasion is an important feature for diagnosing PC.

Answer: A

Explanation: The presence, not the absence, of histologic fibrous bands arranged in a trabecular design is an important characteristic of PC.

18. A surgical team is planning a parathyroidectomy for a patient with PHPT. Regarding localizing studies for preoperative evaluation in cases of parathyroid surgery, which is incorrect?

A. Localizing studies should not be relied on for the diagnosis of PHPT since the diagnosis is entirely by biochemical tests.
B. The preferred localizing imaging studies include sestamibi scintigraphy (MIBI-SPECT imaging), ultrasound, and/or four-dimensional computed tomography (4D-CT).
C. Localizing studies are mandatory before re-exploration.
D. Selection of patients for surgery highly relies on localization studies.
E. Localizing studies help to select patients for minimally invasive surgery and evaluate concurrent thyroid pathology.

Answer: D

Explanation: Localization studies do not confirm the diagnosis of PHPT when positive or rule out the diagnosis when negative. They should not be used as the sole criterion for selecting patients for surgery.

19. A 60-year-old patient with advanced unresectable PC is being considered for targeted therapy. Regarding genetic mutation and parathyroid cancer, which of the following is incorrect?

A. Mutation identification plays a role in advanced unresectable PC.
B. Discovering specific mutations in parathyroid cancer can allow the use of targeted drugs that are already approved for treating other cancers.
C. PIK3CA have a role in PC.
D. MTOR have a role in PC.
E. New drugs, designed for mutations in other tumor types, couldn't be effective in PC.

Answer: E

Explanation: New drugs designed for mutations in other tumor types could be effective in some mutations of PC, emphasizing the potential for targeted therapies.

20. A patient's TNM staging for PC is being discussed. Regional lymph node (LN) involvement by PC, the incorrect answer is:

A. N0: no regional LN metastasis.
B. N1b: metastasis to unilateral, bilateral, or contralateral cervical (level I, II, III, IV, or V).
C. N1b: superior mediastinal lymph nodes (level VII).
D. N1a: metastasis to level VI (pretracheal, paratracheal, and Delphian lymph nodes).

E. N1b: retropharyngeal nodes.

Answer: C

Explanation: Superior mediastinal lymph nodes (level VII) are categorized under N1a, not N1b, in the TNM staging system for PC.

21. A 60-year-old patient who underwent surgery for PC is discussing the possibility of recurrence with their surgeon. Regarding recurrence in PC, which of the following is incorrect?

A. Recurrence is common in patients with PC.
B. Patients with PC should have repeated, lifelong frequent investigations to detect recurrence early.
C. Chemotherapy is successful for persistent or recurrent PC.
D. Reoperation for persistent or recurrent PC has important symptomatic relief and standardizes serum calcium and PTH levels in most patients.
E. Reoperation is associated with some morbidity.

Answer: C

Explanation: Chemotherapy is not successful for the management of persistent or recurrent PC, emphasizing the importance of reoperation in relieving symptoms and eliminating residual disease.

22. A 57-year-old patient is discussing treatment options for PC with their oncologist. Regarding the management for parathyroid tumor, which is incorrect?

A. Chemotherapy is unsuccessful in PC management.
B. Parathyroid cancer is usually radiosensitive.
C. Surgical resection is the best choice for prognosis and therapeutic response.
D. Treatment of choice for inoperable metastatic PC is hypercalcemia control.
E. Intrahepatic and intrapulmonary metastatic tumors and other inoperable distant metastatic lesions can be controlled and ablated transcutaneously with radiofrequency or transcatheter arterial embolization.

Answer: B

Explanation: Parathyroid cancer is usually radioresistant, and chemotherapy is typically not successful in its management.

23. A 70-year-old patient presents with severe hypercalcemia related to malignancy. Which of the following is incorrect regarding the treatment of hypercalcemia of malignancy (HCM)?

A. In patients with HCM, denosumab (Dmab) is the treatment of choice rather than intravenous BP.
B. In patients having HCM > 14 mg/dL, a combination of calcitonin and an intravenous BP or Dmab as initial treatment is better than either treatment alone.
C. In refractory HCM cases on intravenous Dmab, the use of BP is better than without it.
D. PC hypercalcemia treatment is either calcimimetic or an intravenous BP or Dmab.

E. In hypercalcemia due to PC which is uncontrolled on BP or Dmab therapy, the addition of calcimimetic is a better choice.

Answer: C

Explanation: In refractory HCM cases on intravenous BP, the addition of Dmab is typically better than not using it.

24. A 62-year-old patient is diagnosed with hungry bone syndrome following parathyroidectomy for PHPT. Regarding hungry bone syndrome, which of the following is incorrect?

A. Characterized by serum calcium concentration below 8.5 mg/dL.
B. Caused by parathyroid resection for PHPT.
C. Characterized by serum phosphate concentration below 3.0 mg/dL.
D. Risk factors include resected adenoma size, preoperative blood urea nitrogen concentration and alkaline phosphatase concentration, and being of older age.
E. Clinical presentation of the hungry bone syndrome is mostly due to hypophosphatemia than hypomagnesemia.

Answer: E

Explanation: The clinical presentation of hungry bone syndrome is primarily due to hypocalcemia, and the lesser degree is due to hypophosphatemia, hypomagnesemia, and hyperkalemia.

25. A 55-year-old patient is discussing the follow-up care after surgical resection of their parathyroid tumor. Regarding postsurgical resection of the parathyroid tumor, which of the following is incorrect?

A. Hypercalcemia presents before physical symptoms in the majority of patients with recurrent disease.
B. Local recurrences in the neck are easy to identify.
C. Recurrence is usually regional, and it usually happens every (2–5) years.
D. Tumor recurrence occurs in the neck or cervical lymph nodes representing nearly 23% of recurrent cases.
E. Morbidity and mortality of PC mostly result from the metabolic effect of the tumor not directly from malignant growth.

Answer: B

Explanation: Local recurrences in the neck are hard to detect due to being small and multifocal, often obscured by scar tissue from previous surgical procedures.

26. A 63-year-old patient with PC is discussing treatment options for hypercalcemia with their oncologist. Regarding BP in PC, which of the following is incorrect?

A. BP are potent bone resorption inhibitors and are the most useful therapy for hypercalcemia due to malignancy.
B. Zoledronic acid is a type which is more useful than other BP types, including pamidronate.

C. The most common events in patients having cancer and BP are fever, anemia, nausea, constipation, and dyspnea, happened with similar results among zoledronic and pamidronate patients.
D. Renal adverse events happened more in pamidronate patients than in zoledronic acid patients.
E. Zoledronic acid patients have more acceptable mean calcium levels for much more time than patients treated with pamidronate.

Answer: D

Explanation: Renal adverse events occurred more frequently in pamidronate patients than in zoledronic acid patients when used for hypercalcemia management.

27. A 55-year-old patient is diagnosed with PC during surgical evaluation. Regarding the TNM staging system for PC at stage T1N1a, the incorrect statement is:

A. The tumor is localized to the parathyroid gland with extension limited to soft tissue.
B. There is direct invasion into the thyroid gland.
C. Regional lymph node metastasis is present.
D. There is no metastasis to retropharyngeal lymph nodes.
E. No vessel invasion is observed.

Answer: B

Explanation: Direct invasion into the thyroid gland is categorized as T2 in the TNM staging system for parathyroid carcinoma, not T1. The other statements are consistent with T1N1a staging.

28. A 58-year-old patient is diagnosed with a nonfunctional PC and is discussing treatment options with their surgeon. Regarding nonfunctional PC, which of the following is incorrect?

A. Nearly 10% of PC are nonfunctional tumors.
B. Functional or nonfunctional tumors are usually hard to differentiate from benign parathyroid adenoma.
C. Nonfunctional tumors have serum calcium and PTH within the normal range.
D. Most patients present with a neck mass, and its morbidity is due to the systemic effect of the tumor.
E. Nonfunctional tumors are smaller at presentation, are managed through chemotherapy, usually have incomplete excision, and have more locoregional recurrence and metastasis than functional tumors.

Answer: E

Explanation: Nonfunctional tumors are usually larger at presentation, are managed surgically, often have incomplete excision, and have a higher propensity for locoregional recurrence and metastasis compared to functional tumors.

29. A 60-year-old patient with PHPT is discussing treatment options with their surgeon. Which of the following is incorrect as regards the management of PHPT?

    A. Preoperative parathyroid biopsy should be avoided.
    B. Minimally invasive parathyroidectomy is mostly not done in cases of multi-gland disease.
    C. Normal parathyroid gland that is de-vascularized can be autotransplanted.
    D. Drug therapy is more useful than lengthy observation or surgical management.
    E. The histologic diagnosis of PCA depends on having an unequivocal invasion of vessels and the use of biomarkers.

    Answer: D

    Explanation: Surgical management is more successful than lengthy observation or drug therapy in treating PHPT.

30. A 55-year-old patient is diagnosed with advanced PC during surgery. For a tumor staged as T3N1b in PC, the incorrect statement is:

    A. The tumor directly invades the thyroid gland.
    B. The tumor directly invades the recurrent laryngeal nerve.
    C. The tumor invades the esophagus, trachea, and skeletal muscle.
    D. The tumor directly invades the spine.
    E. The tumor has metastasized to contralateral cervical (level V) lymph nodes.

    Answer: D

    Explanation: Direct invasion of the spine would categorize the tumor as T4 in the TNM staging system for parathyroid carcinoma, not T3. The other statements are consistent with T3N1b staging.

31. A 65-year-old male patient with PC is discussing prognostic factors with his oncologist. Understanding which factors affect prognosis is crucial for his treatment plan. Regarding prognostic factors in PC, the incorrect statement is:

    A. Older age at the time of diagnosis is associated with a worse prognosis.
    B. Larger tumor size is associated with a worse prognosis.
    C. Male sex is associated with a worse prognosis.
    D. For patients suspected to have PC, en bloc resection of the parathyroid gland must be done with thyroid lobe excision. Aggressive surgical resection did not improve survival.
    E. Incomplete tumor resection has the same survival rate compared with patients who have no surgical treatment.

    Answer: E

    Explanation: Both complete and incomplete tumor resection provide improved survival compared to patients with no surgical treatment. Incomplete resection is associated with better outcomes than no surgery at all, making the statement incorrect.

32. A 50-year-old patient is considering treatment options for PC. Regarding en bloc resection of the parathyroid tumor, which of the following is incorrect?

    A. En bloc resection has no notable recurrence-free survival advantage in comparison with parathyroidectomy alone.
    B. Can involve resection of the tumor with ipsilateral hemithyroidectomy.
    C. Involves excision of central lymphadenectomy.
    D. En bloc resection should be performed to prolong recurrence-free survival compared with parathyroidectomy alone.
    E. Reoperations are more common in patients having parathyroidectomy alone.

    Answer: A

    Explanation: En bloc resection should be performed to prolong recurrence-free survival compared with parathyroidectomy alone, emphasizing its importance in the management of PC.

33. A 58-year-old patient with PC and metastasis is discussing treatment options with their oncologist. In PC metastasis, which of the following is incorrect?

    A. Parathyroid cancer can metastasize to the lung and liver.
    B. Systemic therapy has minimal effect on the course of the disease and its associated hypercalcemia.
    C. BP drug is another management for metastasis rather than resection but only provides a time-limited calcium-lowering effect.
    D. Aggressive surgical management of pulmonary metastasis is useful for palliation in selected patients.
    E. Chemotherapy is more effective compared to surgical resection in parathyroid tumor metastasis.

    Answer: E

    Explanation: Systemic therapy provides little effect on the disease and hypercalcemia associated with malignancy, emphasizing the limited role of chemotherapy in PC management.

34. Pathology results from a PC surgical specimen are being analyzed using an immunohistochemical panel. Immunohistochemical panels in PC, the incorrect answer is:

    A. Parafibromin, a tumor suppressor protein often lost in parathyroid carcinoma, is included in the panel.
    B. Calretinin, a marker typically associated with mesothelial and some neural tissues, is included in the panel.
    C. Galectin-3, a protein involved in cell growth and apoptosis, is included in the panel.
    D. PGP9.5, a ubiquitin carboxyl-terminal hydrolase, is included in the panel.
    E. Ki67, a nuclear protein associated with cellular proliferation, is included in the panel.

    Answer: B

Explanation: Calretinin has no established role in the immunohistochemical panel for PC, whereas the other markers are relevant for diagnosis and prognosis.

35. A patient with advanced PC is undergoing TNM staging. Regarding T4N1a parathyroid cancer, which of the following is incorrect?

    A. Metastasis to contralateral (level I, II, III, IV, or V) lymph nodes.
    B. Direct invasion into a major blood vessel.
    C. Direct invasion into the spine.
    D. Metastasis to level pretracheal and paratracheal lymph nodes.
    E. Metastasis to level superior mediastinal lymph nodes.

    Answer: A

    Explanation: N1b is defined by metastasis to contralateral (level II, III, IV, V, or I) lymph nodes, while N1a represents metastasis to level VI (pretracheal, paratracheal, and Delphian lymph nodes).

36. A 60-year-old patient presents with symptomatic PHPT. The surgical team discusses the management plan. Which of the following statements regarding the definitive management of PHPT is incorrect?

    A. Surgery is the only definitive management for primary hyperparathyroidism.
    B. Preoperative biopsy of the parathyroid gland is recommended for all patients.
    C. High-volume surgeons tend to achieve better outcomes.
    D. Intraoperative neuromonitoring can help protect the recurrent laryngeal nerve.
    E. Both focused minimally invasive and bilateral exploration surgeries are considered appropriate.

    Answer: B

    Explanation: Preoperative biopsy of the parathyroid gland is recommended for all patients. This statement is incorrect as preoperative parathyroid biopsy should generally be avoided to reduce the risk of seeding and complications.

37. A patient is diagnosed with parathyroid carcinoma. The medical team is considering the genetic aspects of the disease for targeted treatment. Which of the following statements about gene expression in parathyroid carcinoma is incorrect?

    A. Specific genes such as APP, CDH1, KCNJ16, and UCHL1 are differentially expressed in parathyroid carcinoma.
    B. Microarray transcriptome analysis cannot differentiate between parathyroid carcinoma and benign parathyroid adenoma.
    C. Intraoperative PTH monitoring can accurately predict postoperative normocalcemia.
    D. Parathyroid carcinoma is often misdiagnosed as parathyroid adenoma due to overlapping features.

E. Early intraoperative recognition is crucial for a favorable outcome.

Answer: B

Explanation: Microarray transcriptome analysis cannot differentiate between parathyroid carcinoma and benign parathyroid adenoma. This statement is incorrect as microarray analysis has been used to identify differentially expressed genes in parathyroid carcinoma, suggesting its potential in differentiation.

38. A 50-year-old patient with primary hyperparathyroidism is being prepared for surgery. The team discusses localization techniques. Which of the following statements about preoperative and intraoperative localization techniques is incorrect?

A. High-resolution ultrasonography and sestamibi scintigraphy are commonly used for preoperative localization.
B. Carbon nanoparticles are among the methods used to improve the localization of parathyroid glands.
C. Intraoperative localization techniques significantly reduce the risk of damaging parathyroid glands.
D. All reviewed techniques for localization are equally effective and can be interchangeably used in all cases.
E. Indocyanine green has shown promise for the diagnosis of parathyroid adenomas.

Answer: D

Explanation: All reviewed techniques for localization are equally effective and can be interchangeably used in all cases. This statement is incorrect as different techniques have varying degrees of effectiveness and suitability depending on the specific case.

39. A pregnant patient in her third trimester is diagnosed with primary hyperparathyroidism. The medical team considers surgical intervention. Which of the following statements about parathyroidectomy in the third trimester is incorrect?

A. Parathyroidectomy is effective and has a lower risk profile when performed in the third trimester.
B. Delaying surgery until after delivery is the preferred approach to minimize risks to the fetus.
C. Parathyroid adenomas are the most common pathology detected in these cases.
D. Postoperative hypocalcemia is common but manageable with calcium replacement.
E. Hyperparathyroidism is considered a risk factor for preeclampsia.

Answer: B

Explanation: Delaying surgery until after delivery is the preferred approach to minimize risks to the fetus. This statement is incorrect as the study suggests that parathyroidectomy in the third trimester is effective and may carry less risk than delaying surgery.

40. A patient with confirmed parathyroid carcinoma is being discussed for surgical management. Which of the following statements regarding the surgical management of parathyroid carcinoma is incorrect?

    A. Complete excision with negative margins is crucial for a favorable outcome.
    B. Intraoperative recognition of parathyroid carcinoma significantly impacts the surgical strategy.
    C. Postoperative radiotherapy is universally agreed upon as beneficial for all cases of parathyroid carcinoma.
    D. Serum calcium often exceeds 14 mg/dL in patients with parathyroid carcinoma.
    E. Fine needle aspiration is discouraged due to the risk of parathyromatosis.

    Answer: C

    Explanation: Postoperative radiotherapy is universally agreed upon as beneficial for all cases of parathyroid carcinoma. This statement is incorrect as the role of postoperative radiotherapy remains controversial, with some series suggesting benefits while its utility is debated.

Bibliography

1. Wei CH, Harari A. Parathyroid carcinoma: update and guidelines for management. Curr Treat Options in Oncol. 2012;13(1):11–23.
2. Kebebew E. Parathyroid carcinoma. Curr Treat Options in Oncol. 2001;2(4):347–54.
3. Guarnieri V, Scillitani A, Muscarella LA, Battista C, Bonfitto N, Bisceglia M, et al. Diagnosis of parathyroid tumors in familial isolated hyperparathyroidism with HRPT2 mutation: implications for cancer surveillance. J Clin Endocrinol Metab. 2006;91(8):2827–32.
4. Cetani F, Pardi E, Borsari S, Viacava P, Dipollina G, Cianferotti L, et al. Genetic analyses of the HRPT2 gene in primary hyperparathyroidism: germline and somatic mutations in familial and sporadic parathyroid tumors. J Clin Endocrinol Metab. 2004;89(11):5583–91.
5. Marcocci C, Cetani F, Rubin MR, Silverberg SJ, Pinchera A, Bilezikian JP. Parathyroid carcinoma. J Bone Miner Res. 2008;23(12):1869–80.
6. Sharretts JM, Simonds WF. Clinical and molecular genetics of parathyroid neoplasms. Best Pract Res Clin Endocrinol Metab. 2010;24(3):491–502.
7. Busaidy NL, Jimenez C, Habra MA, Schultz PN, El-Naggar AK, Clayman GL, et al. Parathyroid carcinoma: a 22-year experience. Head Neck. 2004;26(8):716–26.
8. Cetani F, Pardi E, Marcocci C. Update on parathyroid carcinoma. J Endocrinol Investig. 2016;39(6):595–606.
9. Erickson LA, Mete O. Immunohistochemistry in diagnostic parathyroid pathology. Endocr Pathol. 2018;29(2):113–29.
10. Ruda JM, Hollenbeak CS, Stack BC Jr. A systematic review of the diagnosis and treatment of primary hyperparathyroidism from 1995 to 2003. Otolaryngol Head Neck Surg. 2005;132(3):359–72.
11. Quinn CE, Healy J, Lebastchi AH, Brown TC, Stein JE, Prasad ML, et al. Modern experience with aggressive parathyroid tumors in a high-volume New England referral Centre. J Am Coll Surg. 2015;220(6):1054–62.
12. Schulte KM, Talat N. Diagnosis and management of parathyroid cancer. Nat Rev Endocrinol. 2012;8(10):612–22.

13. Fancy T, Gallagher D, Hornig JD. Surgical anatomy of the thyroid and parathyroid glands. Otolaryngol Clin N Am. 2010;43(2):221–7.
14. Sadowski SM, Fortuny JV, Triponez F. A reappraisal of vascular anatomy of the parathyroid gland based on fluorescence techniques. Gland Surg. 2017;6(Suppl 1):S30.
15. Villar-del-Moral J, Jiménez-García A, Salvador-Egea P, Martos-Martínez JM, Nuño-Vázquez-Garza JM, Serradilla-Martín M, et al. Prognostic factors and staging systems in parathyroid cancer: a multicenter cohort study. Surgery. 2014;156(5):1132–44.
16. Szalat A, Tamir N, Mazeh H, Newman JP. Successful parathyroidectomy improves cognition in patients with primary hyperparathyroidism: a prospective study in a tertiary medical center and comprehensive review of the literature. Front Endocrinol. 2022;13:1095189.
17. Sawhney S, Vaish R, Jain S, Mittal N, Ankathi SK, Thiagarajan S, et al. Parathyroid carcinoma: a review. Indian J Surg Oncol. 2022;13(1):133–42.
18. Petranović Ovčariček P, Giovanella L, Carrió Gasset I, Hindié E, Huellner MW, Luster M, Piccardo A, Weber T, Talbot JN, Verburg FA. The EANM practice guidelines for parathyroid imaging. Eur J Nucl Med Mol Imaging. 2021;48:2801–22.
19. Pandya C, Uzilov AV, Bellizzi J, Lau CY, Moe AS, Strahl M, et al. Genomic profiling reveals mutational landscape in parathyroid carcinomas. JCI Insight. 2017;2(6):e92061.
20. Kebebew E, Arici C, Duh QY, Clark OH. Localization and reoperation results for persistent and recurrent parathyroid carcinoma. Arch Surg. 2001;136(8):878–85.
21. El-Hajj Fuleihan G, Clines GA, Hu MI, Marcocci C, Murad MH, Piggott T, et al. Treatment of hypercalcemia of malignancy in adults: an Endocrine Society clinical practice guideline. J Clin Endocrinol Metab. 2023;108(3):507–28.
22. Brasier AR, Nussbaum SR. Hungry bone syndrome: clinical and biochemical predictors of its occurrence after parathyroid surgery. Am J Med. 1988;84(4):654–60.
23. Board PA. Parathyroid cancer treatment (PDQ®). In: PDQ cancer information summaries [internet]. National Cancer Institute (US); 2020.
24. Major P, Lortholary A, Hon J, Abdi E, Mills G, Menssen HD, et al. Zoledronic acid is superior to pamidronate in the treatment of hypercalcemia of malignancy: a pooled analysis of two randomized, controlled clinical trials. J Clin Oncol. 2001;19(2):558–67.
25. Amin MB, Greene FL, Edge SB, Compton CC, Gershenwald JE, Brookland RK, et al. The eighth edition AJCC cancer staging manual: continuing to build a bridge from a population-based to a more "personalized" approach to cancer staging. CA Cancer J Clin. 2017;67(2):93–9.
26. Wilkins BJ, Lewis JS Jr. Non-functional parathyroid carcinoma: a review of the literature and report of a case requiring extensive surgery. Head Neck Pathol. 2009;3(2):140–9.
27. Wilhelm SM, Wang TS, Ruan DT, Lee JA, Asa SL, Duh QY, et al. The American Association of Endocrine Surgeons guidelines for definitive management of primary hyperparathyroidism. JAMA Surg. 2016;151(10):959–68.
28. Radu P, Garofil D, Tigora A, Zurzu M, Paic V, Bratucu M, et al. Parathyroid cancer—a rare finding during parathyroidectomy in high volume surgery centre. Medicina [Internet]. 2023;59(3):448. https://doi.org/10.3390/medicina59030448.
29. Asare EA, Sturgeon C, Winchester DJ, Liu L, Palis B, Perrier ND, et al. Parathyroid carcinoma: an update on treatment outcomes and prognostic factors from the National Cancer Data Base (NCDB). Ann Surg Oncol. 2015;22(12):3990–5.
30. Wächter S, Holzer K, Manoharan J, Brehm C, Mintziras I, Bartsch DK, et al. Surgical treatment of parathyroid carcinoma : does the initial en bloc resection improve the prognosis? Chirurg. 2019;90(11):905–12.
31. Obara T, Okamoto T, Ito Y, Yamashita T, Kawano M, Nishi T, et al. Surgical and medical management of patients with pulmonary metastasis from parathyroid carcinoma. Surgery. 1993;114(6):1040–8. discussion 8-9.
32. Truran PP, Johnson SJ, Bliss RD, Lennard TW, Aspinall SR. Parafibromin, galectin-3, PGP9.5, Ki67, and cyclin D1: using an immunohistochemical panel to aid in the diagnosis of parathyroid cancer. World J Surg. 2014;38(11):2845–54.

33. Wilhelm S, Wang TS, Ruan DT, Lee JA, Asa S, Duh Q, Doherty G, Herrera M, Pasieka J, Perrier N, Silverberg S, Solórzano C, Sturgeon C, Tublin M, Udelsman R, Carty S. The American Association of Endocrine Surgeons guidelines for definitive management of primary hyperparathyroidism. JAMA Surg. 2016;151(10):959–68.
34. Adam MA, Untch BR, Olson JA Jr. Parathyroid carcinoma: current understanding and new insights into gene expression and intraoperative parathyroid hormone kinetics. Oncologist. 2010;15(1):61–72.
35. Baj J, Sitarz R, Łokaj M, Forma A, Czeczelewski M, Maani A, Garruti G. Preoperative and intraoperative methods of parathyroid gland localization and the diagnosis of parathyroid adenomas. Molecules. 2020;25(7):1724.
36. Schnatz PF, Thaxton S. Parathyroidectomy in the third trimester of pregnancy. Obstet Gynecol Surv. 2005;60(10):672–82.
37. Goswamy J, Lei M, Simó R. Parathyroid carcinoma. Curr Opin Otolaryngol Head Neck Surg. 2016;24(2):155–62.

Chapter 16
Adrenal Tumors

Haider A. H. Ahmed, Sabah Noori Abdulraheem, and Sajjad G. Al-Badri

1. A 35-year-old woman with a family history of multiple endocrine neoplasia presents with an adrenal mass. In considering familial syndromes associated with adrenal tumors, which of the following statements is incorrect?
   A. Carney's syndrome is due to defects in Ch 2p16 and PRKARIA gene in Ch 17q22.
   B. Von Hippel–Lindau type II is also associated with hemangioblastomas and renal cell carcinoma.
   C. Beckwith–Wiedemann syndrome is also known as the sarcoma, breast, leukemia, and adrenal gland cancer syndrome.
   D. MEN type 1 is associated with parathyroid, pituitary, and pancreatic NETs and adrenal adenomas, as well as carcinomas.
   E. Congenital adrenal hyperplasia is due to a defect in the 21-hydroxylase gene on Ch 6p21.3.

   Answer: C

   Explanation: In surgical oncology, it's important to distinguish between various familial syndromes. The sarcoma, breast, leukemia, and adrenal gland (SBLA) cancer syndrome is associated with Li–Fraumeni syndrome, not Beckwith–Wiedemann syndrome.
2. A 45-year-old woman with a recently discovered adrenal mass is being evaluated for possible adrenocortical carcinoma (ACC). In reviewing the epidemiology of ACC, which of the following statements is incorrect?

H. A. H. Ahmed
Medical City Complex, Baghdad, Iraq

S. N. Abdulraheem
Baghdad Teaching Hospital, Baghdad, Iraq

S. G. Al-Badri (✉)
College of Medicine, University of Baghdad, Baghdad, Iraq

A. S. Mahmood, A. Koulouris (eds.), *MCQs in General Surgical Oncology*,
https://doi.org/10.1007/978-3-031-65738-2_16

A. Incidentalomas are present in approximately 2–4% of individuals.
B. ACC has a reported age-adjusted incidence rate of 0.72–2 persons per million population per year.
C. ACC typically has a bimodal age distribution in the first and fourth decades of life.
D. Most ACCs are confined to the adrenal gland at the time of diagnosis.
E. Most ACCs occur in people with no family history.

Answer: D

Explanation: ACC often presents with advanced disease, and only a minority of cases are confined to the adrenal gland at the time of diagnosis, making this an important consideration in surgical oncology.

3. A 38-year-old woman presents with recent onset of hypertension and signs of virilization. Imaging reveals an adrenal mass. In considering the presentation of adrenal tumors, which of the following statements is incorrect?

A. Around 80% of adrenocortical malignancies present with evidence of steroid hormone excess.
B. Virilizing tumors are usually benign.
C. In patients with hypertension, careful screening will demonstrate primary hyperaldosteronism in 5–13%.
D. Virilizing and feminizing tumors are extremely uncommon.
E. They can present as retroperitoneal hemorrhage.

Answer: B

Explanation: In surgical oncology, it's crucial to recognize that virilizing tumors of the adrenal gland can indeed be malignant, making this statement incorrect and emphasizing the need for vigilance in diagnosis and management.

4. A 47-year-old woman presents with hypertension, hypokalemia, and metabolic alkalosis. Imaging reveals an adrenal mass. In considering clinical syndromes due to adrenal tumors, which of the following statements is incorrect?

A. Around 80% of adrenocortical malignancies present with evidence of steroid hormone excess.
B. The only specific clinical feature of primary hyperaldosteronism is hypertension.
C. No attempt should be made to excise the pheochromocytoma in a pharmacologically unprepared patient.
D. Biochemical findings in Conn's syndrome include hypokalemia and alkalosis.
E. Cushing's disease is adrenocorticotropic hormone (ACTH)-independent.

Answer: E

Explanation: Cushing's disease is due to pituitary oversecretion of ACTH, making it ACTH-dependent. This distinction is crucial in surgical oncology.

5. A 52-year-old woman with a history of hypertension presents with an adrenal mass, and biochemical testing is suggestive of a pheochromocytoma. In

discussing the potential for malignancy in pheochromocytoma, which of the following statements is incorrect?

A. Malignancy in pheochromocytoma is less than 5%.
B. There are no absolute histological criteria to differentiate between benign and malignant pheochromocytomas.
C. Elevated plasma and urinary dopamine and dihydroxyphenylalanine should raise the suspicion of malignancy.
D. S100-positive sustentacular cells indicate malignancy.
E. There are no staging classifications for malignant pheochromocytomas.

Answer: A

Explanation: In surgical oncology, malignancy in pheochromocytoma ranges from 11.6% to 23%, making this statement incorrect and highlighting the potential for malignancy in a significant proportion of cases.

6. A 52-year-old man presents with a 3 cm incidental adrenal mass discovered during imaging for unrelated abdominal pain. He has no history of cancer and no signs of hormonal hypersecretion. In evaluating this suspected adrenal pathology, which of the following statements is incorrect?

A. Nonfunctioning tumors that are not suspicious of malignancy and are smaller than 4 cm warrant no further intervention.
B. Functioning tumors that have a high risk of malignancy (>4 cm) need surgical excision.
C. Biopsy of adrenal tumors is rarely used.
D. Ruling out pheochromocytoma is mandatory.
E. Nonfunctioning adrenal mass in a patient previously treated for cancer should get a biopsy.

Answer: A

Explanation: Nonfunctioning tumor that is not suspicious of malignancy and is smaller than 4 cm should get a repeat CT scan in 6 months to check for any changes in size.

7. A 60-year-old woman with a history of hypertension and weight loss undergoes imaging for an adrenal mass discovered during a routine checkup. When evaluating signs of malignancy in the imaging of adrenal cancer, which of the following statements is incorrect?

A. Enhancement after gadolinium contrast with slow washout indicates malignancy.
B. The maximum diameter of the adrenal mass is predictive of malignancy.
C. Reduced fat content after MRI is an indicator of malignancy.
D. CT attenuation of <10 Hounsfield units (HU) suggests that the likelihood it is a benign adenoma is 80%.
E. MRI is superior to CT in evaluating IVC involvement.

Answer: D

Explanation: In surgical oncology, CT attenuation of a benign adenoma is usually <10 HU on an unenhanced scan, suggesting that the likelihood it is a benign adenoma is nearly 100%, making this statement incorrect and emphasizing the importance of recognizing this diagnostic criterion.

8. A 54-year-old man undergoes an abdominal CT scan for evaluation of nonspecific abdominal pain. An incidental 3 cm adrenal mass is discovered. In considering the management of adrenal incidentalomas, which of the following statements is incorrect?

   A. Approximately 15% of incidentalomas are functional.
   B. The maximum diameter of the adrenal mass is predictive of malignancy.
   C. FNAB is indicated to determine whether it's benign or malignant.
   D. Laparoscopic adrenalectomy is only feasible if the incidentaloma is <10 cm.
   E. A baseline hormonal panel should be repeated annually for 4 years in cases where the initial evaluation is negative.

   Answer: C

   Explanation: In surgical oncology, it's important to recognize that FNA cannot reliably distinguish between a benign cortical adrenal mass and the less common adrenal carcinoma, emphasizing the complexity of diagnosis in such cases.

9. A 52-year-old man is undergoing surgery for an adrenal tumor. The surgical team is reviewing the anatomy of the adrenal glands. Which of the following statements regarding the anatomy of the adrenal gland is incorrect?

   A. The right adrenal gland is smaller and triangular.
   B. The left adrenal gland is crescentic in shape.
   C. The right adrenal gland is located partially behind the inferior vena cava (IVC).
   D. The left adrenal gland is superior and slightly anteromedial to the left kidney, but it is also in close proximity to the pancreas and spleen.
   E. The arterial blood supply for both glands arises from the abdominal aorta.

   Answer: E

   Explanation: While both adrenal glands receive arterial blood supply from multiple sources, this question highlights the importance of recognizing their unique arterial contributions in surgical oncology.

10. A 48-year-old woman is diagnosed with ACC extending into the vena cava. She is being evaluated for potential treatment options. In the management of ACC, which of the following statements is incorrect?

   A. Adrenalectomy is contraindicated in widespread metastatic disease.
   B. Medical therapy is the only treatment in patients with ACC extending into the vena cava.
   C. Open adrenalectomy is the standard surgical approach for localized ACC.
   D. Laparoscopic adrenalectomy can be performed if the ACC is less than 6 cm.
   E. Glucocorticoid coverage may be necessary in patients with hypercortisolism.

   Answer: B

Explanation: In surgical oncology, intracaval extension or tumor thrombus is not a contraindication to surgery; resection may be facilitated by cardiopulmonary bypass. This emphasizes the importance of surgical intervention in certain cases.

11. A 62-year-old man with stage III ACC is undergoing evaluation for surgical resection. In considering the management of ACC metastasis, which of the following statements is incorrect?

    A. Avoiding tumor spillage during resection carries a better prognosis.
    B. The renal hilum is the most common site of lymphatic spread.
    C. Resection is curative in stages I to III.
    D. The role of neoadjuvant therapy is not considered a standard approach.
    E. Some clinicians advocate maximal debulking as a means of improving survival.

    Answer: C.

    Explanation: Resection, while technically possible for most patients with stage I to III disease, is not curative for many, as occult micrometastases are often present at the time of initial presentation, even with stage I disease, emphasizing the challenging nature of ACC management.

12. A 40-year-old woman with an incidentally discovered adrenal mass is undergoing evaluation for potential adrenalectomy. The surgical team is considering a laparoscopic transabdominal approach. Which of the following statements regarding the laparoscopic transabdominal adrenalectomy approach is incorrect?

    A. Can be combined with other transabdominal procedures.
    B. The patient is positioned in lateral decubitus with exposure of the area between the iliac crest and the 11th rib of the affected gland.
    C. More appropriate for obese patients.
    D. Recommended for ACC.
    E. Need to mobilize the abdominal structures.

    Answer: D

    Explanation: In surgical oncology, the laparoscopic transabdominal adrenalectomy approach is not appropriate for highly suspected malignant tumors like ACC or in cases of tumor invasion into adjacent structures. Instead, an open adrenalectomy approach is recommended for such cases, making this statement incorrect.

13. A 45-year-old woman with adrenal tumor is scheduled for adrenalectomy. The surgical team is reviewing the perioperative preparation. Which of the following statements regarding the perioperative preparation of patients with adrenal tumors is incorrect?

    A. Continue aldosterone antagonists postoperatively in patients with Conn's syndrome.
    B. Patients with hypercortisolism need perioperative thromboprophylaxis.
    C. Patients with pheochromocytoma need to be in critical care units post-op.

D. Perioperative steroid supplementation is necessary in patients with Cushing's syndrome to prevent relative adrenal insufficiency.
E. Monitoring for hypoglycemia should be done.

Answer: A

Explanation: In surgical oncology, aldosterone antagonists should be stopped in the postoperative period in patients with Conn's syndrome to prevent hypokalemia and hyperkalemia, making this statement incorrect.

14. A 55-year-old man with a history of multiple abdominal surgeries is scheduled for adrenalectomy due to an adrenal mass. The surgical team is discussing the most suitable approach. Which of the following statements regarding the choice of adrenalectomy approach is incorrect?

A. The transperitoneal approach with the patient in a lateral position is most commonly used.
B. The retroperitoneal approach has a shorter hospital stay and earlier recovery.
C. The transperitoneal approach is better in patients with previous intra-abdominal surgery.
D. The retroperitoneal approach is more useful in those undergoing bilateral adrenalectomy.
E. Trials have found that the two approaches have similar clinical outcomes.

Answer: C

Explanation: The retroperitoneal approach is preferred in patients with previous intra-abdominal surgery as it avoids adhesions and reopening scarred planes. This distinction is important in surgical oncology.

15. A surgical team is preparing for a laparoscopic adrenalectomy in a 47-year-old woman with a left adrenal mass. Which of the following statements regarding the prerequisites for successful adrenalectomy is incorrect?

A. Laparoscopic adrenalectomy success is dependent on correct positioning of the patient and port placement.
B. Careful mobilization of the liver, spleen, and head of the pancreas is important.
C. High insufflation pressures (20–28 mmHg) are considered crucial in the retroperitoneal approach.
D. Grasping the tumor or adrenal gland during operating is not recommended.
E. Not fully removing the gland is associated with a higher risk of recurrence.

Answer: B

Explanation: In the transperitoneal approach, careful mobilization of the liver on the right side and the spleen with the tail of the pancreas on the left side is important. This statement addresses the importance of proper technique in surgical oncology.

16. A 53-year-old woman with advanced ACC is being considered for chemotherapy with mitotane. In discussing the chemotherapy of ACC, which of the following statements is incorrect?

A. The only organ-specific chemotherapeutic drug is mitotane.
B. Mitotane suppresses adrenal steroid secretion and causes adrenal tissue necrosis.
C. Optimal response occurs at blood mitotane concentrations above 14 mg/ml.
D. Mitotane causes a reduction in tumor bulk in the majority of patients.
E. Mitotane causes gastrointestinal and neurologic symptoms.

Answer: D

Explanation: In surgical oncology, it's important to recognize that although mitotane controls excess tumoral hormone secretion in the majority of patients, a reduction in tumor bulk occurs in only 25%, highlighting the limited efficacy in this regard.

17. During a laparoscopic transperitoneal adrenalectomy for a 45-year-old man with an adrenal mass, the surgical team discusses the key steps of the procedure. Which of the following statements regarding laparoscopic transperitoneal adrenalectomy is incorrect?

A. Exposure includes the area between the iliac crest and the 11th rib overlying the kidney.
B. Ports should be placed approximately 9–12 cm apart, with the most lateral port placed through the flank.
C. The medial perirenal adipose tissue should be dissected medially in right adrenalectomy until the lateral border of the IVC is identified.
D. An intraoperative diagnosis of pheochromocytoma indicates conversion to an open procedure.
E. Variation in vascular anatomy is uncommon.

Answer: E

Explanation: In surgical oncology, variation in vascular anatomy is common during laparoscopic adrenalectomy. While the left adrenal vein usually drains into the left renal vein, variations can occur.

18. A 65-year-old man with bilateral pheochromocytomas and a history of cardiovascular disease is being evaluated for adrenalectomy. The surgical team is considering a posterior retroperitoneoscopic approach. Which of the following statements regarding the posterior retroperitoneoscopic adrenalectomy approach is incorrect?

A. Used for patients who require bilateral adrenalectomy.
B. Patient positioned in the prone position with hip and knee flexion at 90°.
C. Not appropriate for obese patients.
D. Does not require abdominal organ mobilization.
E. Cannot be used in patients with cardiovascular compromise due to high insufflation pressure.

Answer: E

Explanation: In surgical oncology, the posterior retroperitoneoscopic adrenalectomy approach does not increase intraperitoneal pressure during insufflation, making it more suitable for patients with cardiovascular or respiratory compromise.

19. A 55-year-old woman with a large ACC is undergoing an open transabdominal adrenalectomy. The surgical team discusses the approach and potential complications. Which of the following statements regarding the open transabdominal adrenalectomy approach is incorrect?

    A. Performed in ACC and malignant pheochromocytoma of any size.
    B. The patient is positioned in the supine position with ipsilateral flank elevation.
    C. Performed through an upper midline or subcostal incision.
    D. It has few complications.
    E. Provides a wide range of accessibility to the intraperitoneal cavity.

    Answer: D

    Explanation: In surgical oncology, the open transabdominal adrenalectomy approach has the disadvantage of having all the morbidity of a major laparotomy, including pain and prolonged ileus postoperatively, making this statement incorrect.

20. A 55-year-old man with a history of adrenocortical carcinoma presents for follow-up. He had undergone adrenalectomy, and recent imaging shows distant metastases. In considering the prognosis of adrenal tumors, which of the following statements is incorrect?

    A. The 5-year overall survival even in patients with distant metastasis is more than 20%.
    B. Small tumors <5 cm that are confined to the adrenal gland have a 5-year overall survival of more than 80%.
    C. Presence of markers of proliferation such as KI-67 indicates a poorer prognosis.
    D. The Weiss histopathologic scoring system is used for adrenocortical cancers.
    E. Hypersecretion of cortisol is associated with a poorer prognosis.

    Answer: A

    Explanation: In surgical oncology, it's crucial to recognize that the 5-year overall survival in patients with distant metastasis is often less than 15%, emphasizing the challenging prognosis associated with advanced disease.

21. A 50-year-old woman underwent surgical resection for stage II ACC. Which of the following statements regarding factors indicating a low risk of recurrence is incorrect?

    A. Microscopically complete (R0) resection indicates a low risk of recurrence.
    B. Stages I–III ACC are associated with a low risk of recurrence.
    C. Lack of MIB-1 staining suggests a lower risk of recurrence.
    D. Ki-67 ≤ 10% is associated with a low risk of recurrence.
    E. Non-mutated β-catenin is associated with a low risk of recurrence.

    Answer: E

    Explanation: Non-mutated β-catenin is not typically associated with a low risk of recurrence.

22. A 60-year-old man with a history of renal cell carcinoma presents with an incidentally discovered adrenal mass. The surgical team is discussing the role of adrenal biopsy. Which of the following statements regarding adrenal biopsy is incorrect?

    A. Most experts do not recommend adrenaloma biopsy.
    B. Radiology literature recommends adrenal biopsy.
    C. Biopsy is contraindicated when metastasis to the adrenals is suspected and a tissue diagnosis is required.
    D. Tissue obtained by a biopsy is rarely adequate to differentiate malignant from benign adrenal lesions.
    E. It can create difficulty with the surgical dissection.

    Answer: C

    Explanation: In surgical oncology, if adrenal metastasis is suspected and a tissue diagnosis is required, biopsy is indicated, especially in patients known or suspected to have lung, breast, renal, and gastrointestinal malignancies, lymphoma, and melanoma. This emphasizes the importance of biopsy in specific clinical situations.

23. A 68-year-old man undergoes a left adrenalectomy for a pheochromocytoma. Postoperatively, he experiences labile blood pressure and is monitored closely in the intensive care unit. In considering the complications of adrenalectomy, which of the following statements is incorrect?

    A. Left adrenalectomy is associated with a higher risk of bleeding than right adrenalectomy.
    B. Left adrenalectomy is associated with a higher risk of bleeding than right adrenalectomy.
    C. Mortality following adrenalectomy is rare.
    D. Extremely labile BP can occur, precipitating a hypertensive crisis.
    E. Pneumothorax can occur either intentionally or inadvertently.

    Answer: B

    Explanation: In surgical oncology, bleeding is more common with right adrenalectomy as it is associated with the risk of IVC injury as well as liver and duodenal injury, making this statement incorrect.

24. A 50-year-old patient is diagnosed with a primary adrenal cancer. The surgical team is considering laparoscopic adrenalectomy. Which of the following statements regarding laparoscopic adrenalectomy for malignant adrenal disease is incorrect?

    A. Laparoscopic adrenalectomy is considered for primary adrenal cancer and metastatic disease.
    B. Careful individual judgment is crucial due to the rarity of prospective data on outcomes.
    C. Laparoscopic adrenalectomy has higher recurrence rates compared to open surgery for malignant adrenal tumors.

D. Advances in surgical techniques have improved the treatment of malignant adrenal tumors.
E. Decision-making regarding laparoscopic resection should account for the malignancy potential of adrenal tumors.

Answer: C

Explanation: Laparoscopic adrenalectomy has higher recurrence rates compared to open surgery for malignant adrenal tumors.

25. A patient with an advanced adrenal carcinoma that has infiltrated the adrenal vein and extended into the inferior vena cava is evaluated for surgery. Which of the following statements about the surgical management of advanced malignant adrenal tumors is incorrect?

A. Advanced adrenal carcinomas may require caval or cavo-atrial thrombectomy.
B. Aggressive surgical approaches justify the poor prognosis without resection or incomplete tumor resections.
C. Radical surgery includes multivisceral resections if necessary.
D. Open surgery is not recommended for tumors with cavo-atrial involvement due to high complication rates.
E. The extent of vascular involvement classifies into four types, requiring increasingly challenging surgical procedures.

Answer: D

Explanation: Open surgery is not recommended for tumors with cavo-atrial involvement due to high complication rates.

26. A 45-year-old patient with a small benign adrenal tumor is discussing surgical options. Which of the following statements about the surgical approach to adrenal tumors is incorrect?

A. Laparoscopic adrenalectomy is the first-choice treatment for small-to-medium benign adrenal tumors.
B. Robotic adrenalectomy has gained popularity and has outcomes comparable to laparoscopy.
C. The open approach is the preferred method for treating adrenocortical cancer, especially with neighbor tissue involvement.
D. Minimally invasive techniques are favored for large malignant adrenal tumors without any radiological signs of malignancy.
E. Recent evidence suggests caution in treating localized adrenocortical carcinoma with laparoscopy due to higher rates of local or peritoneal recurrence.

Answer: D

Explanation: Minimally invasive techniques are favored for large malignant adrenal tumors without any radiological signs of malignancy. This statement is incorrect as the open approach is preferred for large tumors and adrenocortical cancer with potential neighbor tissue involvement.

27. A patient with a large adrenal tumor is being evaluated for potential surgery. Which of the following statements regarding the approach to large adrenal tumors is incorrect?

A. Recent guidelines recommend an individual approach rather than a clear size cutoff for surgery.
B. Tumor size of more than 4 cm in diameter represents high specificity for the diagnosis of a malignant tumor.
C. The decision about surgery should not be based only on the size of a tumor.
D. Imaging studies, growth patterns, and urine/serum steroid metabolomics are important in assessing the risk of malignancy.
E. Patients with LATs should be managed by an expert multidisciplinary team.

Answer: B

Explanation: Tumor size of more than 4 cm in diameter represents high specificity for the diagnosis of a malignant tumor. This statement is incorrect as the specificity for malignancy based on size alone is relatively low, indicating the importance of a comprehensive assessment.

28. A surgical team is considering laparoscopic adrenalectomy for a patient with a metastatic tumor to the adrenal gland. Which of the following statements about laparoscopic adrenalectomy for malignancy is incorrect?

A. Laparoscopic adrenalectomy is safe and effective for metastatic colorectal, lung, and renal tumors.
B. Radical resections for primary adrenal malignancies can be effectively performed laparoscopically.
C. The laparoscopic technique is recommended for all primary adrenal malignancies to ensure minimal invasiveness.
D. Technical advances and increased experience have expanded the indications for laparoscopic surgery in malignant cases.
E. Long-term follow-up is needed to establish the minimally invasive technique as the preferred approach for primary adrenal malignancies.

Answer: C

Explanation: The laparoscopic technique is recommended for all primary adrenal malignancies to ensure minimal invasiveness. This statement is incorrect as the article suggests cautious consideration of laparoscopic surgery for primary adrenal malignancies, ensuring complete tumor resection with an intact capsule.

Bibliography

1. Kamilaris CDC, Hannah-Shmouni F, Stratakis CA. Adrenocortical tumorigenesis: lessons from genetics. Best Pract Res Clin Endocrinol Metab. 2020;34(3):101428. https://doi.org/10.1016/j.beem.2020.101428. Epub 2020 May 23. PMID: 32507359; PMCID: PMC7427505
2. Fassnacht M, Allolio B. Epidemiology of adrenocortical carcinoma. In: Hammer GD, Else T, editors. Adrenocortical carcinoma: basic science and clinical concepts. New York: Springer; 2010. p. 23–9.
3. Allolio B, Fassnacht M. Adrenocortical carcinoma: clinical update. J Clin Endocrinol Metab. 2006;91:2027–37.

4. Mete O, Erickson LA, Juhlin CC, de Krijger RR, Sasano H, Volante M, Papotti MG. Overview of the 2022 WHO classification of adrenal cortical tumors. Endocr Pathol. 2022;33(1):155–96. https://doi.org/10.1007/s12022-022-09710-8. Epub 2022 Mar 14. PMID: 35288842; PMCID: PMC8920443
5. Zarnegar R, Kebebew E, Duh QY, Clark OH. Malignant pheochromocytoma. Surg Oncol Clin N Am. 2006;15(3):555–71. https://doi.org/10.1016/j.soc.2006.05.009.
6. Elsayes KM, Emad-Eldin S, Morani AC, Jensen CT. Practical approach to adrenal imaging. Radiol Clin North Am. 2017;55(2):279–301. https://doi.org/10.1016/j.rcl.2016.10.005. Epub 2016 Dec 12
7. Szolar DH, Korobkin M, Reittner P, Berghold A, Bauernhofer T, Trummer H, Schoellnast H, Preidler KW, Samonigg H. Adrenocortical carcinomas and adrenal pheochromocytomas: mass and enhancement loss evaluation at delayed contrast-enhanced CT. Radiology. 2005;234(2):479–85. https://doi.org/10.1148/radiol.2342031876.
8. Mazzaglia PJ, Monchik JM. Limited value of adrenal biopsy in the evaluation of adrenal neoplasm: a decade of experience. Arch Surg. 2009;144(5):465–70. https://doi.org/10.1001/archsurg.2009.59.
9. Barszcz K, Przespolewska H, Olbrych K, Czopowicz M, Klećkowska-Nawrot J, Goździewska-Harłajczuk K, Kupczyńska M. The morphology of the adrenal gland in the European bison (Bison bonasus). BMC Vet Res. 2016;12(1):161. https://doi.org/10.1186/s12917-016-0783-8. PMID: 27487830; PMCID: PMC4972984
10. Laan DV, Thiels CA, Glasgow A, Wise KB, Thompson GB, Richards ML, Farley DR, Truty MJ, McKenzie TJ. Adrenocortical carcinoma with inferior vena cava tumor thrombus. Surgery. 2017;161(1):240–8. https://doi.org/10.1016/j.surg.2016.07.040. Epub 2016 Nov 17
11. Allolio B, Fassnacht M. Clinical review: Adrenocortical carcinoma: clinical update. J Clin Endocrinol Metab. 2006;91(6):2027–37. https://doi.org/10.1210/jc.2005-2639. Epub 2006 Mar 21
12. Del Pizzo JJ. Transabdominal laparoscopic adrenalectomy. Curr Urol Rep. 2003;4(1):81–6.
13. Schreiner F, Anand G, Beuschlein F. Perioperative management of endocrine active adrenal tumors. Exp Clin Endocrinol Diabetes. 2019;127(2–03):137–46. https://doi.org/10.1055/a-0654-5251. Epub 2018 Aug 14
14. Assalia A, Gagner M. Laparoscopic adrenalectomy. Br J Surg. 2004;91:1259–74.
15. Walz MK, Alesina PF, Wenger FA, et al. Posterior retroperitoneoscopic adrenalectomy result of 560 procedures in 520 patients. Surgery. 2000;140(6):943–8. discussion 948–50
16. Hahner S, Fassnacht M. Mitotane for adrenocortical carcinoma treatment. Curr Opin Investig Drug. 2005;6:386–94.
17. Howe JR. Laparoscopic adrenalectomy. In: Scott-Conner CEH, Dawson DL, editors. Operative anatomy. Philadelphia: Wolters Kluwer/Lippincott Williams & Wilkins; 2009. p. 614.
18. Perrier ND, Kennamer DL, Bao R, Jimenez C, Grubbs EG, Lee JE, Evans DB. Posterior retroperitoneoscopic adrenalectomy: preferred technique for removal of benign tumors and isolated metastases. Ann Surg. 2008;248(4):666–74.
19. Godellas CV, Prinz RA. Surgical approach to adrenal neoplasms: laparoscopic versus open adrenalectomy. Surg Oncol Clin N Am. 1998;7(4):807–17.
20. Wagnerova H, Lazurova I, Felsoci M. Adrenal metastases. Bratisl Lek Listy. 2013;114(4):237–40. https://doi.org/10.4149/bll_2013_049.
21. Edgren M, Eriksson B, Wilander E, Westlin JE, Nilsson S, Oberg K. Biological characteristics of adrenocortical carcinoma: a study of p53, IGF, EGF-r, Ki-67 and PCNA in 17 adrenocortical carcinomas. Anticancer Res. 1997;17(2B):1303–9.
22. Zhang CD, Delivanis DA, Eiken PW, Atwell TD, Bancos I. Adrenal biopsy: performance and use. Minerva Endocrinol. 2019;44(3):288–300. https://doi.org/10.23736/S0391-1977.19.02969-9. Epub 2019 Feb 6
23. Bergamini C, Martellucci J, Tozzi F, Valeri A. Complications in laparoscopic adrenalectomy: the value of experience. Surg Endosc. 2011;25(12):3845–51. https://doi.org/10.1007/s00464-011-1804-0. Epub 2011 Jun 17

24. Saunders B, Doherty G. Laparoscopic adrenalectomy for malignant disease. Lancet Oncol. 2004;5(12):718–26.
25. Musholt T. Surgical management of advanced malignant adrenal tumours. Eur Surg. 2003;35:97–101.
26. Fiori C, Checcucci E, Amparore D, Cattaneo G, Manfredi M, Porpiglia F. Adrenal tumours: open surgery versus minimally invasive surgery. Curr Opin Oncol. 2019;31(1):7–12.
27. Ambroziak U. Approach to large adrenal tumors. Curr Opin Endocrinol Diabetes Obes. 2021;28(3):271–6.
28. Cobb WS, Kercher KW, Sing RF, Heniford BT. Laparoscopic adrenalectomy for malignancy. Am J Surg. 2005;189(4):405–11.

MIX
Papier aus verantwortungsvollen Quellen
Paper from responsible sources
FSC® C105338

If you have any concerns about our products,
you can contact us on
ProductSafety@springernature.com

In case Publisher is established outside the EU,
the EU authorized representative is:
Springer Nature Customer Service Center GmbH
Europaplatz 3, 69115 Heidelberg, Germany

Printed by Libri Plureos GmbH
in Hamburg, Germany